Recent Results in Cancer Research

Fortschritte der Krebsforschung

Progrès dans les recherches sur le cancer

36

Edited by

Editor in chief

P. Rentchnick, Genève

Springer-Verlag Berlin · Heidelberg · New York 1971

Current Concepts in the Management of Lymphoma and Leukemia

Edited by

J. E. Ultmann · M. L. Griem · W. H. Kirsten · R. W. Wissler

With 46 Figures

Springer-Verlag Berlin · Heidelberg · New York 1971

Symposium on Current Concepts in the Management of Lymphoma and Leukemia
The University of Chicago Pritzker School of Medicine, March 7th and 8th, 1970

Sponsored by the Swiss League against Cancer

ISBN-13: 978-3-642-46261-0 e-ISBN-13: 978-3-642-46259-7
DOI: 10.1007/978-3-642-46259-7

Preface

This volume summarizes the Proceedings of the fourth biennial Cancer Teaching Symposium held on March 7 and 8, 1970, at the University of Chicago Pritzker School of Medicine. The program was prepared by Drs. LAWRENCE ALLEN, MELVIN GRIEM, WERNER KIRSTEN, LEON JACOBSON, JOHN ULTMANN, ROBERT WISSLER, and STANLEY YACHNIN. The purpose of the Symposium was to present current advances in the area of lymphoma and leukemia to the staff and students of this medical center and to students and interested physicians from other institutions in the Chicago area. Like the other teaching symposia held in 1964, 1966, and 1968, this Symposium attracted over 450 physicians and scientists. In the course of one and a half days the audience had the opportunity to listen to the twenty-four invited speakers and to lively discussions. The formal presentations as well as discussions are recorded in these pages.

This Teaching Symposium could not have been undertaken without the faithful assistance of the Program Committee, the Cancer Training Grant Advisory Committee, the staff who recorded and transcribed the Proceedings, and the editorial assistants. We wish to thank the following for their efforts: DOROTHY A. WILLIS, Administrative Secretary for Institutional Cancer Training Grant, Dr. ROBERT L. HUNTER, Dr. ROBERT H. KIRSCHNER, Dr. ROBERT A. ORLANDO, Dr. STEPHEN STRUM, RANDOLPH HUGHES, JULIA KANT, GEORGIA MOHR, TERRY PEARSON, FRIEDA RANNEY, and CAROL REESE.

This Symposium received financial support from the Cancer Training Program T12 CA 08077-04 and The Chicago Tumor Institute.

JOHN E. ULTMANN, M.D.
ROBERT W. WISSLER, Ph.D., M.D.

Introduction

During the past decade, great strides have been made in the diagnosis and management of patients with lymphoma and leukemia. Stimulated by advances in radiotherapeutic techniques, clinicians have looked for new ways to classify and stage the disease in patients with lymphoma to determine curability. In so doing, they have re-examined previous staging procedures and have expanded the approach to staging by the introduction of new techniques, including lung tomography, inferior venacavography, lower extremity lymphography, and isotope scanning of liver, spleen, and bone. These approaches have led to revisions of clinical staging criteria. More recently, laparotomy and splenectomy have been introduced as part of the work-up of patients with lymphoma in an attempt to delineate further the criteria for curability.

Pathologists re-examining histologic features useful for the diagnosis and classification of lymphoma have developed precise diagnostic criteria permitting more meaningful differentiation of these tumors than heretofore possible. The advances in the clinical and pathologic diagnosis of lymphoma were summarized in the present symposium by Drs. Henry Rappaport, chairman, and Robert Lukes, William Sheehan, Saul Rosenberg, and Lawrence Allen.

Review of treatment failures and modern considerations of radiobiology have resulted in new approaches to the cure of lymphoma by means of radiotherapy. Wide field, intensive radiotherapy appears to offer an opportunity for cure to a significant number of patients with lymphoma. Current concepts in radiotherapy of lymphoma were reviewed by Drs. Vera Peters, chairman, Robert Bruce, Henry Kaplan, Ralph Johnson, Melvin Griem, and Eugene Cronkite.

During the past few years, laboratory data in animals with acute leukemia demonstrated the possibility of achieving cure by application of intensive chemotherapy. The prerequisites for understanding current therapy of patients with acute leukemia are an understanding of the biochemical and pharmacologic properties of agents used in the managment of acute leukemia and considerations of the cell cycle applicable in the chemotherapy of this disease. These subjects, together with the current status of clinical therapy, were reviewed by Drs. Gordon Zubrod, chairman, Alan Sartorelli, Emil Freireich, Bayard Clarkson, and Paul Carbone.

Profiting from the lessons apparent from the management of patients with acute leukemia, new strides have been made in the chemotherapy of the chronic leukemias and in the management of patients with lymphoma who cannot be cured by radiotherapy. A review of this area was presented under the chairmanship of Dr. Stanley Yachnin, by Drs. Glynn Wheeler, David Galton, and Vincent DeVita.

The final portion of the Symposium was devoted to the presentation of new approaches to the management of lymphoma and leukemia. Particular emphasis was placed on understanding of the immunological reactivity against tumor specific antigens and on experimental approaches to the immunotherapy of lymphoma. These areas were discussed by Drs. THOMAS HALL, chairman, KARL ERIC HELLSTRÖM, and ALEXANDER FEFER.

The editors are grateful to all the participants in this conference who permitted publication of their manuscripts.

J. E. ULTMANN, M. L. GRIEM,
W. H. KIRSTEN, R. W. WISSLER

Contents

Welcoming Remarks. LEON O. JACOBSON 1

Keynote Address. CARL G. BAKER 2

Diagnosis of Lymphoma

Chairman: HENRY RAPPAPORT

Malignant Lymphoma: Histologic Considerations. ROBERT J. LUKES 6

Discussion: The Relationship between Lymphocytic Leukemias and Lymphomas. WILLIAM W. SHEEHAN 24

The Clinical Evaluation and Staging of Patients with Malignant Lymphoma. SAUL A. ROSENBERG 32

Discussion: The Staging of Lymphoma. LAWRENCE W. ALLEN, STEPHEN B. STRUM, JOHN E. ULTMANN, HENRY RAPPAPORT 43

Radiotherapy of Lymphoma

Chairman: VERA M. PETERS

An Empirical Cellular Approach to the Improvement of Cancer Chemotherapy. WILLIAM R. BRUCE, H. LIN 47

Radiation Therapy with Curative Intent in the Malignant Lymphomas. HENRY S. KAPLAN 52

Discussion: The Curative Radiotherapy of Lymphomas. RALPH E. JOHNSON . 57

Discussion: Reasons for Failure of the Curative Radiotherapeutic Management of Patients with Lymphomas. MELVIN L. GRIEM 63

Extracorporeal Irradiation of Blood in the Treatment of Chronic Lymphocytic Leukemia. EUGENE P. CRONKITE 67

Therapy of Acute Leukemia

Chairman: C. GORDON ZUBROD

Some Biochemical and Pharmacologic Considerations of Agents in the Management of Acute Leukemia. ALAN C. SARTORELLI 74

Consideration of the Cell Cycle in Chemotherapy of Acute Leukemia. BAYARD CLARKSON, AKIO TODO, MAKOTO OGAWA, TIMOTHY GEE, JERROLD FRIED . 88

Current Status of Therapy for Acute Leukemia. EMIL J FREIREICH, GERALD P. BODEY, JACQUELINE S. HART, JOHN P. WHITECAR, JR., KENNETH B. MCCREDIE 119

Burkitt's Tumor: A Comparative Study in Africa and the United States. PAUL P. CARBONE, JOHN L. ZIEGLER, RICHARD MORROW, SEBASTIAN KYALWAZI, CLARENCE H. BROWN, VINCENT T. DEVITA, COSTAN BERARD 126

Chemotherapy of Chronic Leukemias and Lymphoma

Chairman: STANLEY YACHNIN

Pharmacological Considerations of Alkylating Agents. GLYNN P. WHEELER . . 137

Management of the Chronic Leukaemias. DAVID A. G. GALTON 147

Chemotherapy of the Lymphomas. VINCENT T. DEVITA 159

Discussion: Treatment of Chronic Lymphocytic Leukemia. RALPH E. JOHNSON . 172

New Approaches to Management of Leukemia and Lymphoma

Chairman: THOMAS HALL

Immunity to Human Tumor Antigens. KARL E. HELLSTRÖM, INGEGERD HELLSTRÖM 175

Experimental Approaches to Immunotherapy of Cancer. ALEXANDER FEFER . 182

Summary of Conference. C. GORDON ZUBROD 193

List of Participants

Allen, Lawrence W., Department of Medicine, University of Chicago, Chicago, IL

Baker, Carl G., National Cancer Institute, National Institutes of Health, Bethesda, MD

Bruce, W. Robert, University of Toronto, Princess Margaret Hospital, Toronto, Ontario, Canada

Carbone, Paul P., Medicine Branch, National Cancer Institute, National Institutes of Health, Bethesda, MD

Clarkson, Bayard, Division of Chemotherapy Research, Sloan Kettering Institute for Cancer Research, New York, NY

Cronkite, Eugene P., Medical Department, Brookhaven National Laboratory, Upton, NY

DeVita, Vincent T., Solid Tumor Service, Medicine Branch, National Cancer Institute, National Institutes of Health, Bethesda, MD

Fefer, Alexander, Division of Oncology, Department of Medicine, University of Washington, Seattle, WA

Freireich, Emil J, Department of Developmental Therapeutics, M. D. Anderson Hospital, University of Texas, Houston, TX

Galton, David A. G., Institute of Cancer Research and Royal Postgraduate Medical School, London, England

Griem, Melvin L., Department of Radiology, University of Chicago, Chicago, IL

Hall, Thomas, School of Medicine and Dentistry, The University of Rochester, Rochester, NY

Hellström, Karl Erik, Department of Pathology, University of Washington, Seattle, WA

Jacobson, Leon O., Division of Biological Sciences, University of Chicago, Chicago, IL

Johnson, Ralph E., Radiation Branch, National Cancer Institute, National Institutes of Health, Bethesda, MD

Kaplan, Henry S., Department of Radiology, Stanford University Medical Center, Stanford, CA

Lukes, Robert J., Department of Pathology, University of Southern California, Los Angeles, CA

Peters, M. Vera, Radiotherapy Department, Princess Margaret Hospital, University of Toronto, Toronto, Ontario, Canada

Rappaport, Henry, Department of Pathology, University of Chicago, Chicago, IL

Rosenberg, Saul A., Departments of Medicine and Radiology, Stanford University, Stanford, CA

SARTORELLI, ALAN C., Department of Pharmacology, Yale University School of Medicine, New Haven, CT

SHEEHAN, WILLIAM W., Pathology Division, US Army Biological Defense Research Center, Fort Detrick, Frederick, MD

ULTMANN, JOHN E., Department of Medicine, University of Chicago, Chicago, IL

WHEELER, GLYNN P., Biochemistry Department, Southern Research Institute, Birmingham, AL

WISSLER, ROBERT W., Department of Pathology, University of Chicago, Chicago, IL

YACHNIN, STANLEY, Department of Medicine, University of Chicago, Chicago, IL

ZUBROD, C. GORDON, National Cancer Institute, National Institutes of Health, Bethesda, MD

Welcoming Remarks

Leon O. Jacobson

As I look around, it's easy to recognize a large number of distinguished guest speakers from around the world and many of my former colleagues throughout the country. I also recognize faculty and students in the room.

It is a great pleasure to welcome you here to the University, especially for a conference such as this. There are a few who are as old as I am and have been involved in the lymphoma-leukemia field for many years. Some of you were working in the endeavor in the early 40's. Many of us shared in the introduction of nitrogen mustard with a great deal of fear and trepidation as we applied it to those first few patients.

I know that this conference is going to be most interesting and rewarding and, as is true with most conferences that are led by the kinds of people that are speaking here, surely new ideas will come through. I do hope you enjoy these two days with us and will profit from these deliberations.

Keynote Address

Carl G. Baker

First, I want to thank Dean Jacobson for his kind hospitality and for the invitation of the Program Committee to participate in this symposium. I anticipate learning new things along with those of you in the audience. I thought perhaps you might be interested in some comments regarding the fiscal stresses we face these days, about problems of priorities, and how these priorities look from the point of view of scientists and of laymen, including members of Congress. Perhaps we can gain a little insight on how the Congress and the public may now be looking at these priorities, which seems to me to be very germane to the present situation on funding. I will try to use examples from the lymphoma and leukemia areas to illustrate some of the aspects of priority decision making.

This meeting itself represents an important link in a complex chain of forces and events that deal with the question of priorities. Meetings such as this symposium are important for bringing together the latest information, summarizing the state of the art, and indicating where the research leads are. At times, we develop important syntheses from such meetings. We are here to learn and to teach, and to stimulate each other, particularly in obtaining new perspectives and new concepts. I hope we succeed in those aims.

If one looks at the relative amounts of fundings in different areas of cancer research, it is notable that the area of leukemias and lymphomas has been for some time one of the areas of high priority, receiving relatively higher funding than most other cancer research areas. For example, of the total budget of the National Cancer Institute of $ 184 million last year, leukemia and lymphoma research accounted for somewhere in the neighborhood of $ 40 to $ 50 million. Why should this kind of research consume, so to speak, that high a proportion of the dollar resources? What are the events that led to this situation? Certainly in terms of the number of cases of leukemias and lymphomas, even taken together, this amount is out of proportion to the other problems of the cancer field as a whole. Why is the public willing to support this area? Why does science put that much stress on it? What are the elements that lead to priority decisions?

It seems to me that there are three main elements in making priority decisions. One element is the *importance of the problem.* Although leukemia is not as important as colon cancer or lung cancer in terms of the number of cases, the fact that many leukemias occur in children has given an impetus to this area of research in public interest that goes beyond the mere numbers. Or, to say it in another way, in our cultural system, the value of children is placed at a high level. I might remind you that not all cultural systems look at children in this way. This value judgment has led the public to provide relatively generous support to leukemia efforts, and this is reflected not only in the Congressional appropriations, but also in the leukemia societies and activities of the American Cancer Society. Importance is also ascribed to the problem because prevention or cure of fatal disease in *young* people means longer lives than similar successes with older diseased subjects. Perhaps also, more significance is afforded leukemia because surgery and radiation are not effective therapeutic means.

A second element in priority decision making is the assessment of *the state of the art,* or the *maturity of the field,* and the extent of richness of research leads. Some of the most important recent progress in cancer research lies in the area of leukemias and lymphomas. Not only are we beginning to see concrete statistical evidence of therapeutic improvement, but developments that we see today are providing new insights into the treatment of these diseases which in turn will have important ramifications, not only to leukemias and lymphomas themselves, but for other kinds of cancers as well. Moreover, studies on etiology are moving very rapidly and many leads are ready for development which can occur quickly with the present program capability. Thus, from the standpoint of the scientist, one reason we have high emphasis on leukemias and lymphomas is that most cancer investigators see the possibilities for further development because of maturity of concepts and knowledge of the field. Most of these scientists see this as an area with more opportunity than, say, the lung cancer or colon cancer areas. In other words, we know more, at least we think we know more, about what to do.

The third element is the *probability that successses will be attained if additional investments are put into the field.* While this element is related to the previous one, it differs in the same sense that the *closeness* to one's destination differs from the *rate* at which one is moving along.

A layman, I believe, looks at these same three elements with a somewhat different perspective than the scientist does. The layman is primarily concerned with practical solutions to real life problems of cancer patients, either with successful treatment of those diseases already in being, or with an area which has not received as much emphasis: cancer prevention. If you solve the problem, will it lead to practical results in terms of patients? The scientist often considers, I think, the importance of the problem in terms of whether the area is ready for a new conceptual development. The problem area is important if we can obtain new conceptual advances in science.

How these two viewpoints are welded together is a complex subject. Part of the problem is to communicate with the layman as to why scientists think certain areas are of high priority. We as members of the scientific community need to devote more effort to understanding what the layman expects to obtain for providing funds through appropriations and voluntary organizations. Regarding the question of state of the art, the laymen in Congress have to depend on testimony from experts. Occasionally, a problem results from experts with perfectly equal high-quality credentials before the committee giving opposite views in answer to important questions posed at the Hearings. And if you were the Congressman listening to that in an area you did not understand in detail, I think you would conclude — "Well, I guess they don't know what the answer is on this point." We may need to admit we don't know more than we have on occasion in the past. I think the Congressmen also are quite interested nevertheless in having expert opinion: "All right, suppose we give you funds, what are the chances of having success?" They mean success, I think, again in terms of will there be a better cure rate. For example, will there be fewer patients?

This blending of these two broad points of view plus many others becomes crystallized in the development of budget put together each year and in the actions taken on each budget. The number of forces that are brought to bear in this process are many and complex. Forces afoot today in society, such as new interest in urban development, transportation, race problems, and so on, have brought forth a whole array of new elements in competition with funds for health research. These forces were not present with the same degree of insistence three or four years ago. Congressman have to face up to the difficult question of allocating money. The first kind of decision many Congressman, I think, try to make is: Of the total resources available from appropriations, how much should be devoted to *health?* Then once that decision is roughly settled, there are a series of forces competing for dollars within the total area to determine the proportion for health *research.* In earlier times, medical *research* was certainly one of the more popular parts of competition within the total health dollar category. Nowadays, health *care* is getting much more attention. Medical research is faring somewhat less well in this competition now than has been the case over the last several years.

There are many other forces involved, some of which are political, and I don't mean this in a derogatory sense. The job of politics really, it seems to me, is to decide among various points of view as to where priorities ought to lie. The Congress is a main force in settling this kind of question. How much should go into cancer research is primarily a political question, not a scientific one. What proportions of that money should go into different areas of cancer research, however, is primarily a scientific question. I think most of us would hope that the Congress would not place too many earmarkings on these categories of cancer investigation. Nevertheless, there are occasions when Congressional committees will put very stringent constraints or strong earmarkings in a particular appropriation.

The question of communicating then between the scientific community and the Congress and public may become more insistent now with these tighter priorities. One of the points I would like to leave with you is some considerations of how all of us can do a better job in communicating to the public and to Congress why we think certain areas in medical research are important, or even, why medical research should compete successfully in the complex arena of determining priorities. This can be done in part by many of us devoting a little more attention to the problem than we have in the past. The question of letting your Congressman know about the kinds of problems that you face in your own institution is certainly legitimate and the proper thing to do. Congressmen are looking for information on the effects produced by what they do in the Congress. Perhaps we need to devote a little more attention to our relationship with the press, i. e., the magazines and the printed and TV news media that are trying to communicate with the public. How we convey some of these complex ideas to laymen is not the simplest thing in the world, but I think perhaps we haven't devoted enough attention to that. In view of the present situation, we may need to do more of that.

Once priorities get settled, the question, of course, arises on the means of implementation. The various sections of this symposium illustrate major components in the fields of leukemia and lymphomas. I would like to make just a few remarks on some of those features. In reference to the first section on diagnosis of lymphoma, I want to put in a plug for things that some people consider mundane. I'm talking about things like *definitions, terminology, classification* and *standardization.* Counting seems to be a very simple matter, but unless we have our standards set fairly clearly in such complex things as the different kinds of lymphomas, counting cannot be done appropriately. We often fail to pay enough attention to these more mundane things of struggling with clear definitions and clear terminology and settling on classifications we can agree on and live with. Careful attention to these more mundane things, coupled with the idea of sound experimental design of the studies, are really the foundation stones for the good use of computers. Too often people are trying to jump in and use computers without having gone through the more laborious clarifying definitional problems. Many people are bored to tears in developing clear definition, but it's essential that we pay considerable attention to these areas, and I'm glad to see that the symposium starts out with this subject. I know Dr. RAPPAPORT has been a leader in defining some of the problems in lymphoma.

I do not have time to comment on the other areas of the symposium very much. I do want to put in one more plug for the value of empiricism in the area of chemotherapy. We now have a number of drugs that are active and we are beginning to see cures. We are moving out to a new phase of gaining a deeper insight into how these drugs are acting. But before we had the drugs we were not able to do that. And how do we get the drugs or how do we find new drugs? I believe that basically we're still in a phase of having to do it with a heavy element of empiricism. I think we will keep on finding drugs that way. It seems to me that the history of drug development by and large has shown that most new drugs come from empiricism; it is only after the drugs are available that we begin to get insight into the mechanisms of action. However, once a critical mass of compounds is reached, we are quite hopeful that new drugs can be developed based on the understanding of the activities of those first few drugs that we picked up by empiricism. An area of shortage in this regard is manpower in pharmacology and chronic toxicology, both in cancer chemotherapy and in carcinogenesis investigations. I will make a plea for attention in medical schools in this area along with perhaps trying to make preventive medicine a little more respectable. In medical schools, we have not given due attention to the areas of prevention and causation. Too often the whole area of preventive medicine in medical schools is looked down upon, and it doesn't seem to get attention commensurate with its importance. So I will ask those of you in the medical schools to give considerations to perhaps helping out in that area.

These are the main points I will leave with you. I hope that we will have the successful symposium which I anticipate from looking at the program. Thank you very much for the opportunity of being here with you.

Malignant Lymphoma: Histologic Considerations

ROBERT J. LUKES

With 9 Figures

Introduction

The morphologic identification and classification of malignant lymphomas have been the subjects of confusion and controversy for decades. The remarkable diversity of the histologic and cytologic manifestations of the malignant lymphomas and the difficulty of precise cytologic identification in tissue sections, particularly of poorly differentiated cells, have produced a unique terminologic maze that has precluded effective comparison of case series from different centers. The traditional classifications of malignant lymphoma have been employed in an unappreciated, extraordinarily variable fashion and have proved ineffective in prognostication and communication in my experience.

In the past decade evidence of disenchantment has appeared in the literature, but much of it has past unnoticed. The meaningless status of the term *reticulum cell sarcoma* has been demonstrated by GALL [1]. The existence of follicular lymphoma has been challenged by RAPPAPORT, WINTER and HICKS [2], and I have recently demonstrated the extreme variability in the use of the term *lymphosarcoma* [3]. The superiority of clinical staging over traditional cytologic classifications in prognosis has been demonstrated by PETERS [4]. Finally we have challenged the position of Hodgkin's disease in the scheme of malignant lymphoma [5—7].

This presentation will be limited to a brief consideration of (1) the terminologic and conceptual problems; (2) the definition of 4 cytologic groups of malignant lymphomas; (3) the interrelationship of leukemias and lymphomas and the significance of the distribution of involvement; and (4) the position of Hodgkin's disease, mycosis fungoides and macroglobulinemia in the scheme of malignant lymphoma.

Terminologic Problems

Communication in the field of malignant lymphoma has become increasingly difficult during the past few decades because of terminologic confusion resulting from the problem of precise cytologic identification, particularly of poorly differentiated cells in tissue sections and the lack of correlative histologic and cytologic studies on lymphomas and leukemias.

The majority of pathologists in the United States generally agree that malignant lymphoma be defined as a malignant neoplasm of lymphoid tissue derivatives; but beyond this there is little accord. The lack of agreement on cytologic types, the related character of distribution, the relationship to leukemia, the site of origin, all have permitted wide divergence in basic concept, led to marked differences in terminology, and in essence, accommodated any pathologist's personal viewpoint.

The following is a definition which I have employed for a number of years and includes these basic features of lymphomas. *Malignant lymphoma* is a neoplastic proliferative process of lymphoreticular tissue involving stem cells (undifferentiated cells) and lymphocytes or histiocytes in varying degrees of differentiation. It occurs essentially in a homogeneous population of a single cell type; when mixtures are found, they appear to represent variations in the size or configuration of a single cell type. The character of histologic involvement is either diffuse (uniform) or nodular, and the distribution of involvement may be irregular or systemtic (generalized). Leukemias and lymhomas of stem cells, lymphocytes and histiocytes are fundamentally identical processes for each cell type. The occurrence of lymphoma cells in the peripheral blood seems to be related to the character of the distribution of the cellular proliferation.

From this definition of malignant lymphoma terminologic problems are inherent in the nature of the process. Upon comparative evaluation of a few of the most commonly used classifications of malignant lymphoma recorded in Table 1, there seems to be little difference between the classifications. Upon closer examination we see that many terms are used for poorly differentiated cells; at times identical terms are employed in a different fashion in the various classifications. Furthermore, the term *lymphosarcoma* has been used with extreme variability from a specific cell type to a synonym for malignant lymphoma. It is commonly employed to refer to all lymphoma cells with scanty cytoplasm in histologic sections including well differentiated lymphocytes, poorly differentiated lymphocytes, stem cells, leukemias of poorly differentiated types, and erroneously at times, tumor cells of nonreticuloendothelial origin where the cytoplasm is scanty or the cytologic details are obscured by technical factors. From this comparative evaluation of the classification of lymphomas of lymphocytes and poorly differentiated reticulum cells or stem cells listed in Table 1, it is obviously necessary to specify the classification employed and require the definition of the term. The lymphosarcoma of Jackson and Parker [8] is not equivalent to the lymphosarcoma of Custer and Bernhard [9], since the latter includes lymphocytoma and lymphoblastoma of Jackson and Parker [8], and possibly the stem cell of Gall and Mallory [10]. The lymphoblastic lymphoma of Gall and Mallory [10] is not equivalent to that of Berman [11], since Gall and Mallory [10] have separated and identified the stem cell as a distinctive type of lymphoma.

From an evaluation of Table 1, *reticulum cell sarcoma* does not seem to present a terminologic problem, but its usage is more variable than the term *lymphosarcoma.* The marked variation in the use of the term *reticulum cell sarcoma* in the literature was pointed out by Gall [1] who demonstrated the meaningless status and undesirability of this term in his comparative evaluation of the major reports of the

Table 1. *Comparison of classification of malignant lymphoma*

GALL and MALLORY [10]	JACKSON and PARKER [8]	CUSTER and BERNHARD [9]	BERMAN [11]
Lymphocytic	Lymphocytoma		Lymphocytic
Lymphoblastic	Lymphoblastoma		Lymphoblastic
	Lymphosarcoma	Lymphosarcoma	
Stem cell			
	Reticulum cell sarcoma	Reticulum cell sarcoma	Reticulum cell
Clasmatocytic			
Follicular	Giant follicle lymphoma	Follicular	
			Mixed types (a) Follicular (b) Hodgkin's disease
Hodgkin's lymphoma	Hodgkin's disease Paragranuloma Granuloma Sarcoma	Hodgkin's disease Paragranuloma Granuloma Sarcoma (Reticulum cell sarcoma)	

literature in which a detailed definition was provided. The definitions in the literature of reticulum cell sarcoma indicated that the cells may be small or large, vary widely in configuration, and in the quantity and character of cytoplasm. Similar marked variations in size and configuration were noted in the definition of the nuclear characteristics with vesicular nucleus and a prominent nucleolus the only consistently recorded features. In addition however the nucleus was often defined as hyperchromatic and at times the nucleolus was recorded as absent or not prominent. From this summation of the cytologic criteria employed for the reticulum cell sarcoma, it is uncertain whether the primitive reticulum cell (stem cell) usually is included within this category. This broad application of the term *reticulum cell sarcoma* demonstrated in the literature indicates that the term is employed for almost any cell type. This situation is partially a reflection of the pathologist's conceptual concern for the multipotential character of the reticulum cell. From my experience with consultative cases, the term is used for the most part in an essentially nonspecific fashion for lesions that cannot be readily classified elsewhere.

The futility of communications with the term *reticulum cell sarcoma* led GALL [1] to recommend discontinuing its use and utilizing more specific cytologic types. The term *clasmatocyte* originally suggested by GALL and MALLORY [10] in 1942 for the phagocytic reticulum cell sarcoma was modified in the above report [1] to the more appropriate term *histiocytic lymphoma* for the various degrees of differentiation of the reticulum cell beyond the stem cell, regardless of the presence or absence of phagocytosis. Retention of the term *stem cell* for the primitive reticulum cell was recommended. Fibril production, formerly one of the major criteria for the diagnosis of *reticulum cell sarcoma* [12] is not a prominent feature of the stem cell or the poorly differentiated histiocytic lymphoma, and is observed in prominent degrees in only a small proportion of cases with histiocytic lymphoma, in my experience. Similarly the pleomorphic lymphomas of histiocytes which may at times be indistinguishable from Hodgkin's sarcoma of JACKSON and PARKER [8] in individual specimens, may deserve separate designation as a pleomorphic variant of histiocytic lymphoma.

Elimination of the terminologic problem may never be achieved, but it can be minimized by careful attention to technical factors, essential for accurate cytologic identification. Improperly fixed and thick, overstained sections represent the major cause of problems in cytologic identification and diagnostic difficulties on lymph node lesions. Unquestionably, extensive experience is required to be familiar with the extraordinary variations in lesions, but ideally fixed and stained sections together with excellent tissue imprints (touch preparation) will permit resolution of the majority of the problems.

Conceptual Problems

The malignant lymphomas have provided one of the most fertile fields for conceptual disputes during recent decades primarily because of the remarkable variability of clinical and histologic manifestation and the difficulty in precise cytologic identification and classification. The simulation of malignant lymphoma by severe reactive processes undoubtedly has contributed to conceptual differences and accounts for the appearance of prolonged survival cases and apparent cures in many malignant lymphoma case series, particulary following regional therapy of Stage I disease in lymph nodes or localized extranodal masses.

Origin of Malignant Lymphoma: The dispute over the unicentric or multicentric origin of malignant lymphomas remains unresolved. The extranodal lymphoid tissue proliferations in the past often have been designated as primary lymphomas. In my experience these lesions on careful examination often have presented features of lymphoid reaction and the process has followed a benign course, all of which has encouraged me to use the terms *pseudolymphoma* or *pseudolymphomatous reaction.*

Whether these lesions represent severe reactive lymphoid proliferations or primary lymphomas of unicentric type is difficult to establish with certainty on a histologic basis. The reports on the evaluation of lymphoid lesions of the stomach [13—14] and the lung [15] provide evidence of the frequent benign course of extranodal lymphoid lesions in these locations. My experience with extranodal lesions from almost every anatomical site is essentially similar.

For this reason it is my belief that all extranodal lymphoid proliferations should be evaluated with extreme caution and primary consideration given to the possibility of a pseudolymphoma or pseudolymphomatous reaction, particularly if it is composed of small lymphocytes. Whether or not malignant lymphomas originate in lymph nodes and extranodal sites as unicentric focus and are resectable, remains unresolved and is difficult to clarify. In Hodgkin's disease, however, evidence from radiotherapy studies [16] is now available that provides at least some support for the unicentric concept.

Follicular Lymphoma: Through the decades, follicular lymphoma has provided the major source of controversy in the field of malignant lymphomas and received a special designation of Brill-Symmers disease because of the dispute over the significance of its nature. This controversy was concerned with the malignant potential of giant follicle hyperplasia for transition into follicular lymphoma and the differential diagnostic problem between the two lesions. The malignant neoplastic character of the process from its inception was proposed by CALLENDER [17] and its distinctiveness as an entity by GALL, MORRISON and SCOTT [18]. Insight into the nature of the process was provided by RAPPAPORT, WINTER and HICKS [2] who proposed that the process represented the tendency of lymphoma cells to aggregate in nodular fashion without origin in follicular hyperplasia. On the basis of this concept, these authors proposed that malignant lymphomas have both diffuse and

Table 2. *Classification of malignant lymphoma* (GALL and RAPPAPORT) [19]

"Follicular" (Nodular)	Diffuse
Lymphocytic type, well differentiated (W. D.)	
Lymphocytic type, poorly differentiated (P. D.)	
Stem cell type } "Reticulum cell sarcoma"	
Histiocytic type }	
Histiocytic-lymphocytic (mixed cell type)	
Hodgkin's type (paragranuloma, granuloma and sarcoma)	

nodular expressions, and the natural evolution of a lymphomatous process is from the nodular to diffuse type. This concept provided the basis for reclassification of lymphomas proposed initially by RAPPAPORT, WINTER and HICKS [2] that combined the cytologic types of GALL and MALLORY [10], and the nodular concept of lymphoma. It was later refined by GALL and RAPPAPORT [19] and is recorded in Table 2. According to this classification, all cytologic types of malignant lymphoma occur in either diffuse (Fig. 1) or nodular form (Fig. 2). A lymphoma is designated by the cell type followed by an indication whether it exhibits a diffuse or nodular histologic pattern; e. g. lymphocytic lymphoma, poorly differentiated, nodular. The diagnostic value of this concept is the emphasis on the lack of developmental relationship between nodular lymphomas and reactive follicles. This view is based on the lack of evidence of transition from follicular hyperplasia to follicular lymphoma in the study of RAPPAPORT et al. [2].

Transitions in Malignant Lymphoma: The potential for transitions between the cytologic types of malignant lymphoma was presented by CUSTER and BERNHARD [9] in 1948. From their extensive experience at the Armed Forces Institute of Pathology during World War II, these authors indicated that a wide range of changes in the type of lymphoma occurred in their cases, 31% in sequential biopsy specimens and 37% between biopsy and autopsy. This observation remains unchallenged by a detailed study based upon a large autopsy population. Although a wide variation in lymphoma was reported by CUSTER and BERNHARD [9], they acknowledged that three principal changes were observed: (1) the change between follicular lymphoma and the various cytologic types of malignant lymphoma, including reticulum cell sarcoma and Hodgkin's sacroma; (2) the change in Hodgkin's disease with progression from paragranuloma to granuloma to sarcoma, but most commonly from granuloma to sarcoma; (3) the development of leukemic manifestations.

From my own experience with over 5000 autopsy cases of malignant lymphomas, leukemias and Hodgkin's disease it is acknowledged that changes in the histologic expression are relatively frequent with the progression of the disease, but these changes are believed to represent different expressions of the evolving process rather than a true transition in the basic process. The majority of changes observed are similar to those recorded by CUSTER and BERNHARD [9] with only a rare case exhibiting a true transition in cell type with the appearance of a new or second type of lymphomatous cellular proliferation.

Simulation of Malignant Lymphoma: The simulation of malignant lymphoma by severe reactive processes in both normal individuals and abnormal reactors undoubtedly accounts for at least part of the disagreement on terminology and concepts. It appears likely that the survival data in many case series through the decades and in the recent studies evaluating the effectiveness of therapeutic agents are distorted by this factor through the erroneous inclusion of benign cases. All the commonly used general criteria for the establishment of the diagnosis of malignant lymphoma may be observed in severe reactive processes from my experience including (1) the obliteration of lymph node architecture, (2) infiltration of the capsule, and (3) cellular atypia.

Because of the severe and diversified benign reactions of normal lymphoid tissue and the essentially unknown expressions of abnormal reactors, it is my belief that the diagnosis of malignant lymphoma should be established only on the basis of positive morphologic criteria, consisting primarily of the identification of specific cytologic types of malignant lymphoma, rather than as an exclusion diagnosis.

Classification and Cytologic Types

At the present time there is no general agreement among pathologists on the classification of malignant lymphoma. If any classification has gained favor, it is that of GALL and MALLORY [10] recorded in Table 1. Its modified descendant, the classification of GALL and RAPPAPORT [19], Table 2, combines the cytologic types of GALL and MALLORY [10] and the nodular concept of lymphoma proposed by RAPPAPORT et al. [2]. Because of its striking and fundamental departure from previous classifications, particularly the concept of nodular lymphoma, it has not gained widespread acceptance and only the study of DORFMAN [21] has provided support for this concept. At the present time we are engaged in a study evaluating this concept using a relatively large population of malignant lymphomas. Unfortunately, our findings are too incomplete at the present time to permit a definite conclusion. Nevertheless, the simplicity of the concept proposed by RAPPAPORT et al. [2] in general is appealing.

Whether or not all the variations in cytologic types proposed by RAPPAPORT et al. [2] on detailed reevaluation can be substantiated to occur in nodular as well as diffuse pattern and the possibility of a relationship of the cytologic types to follicular center cells can be excluded, must await completion of the study now in progress.

The classification that I presently use (Table 3) is based on the classification of Gall and Rappaport [19], but with several significant differences. The mixed lymphocytic and histiocytic type of lymphoma is omitted because it appears that this proliferation represents a variation in a single large cell type, which Rappaport designated, the histiocyte. In addition Hodgkin's disease is placed in a questionable position because of its uncertain nature which will be considered in a subsequent discussion. Each cytologic type may occur in either diffuse (Fig. 1) or nodular (Fig. 2) form.

Table 3. *Classification of malignant lymphoma*

A-Diffuse	B-Nodular
1. Lymphocytic, well differentiated (W. D.)	
2. Lymphocytic, poorly differentiated (P. D.)	
3. Stem cell	
4. Histiocytic	
? Hodgkin's disease [a]	

[a] Hodgkin's disease is included within the classification in a questionable position indicating its unestablished nature.

Cytologic Types: The cytologic types employed in these classifications were defined originally in detail by Gall and Mallory [10] and from a histochemical and enzymatic standpoint by Braunstein and Gall [20] and Dorfman [21]. They have been recently reviewed in detail and beautifully illustrated by Rappaport [22]. Although only 4 cell types are included, there are admittedly a number of variations within 2 groups, lymphocytic lymphoma, poorly differentiated type and histiocytic lymphoma. It appears impossible at the present time to subclassify these types effectively from either a cytologic or prognostic standpoint. Accurate, reproducible classification of malignant lymphomas into these 4 cytologic groups, at times may be difficult and attention to histologic preparations is essential for precise cytologic identification. Unquestionably, tissue imprints (touch preparations) will aid immeasureably in the cytologic evaluation.

Lymphocytic Lymphoma, Well Differentiated: This lymphoma (Fig. 3) consists essentially of a proliferation of small to medium-sized lymphocytes with scanty or indiscernible cytoplasm that are characteristically of uniform size and configuration, but are indistinguishable individually from normal lymphocytes. The most distinctive features of this lymphocytic proliferation in H & E stained sections are the uniformity in the appearance of the lymphocytes with a rarity of reticulum cells and essentially an absence of plasma cells. The process is indistinguishable from the histologic manifestations of chronic lymphocytic leukemia, and in the opinion of the author, the processes are identical.

Lymphocytic Lymphoma, Poorly Differentiated: This lymphoma (Fig. 4) consists of a proliferation of medium-sized cells of distinctly variable size and configuration;

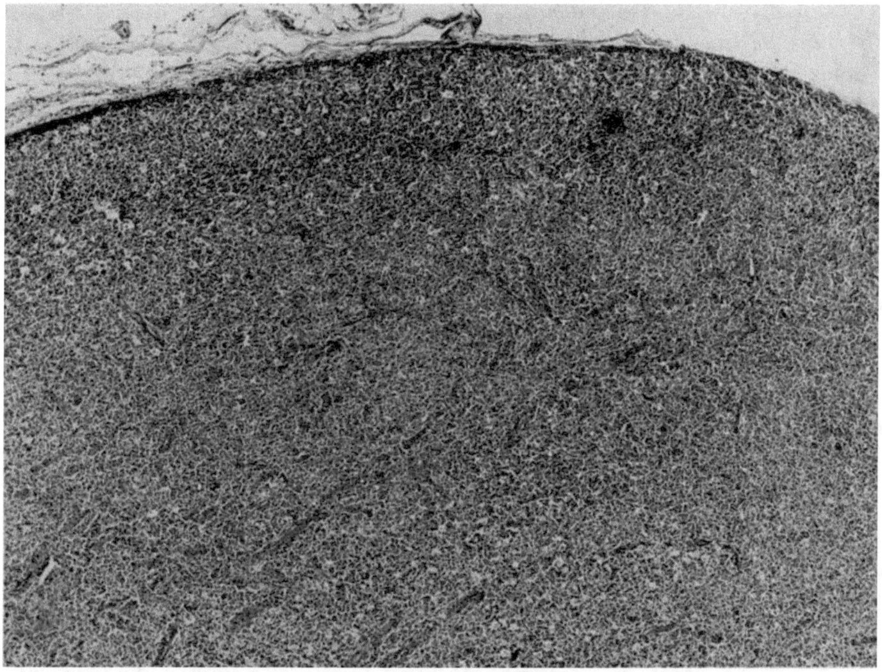

Fig. 1. Malignant lymphoma, diffuse histologic pattern. AFIP access, No. 747 054. H & E, ×30

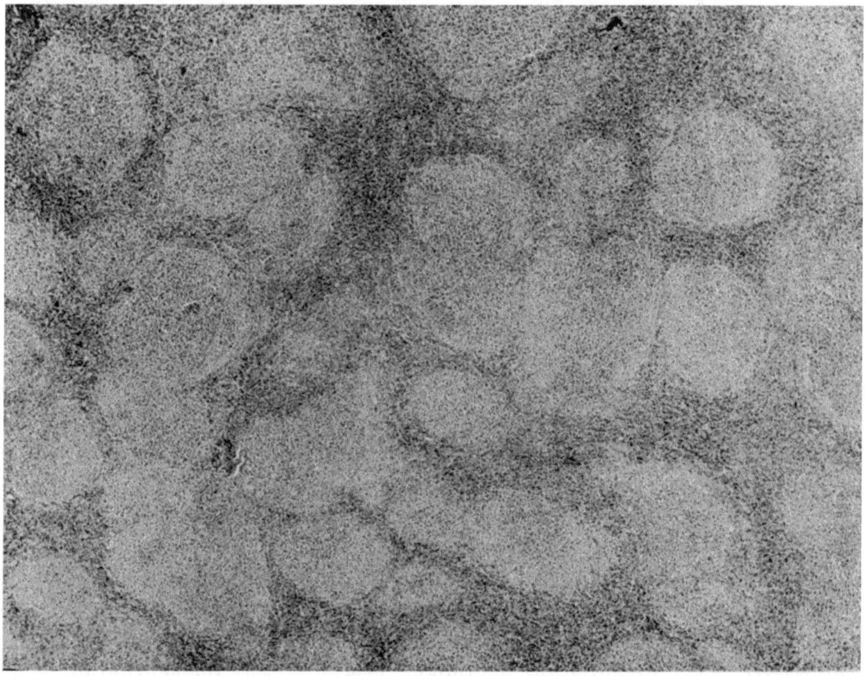

Fig. 2. Malignant lymphoma, nodular pattern. AFIP access. No. 915 320. H & E, ×30

the cytoplasm is scanty to indistinct, and the nucleus is characteristically irregular, with areas of linear subdivisions representing cleavage planes. At times a small nucleolus is apparent. The most distinctive feature of this process is the inconsistency in size and configuration of the nucleus associated with cleavage planes. This cellular proliferation is associated commonly with evidence of a nodular histologic pattern and represents the most common type of nodular lymphoma.

Stem Cell (Undifferentiated Cell) Lymphoma: This lymphoma (Fig. 5) in tissue sections is composed of relatively uniform-appearing medium-size cells with round

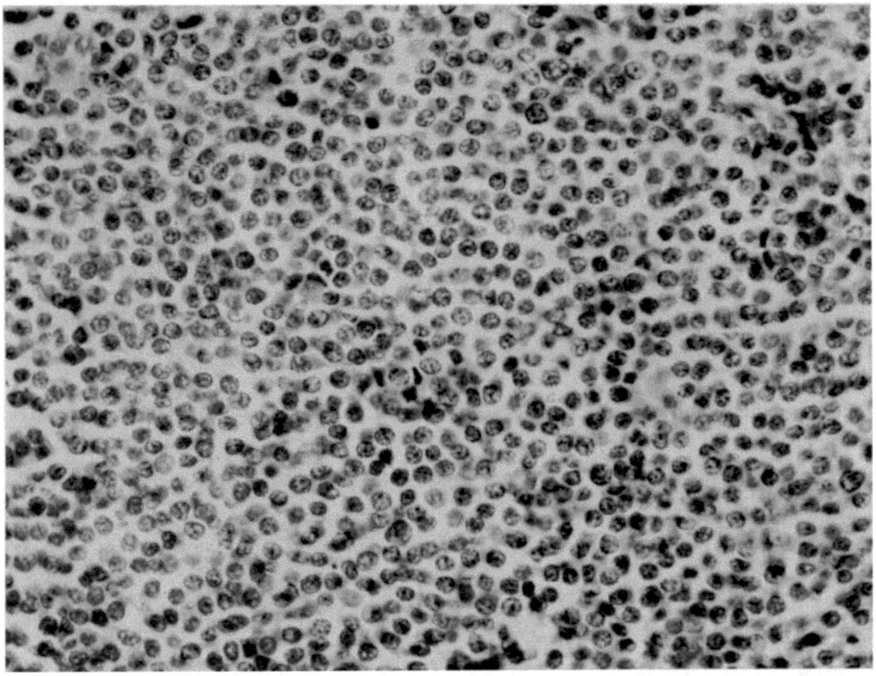

Fig. 3. Lymphocytic lymphoma, well differentiated. LACH No. 59-7876. H & E, ×500

to oval nuclei with finely stippled, uniformly distributed chromatin. The nucleoli are small and inconspicuous. The cytoplasm is amphophilic and slight to moderate in amount. The cellular borders are commonly indistinct because of the cohesive character of the cells. Large, pale histiocytes with abundant cytoplasm and phagocytized debris presenting the so-called "starry-sky appearance" are commonly interspersed in varying frequency, but are not an essential feature for the identification of this type of malignant lymphoma. The Burkitt lymphoma most typically exhibits the cytologic features of the stem-cell lymphoma.

Histiocytic Lymphoma: Included within this type of lymphoma (Figs. 6—8) are a number of cytologic variants with varying degrees of cytoplasm and wide variation in nuclear size and configuration. These variations appear to represent different degrees of differentiation, cytologic behavior, and pleomorphism of the tumor. The nucleus is generally large and oval, though at times it may be extremely

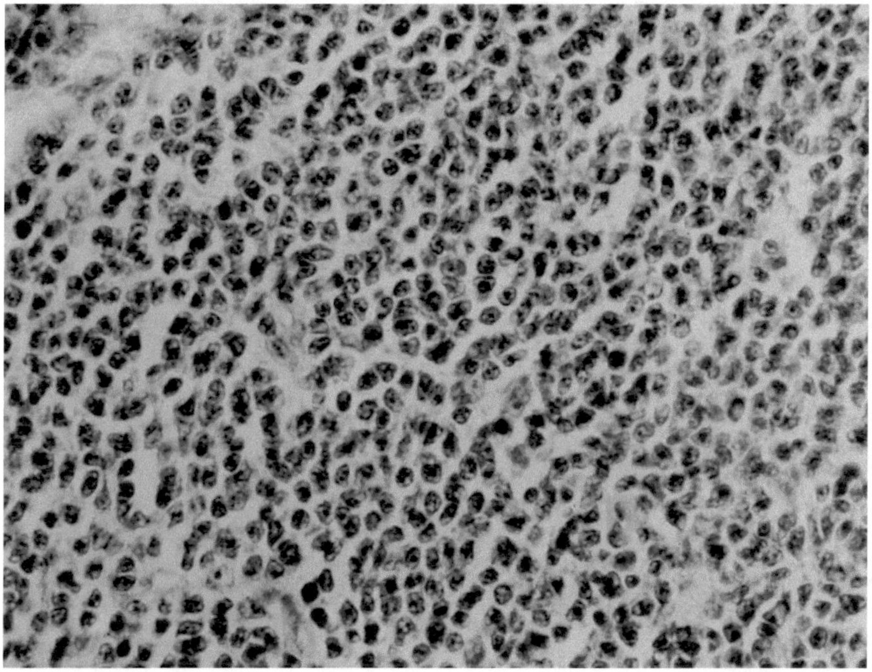

Fig. 4. Lymphocytic lymphoma, poorly differentiated. LACH No. 64-6423. H & E, ×500

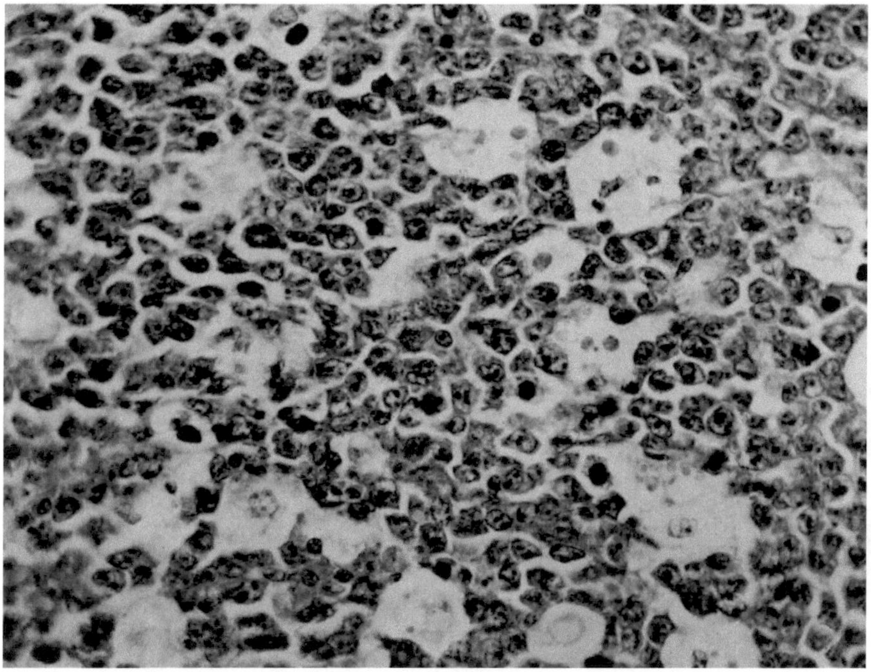

Fig. 5. Stem cell lymphoma. LACH No. 56-2334. H & E, ×500

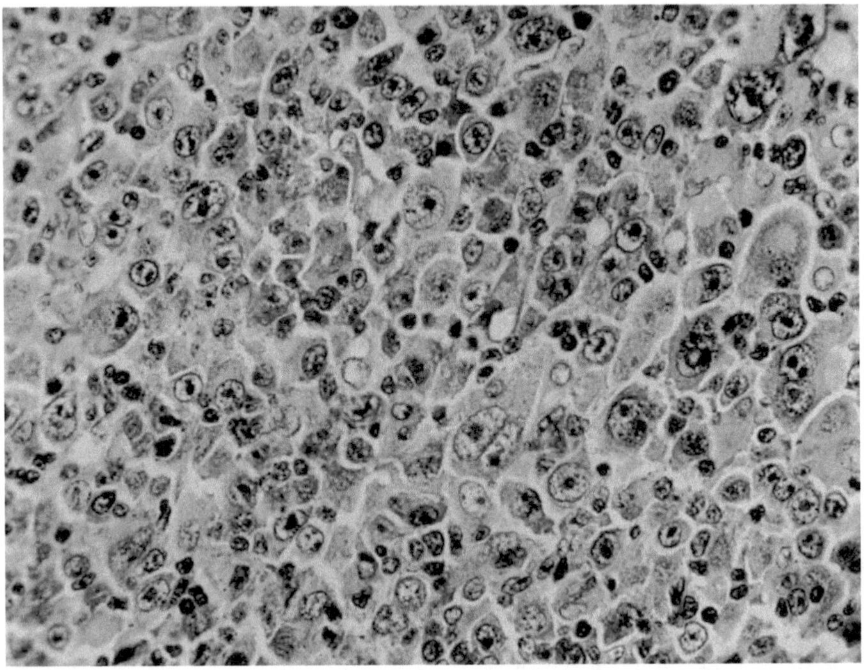

Fig. 6. Histiocytic lymphoma, moderately well differentiated. AFIP Access. No. 955 188. H & E, ×500

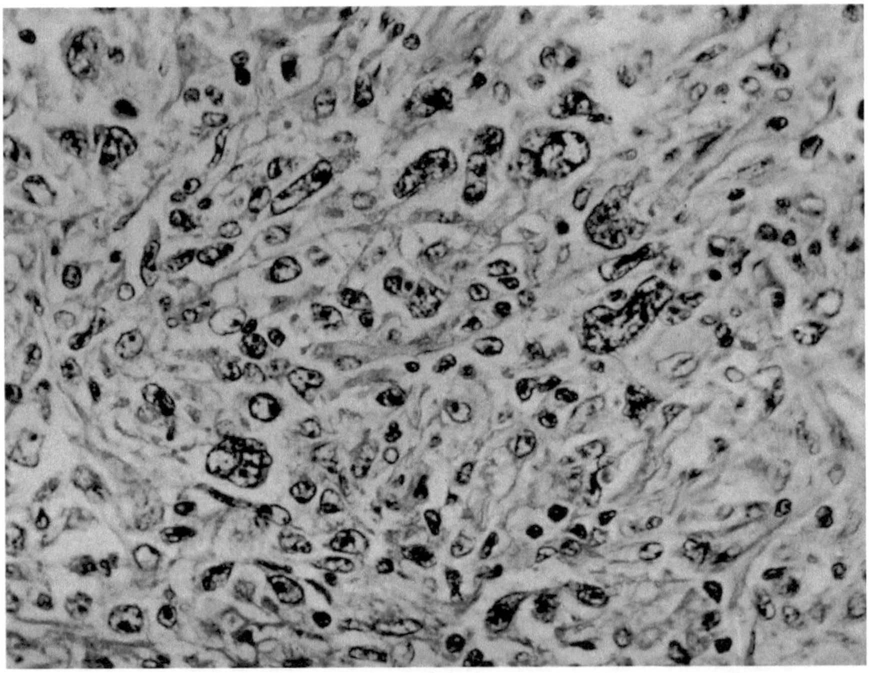

Fig. 7. Histiocytic lymphoma, pleomorphic. AFIP Access. No. 1 155 957. H & E, ×500

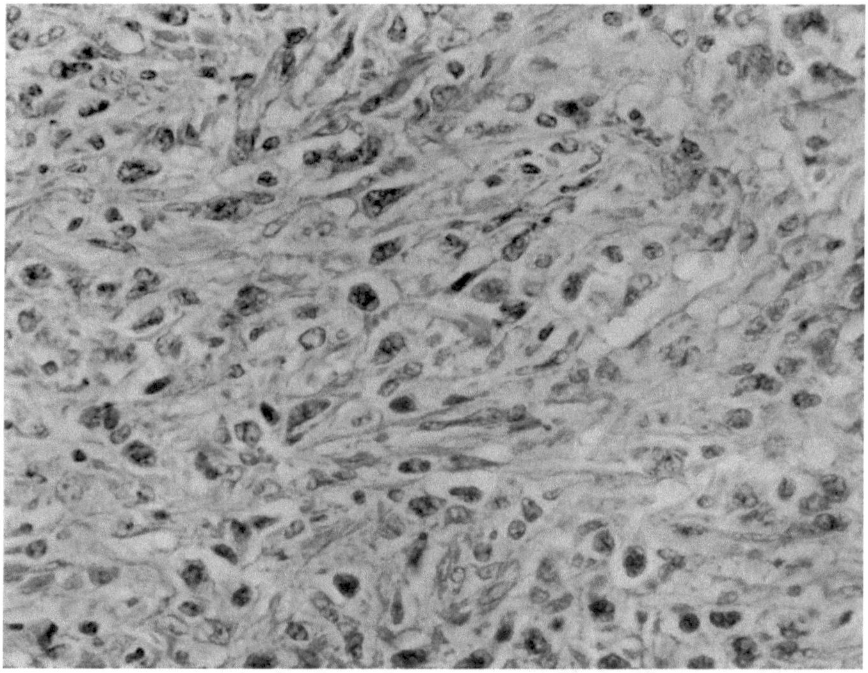

Fig. 8. Histiocytic lymphoma, fibrile producing. Note that pleomorphic and fibrile producing variants of histiocytic lymphoma may occur in the same lesion. AFIP Access. No. 1 155 957. H & E, ×500

variable and pleomorphic. The character of the chromatin varies from finely reticulated to vesicular and the nucleolus is often prominent and large, and on occasions may resemble an inclusion body. The cytoplasm, though variable in quantity and appearance, is commonly finely granular and acidophilic, and on occasions contains phagocytic material. At times the pleomorphic cells are binucleated or multinucleated resembling Reed-Sternberg cells and Hodgkin's sarcoma. Through the years I have regarded this type as histiocytic type, pleomorphic unless there is evidence elsewhere of one of the other histologic manifestations of Hodgkin's disease. In a relatively small proportion of the cases, reticulum fibril production is prominent and intimately associated with individual cells. Although there are numerous cytologic variants included within the histiocytic type, it seems reasonable to designate these as descriptive sub-types until more meaningful evidence becomes available to justify further separation.

The Relationship of Leukemias and Lymphomas

Although the relationship of lymphomas and leukemias will be considered in detail elsewhere on this program, a few brief comments on the comparative distributions of leukemic and lymphoma cells may be of assistance in understanding these processes. Lymphomas and leukemias have been regarded generally, as distinctive and separate processes in the past, even though it has been generally acknowledged that lymphoma cells may be observed at times in the course of the disease in the peripheral blood in varying numbers. The distinction between leukemias and lymphomas fundamentally appears to be related to factors that influence the distribution of the cellular proliferation.

By tradition the term *leukemia* has been applied to all processes with numerous abnormal or neoplastic cells in the peripheral blood. The widely accepted definition of leukemia, however, is based upon diffuse involvement of the bone marrow by specific types of neoplastic cellular proliferation which is typically associated with uniform involvement of spleen, liver and lymph nodes. The distribution of lymphomas by contrast is irregular and variable, and may be limited to a single group of lymph nodes or a mass, and the marrow, spleen or liver may be uninvolved or exhibit irregular nodular involvement. The distribution of leukemias and lymphomas is schematically compared in Fig. 9, with the distribution in the leukemias designated as *systemic* and in the lymphomas as *irregular*.

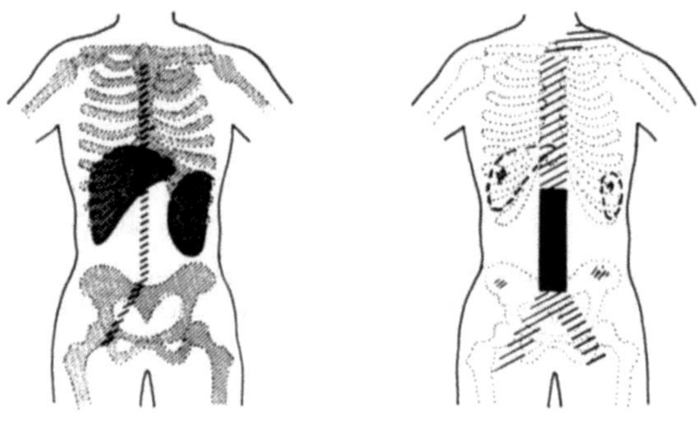

Fig. 9. Comparison of distribution of involvement in leukemia and lymphoma. In leukemia the distribution typically is widespread (systemic), uniformly involving bone marrow, spleen, liver and lymph nodes. In lymphomas it is irregular, initially manifested in a limited area (e. g. the retroperitoneum dark area), with extension to adjacent lymph node regions (striped areas), and later to nodular areas in spleen, liver and bone marrow

Lymphoma cells may be found in the peripheral blood in each cytologic type, particularly if the blood is repeatedly examined in the later stages of the disease, even though the distribution of the process at the time is not systemic in character. The cytologic type of lymphoma appears to be related to the histologic pattern (nodular or diffuse), the type of distribution (system or irregular), and the occurrence of lymphoma cells in the peripheral blood [23].

Hodgkin's Disease

Hodgkin's disease is generally regarded as a malignant neoplasm by both clinicians and pathologists in the United States. The results of our recent study [5—7] of 377 U. S. Army cases of Hodgkin's disease (World War II) have raised serious questions regarding the position of Hodgkin's disease in the scheme of malignant lymphoma and the fundamental nature of the disease process. The remarkable variation in the histologic features associated with the Reed-Sternberg cells were interpreted as different expressions of the response of the host and were related to the immunologic state. An inverse relationship between the frequency of lymphocytes and Reed-Sternberg cells was emphasized and the relationship between the wide variation in the histologic findings and the clinical stages of Peters [24] was demonstrated. On the basis of these observations, it was proposed that the Hodgkin's disease process may represent the attempted induction of malignant neoplasia. It was suggested that Hodgkin's disease may not be a malignant neoplasm from its inception, since only a small proportion of cases in the terminal phase of the disease appear to achieve a convincing malignant neoplastic state as a pleomorphic pro-

Table 4. *Comparison of classifications of Hodgkin's disease*

Jackson and Parker [8]	Lukes, Butler and Hicks [6]	Lukes et al. [25]
	Lymphocytic and/or histiocytic	Lymphocyte predominance
Paragranuloma	(a) Nodular	
	(b) Diffuse	
	Nodular sclerosis	Nodular sclerosis
Granuloma	Mixed	Mixed cellularity
	Diffuse fibrosis	
Sarcoma	Reticular	Lymphocyte depletion

liferation of Reed-Sternberg cells. The latter state would be classified as the sarcoma type according to Jackson and Parker [8]. If Hodgkin's disease is a neoplastic proliferation, according to this view, whether benign or malignant, it involves only the Reed-Sternberg cell and the associated proliferation represents the host's response. This interpretation emphasized the necessity of requiring the identification of a typical Reed-Sternberg cell for the diagnosis of Hodgkin's disease.

In our study [5—7] six new histologic types were described based on the predominant histologic features and the relative frequency of Reed-Sternberg cells. These histologic types are listed in Table 4, in comparison with histologic types of Jackson and Parker [8] and an abbreviated version of our classification proposed at the National Cancer Institute-American Cancer Society-sponsored conference on "Obstacles to the Control of Hodgkin's disease" at Rye, New York in 1965 [25].

The lymphocytic and histiocytic (L & H) nodular and diffuse types reflect the common association of L & H proliferation in Hodgkin's disease, although either cell type may predominate or occur as a relatively pure cellular proliferation. Comparative classification with the types of Jackson and Parker [8] demonstrated that the number of cases in the prognostically favorable L & H groups more than doubled those in the paragranuloma group. Nodular sclerosis presents 2 distinctive histologic features: (1) variable degrees of fibrosis in the form of birefringent collagen bands that frequently isolated nodules of abnormal lymphoid tissue, and (2) large distinctive variants of Reed-Sternberg cells with abundant cytoplasm and sharply demarcated cellular borders presenting the appearance of a cell situated in a lacuna. The remarkably high incidence of mediastinal involvement in nodular sclerosis was interpreted as a regional histologic expression of Hodgkin's disease in the mediastinum. The mixed type consists of a variety of cell types associated with disorderly fibrosis of limited degree. Diffuse fibrosis is composed predominantly of disorderly nonbirefringent fibrillar connective tissue associated with cellular depletion, particularly of lymphocytes, with a variable number of residual Reed-Sternberg cells. The reticular type consists predominantly of Reed-Sternberg cells with only a small

Table 5. *Hodgkin's disease. Relationship of histologic types and clinical stages to survival*

Histologic types	No. of cases	No. of survivors at 15 yrs.	Median survival, years			
			All stages	I	II	III
L & H						
Nodular	23	10	12.4	16.0	12.0 [a]	4.3 [b]
Diffuse	40	11	7.4	9.5	4.8	5.5 [b]
Nodular sclerosis	149	23	4.2	11.0	3.2	1.8
Mixed	97	10	2.5	4.8	2.5	1.2
Diffuse fibrosis	47	1	0.9	1.1	3.2	0.4
Reticular	21	1	2.3	5.7	2.7	0.6

L & H is used to designate lymphocytic and histiocytic types.
[a] Only 2 cases in this group; therefore an average was used.
[b] Only 3 cases in each of these groups; an average was recorded as most representative.

proportion of the cases exhibiting marked pleomorphism of Reed-Sternberg cells similar to the sarcoma type of JACKSON and PARKER [8].

A significant relationship between the histologic types, clinical stages and survival was demonstrated. The relationship of histologic types and clinical stages to survival are recorded in Table 5. The L & H types were observed primarily in clinical Stage I disease and had a prolonged median survival that ranged from 9.5 to 16 years. By contrast diffuse fibrosis and reticular types with depletion of lymphocytes were most commonly observed with Stage III disease of PETERS [24] and had short median survivals of 0.4 and 0.6 years respectively. Nodular sclerosis was observed with equal frequency in each stage. It was, however, the most common histologic type observed in Stage I where it had prolonged median survivals that fell within the range of the L & H types. The mixed type was also found with equal frequency in each stage, but appears to represent changing disease, even in Stage I, with limited duration of median survival.

From recent studies [26—28] the new histologic types appear to be readily applicable and of considerable prognostic value. The L & H types are associated predominantly with clinical Stage I disease and have remarkable prolonged median survivals. In addition, nodular sclerosis has emerged as a lesion of major prognostic significance and is the most common histologic type. The association of diffuse fibrosis and reticular types primarily with progressive disease and short median survivals also has received support [24].

On the basis of the association of the histologic types with clinical stages, an evolution of the morphologic findings in Hodgkin's disease was proposed in our earlier report [6] with nodular sclerosis excluded because of its regional association with the mediastinum. With lymphocytic and/or histocytic proliferation, the clinical disease is usually quiescent and manifested as clincal Stage I. If the proliferation is nodular, it is likely to remain unchanged and quiescent. With loss of lymphocytes and the addition of other cell types, including the appearance of disorderly connective tissue and an increase in Reed-Sternberg cells, the appearance of the mixed type is indicated. This is associated with the change to progressive disease, commonly with clinical Stage II or III of PETERS [24]. Further loss of lymphocytes and marked increase in Reed-Sternberg cells or the extensive formation of disorderly fibrillar connective tissue indicates the reticular and diffuse fibrosis types which are associated with clinical Stage III of PETERS [24], systemic symptoms, lymphocytopenia and rapidly progressive disease.

Comparative classification with the histologic types of JACKSON and PARKER [8] demonstrates that the overwhelming majority of cases exhibit the features of the heterogeneous granüloma type, representing approximately 90% of the cases in the majority of studies. In our recent study 91% presented features of granuloma, 8% paragranuloma and 1% sarcoma. From a review of Table 4, it is evident that the granuloma type has numerous histologic expressions and the paragranuloma and sarcoma types represent extremes of a spectrum of histologic findings in Hodgkin's disease.

At the conference on "Obstacles to the Control of Hodgkin's Disease", sponsored by the National Cancer Institute and American Cancer Society at Rye, New York, a new classification was proposed [25]. It is based on the classification of LUKES, BUTLER and HICKS [6], and represents an abbreviated form with 4 types, lymphocyte predominance, nodular sclerosis, mixed cellularity and lymphocyte depletion. These are listed for comparison in Table 4, with our orginally described histologic types and those of JACKSON and PARKER [8]. It was the belief of the members of the Nomenclature Committee on Morphology that 4 types would prove useful to clinicians and could be easily related to the clinical hematologic and immunologic manifestations. It appears, however, that the originally proposed descriptive histologic types may be more useful to the pathologist because of their descriptive connotations, which was the original design.

Relationship of Other Proliferative Disorders to Malignant Lymphoma

The position in the scheme of malignant lymphoma of a number of proliferative processes involving the reticuloendothelial system remains controversial. Mycosis fungoides has gained a position similar to that proposed for Hodgkin's disease, with general acceptance of its malignant neoplastic character in the tumor phase. The process from my experience should not be included within the systemic malignant lymphomas in agreement with the view of RAPPAPORT [22]. It may arise from a distinctive cell type, possibly the mesenchymal cells of the dermis. The relationship of mycosis fungoides to Sezary's syndrome is unestablished at this time. Evidence of systemic involvement of lymphoid tissue in mycosis fungoides in validated cases has been rare, although BLOCK et al. [29] recently have claimed frequent visceral involvement. In my experience, most cases purported to represent examples of mycosis fungoides with visceral involvement upon critical evaluation, however, present features of systemic lymphomas in advanced stages of the disease where the initial apparent manifestation appeared in the skin. The lymphoid tissue proliferation associated with the macroglobulinemia of Waldenstrom appears to represent a closely related variant of lymphocytic leukemia and lymphocytic lymphoma because of the plasmacytoid lymphocytic character of the cellular proliferation. Multiple myeloma with the predominant involvement of the bone marrow and essentially secondary lymph-node involvement seems unrelated and justifies exclusion from the malignant lymphomas to a group of allied disorders. *Lymphoepithelioma* an unfortunate term has been definitely established as a primary carcinoma arising in the nasopharynx or paranasal sinuses.

Summary

The terminologic maze and conceptual disputes that characterized this field for decades have been reviewed and are believed to limit valid comparison of the results of various lymphoma studies from either a clinical or a morphologic viewpoint. The present meaningless status of the terms *reticulum cell sarcoma* and *lymphosarcoma* has been emphasized. There is encouraging evidence recently of enlightment on the nature of follicular lymphoma that provides the basis for a simplified terminologic and morphologic classifications.

The important relationship of cytologic types to the histologic pattern, the character of the distribution of the cellular proliferation, and the occurrence of leukemic manifestations has been presented. Our recent work on Hodgkin's disease has been reviewed and a questionable status for Hodgkin's disease in the scheme of malignant lymphoma has been recommended because the majority of histologic components in the process appear to represent host factors, rather than a neoplastic proliferation.

Published in part as presentation for the Proceedings of the International Symposium on Lymphology in Zurich, Switzerland, July 19—23, 1966. Progress in Lymphology. Ed.: A. RUTTIMANN. Stuttgart: G. Thieme 1967, p. 109.

Also published in part as presentation for the Proceedings of the International Conference on Leukemia-Lymphoma in Ann Arbor, Michigan, October 9—13, 1967. Ed.: C. J. D. ZARAFONETIS. Philadelphia: Lea & Febiger 1968, p. 331.

References

1. GALL, E. A.: Enigmas in lymphoma. Reticulum cell sarcoma and mycosis fungoides. Minnesota Med. **38**, 674 (1955).
2. RAPPAPORT, H., WINTER, W. J., HICKS, E. B.: Follicular lymphoma: re-evulation of its position in the scheme of malignant lymphoma based on survey of 253 cases. Cancer **9**, 792 (1956).
3. LUKES, R. J.: A review of the American concept of malignant lymphoma. In: Progress in Lymphology. Ed.: A. RUTTIMANN. Stuttgart: G. Thieme 1967, p. 109.

4. PETERS, M. V.: The contribution of radiation therapy in the control of early lymphomas. Amer. J. Roentgenol. **90**, 956 (1963).
5. LUKES, R. J.: Relationship of histologic features to clinical stages in Hodgkin's disease. Amer. J. Roentgenol. **90**, 944 (1963).
6. — BUTLER, J. J., HICKS, E. B.: The natural history of Hodgkin's disease as related to its pathologic picture. Cancer **19**, 317 (1966).
7. — — The pathology and nomenclature of Hodgkin's disease. Cancer Res. **26**, 1063 (1966).
8. JACKSON, H., PARKER, F.: Hodgkin's disease and allied disorders. New York: Oxford University Press 1947.
9. CUSTER, R. P., BERNHARD, W. G.: Interrelationship of Hodgkin's disease and other lymphatic tumors. Amer. J. med. Sci. **216**, 625 (1948).
10. GALL, E. A., MALLORY, T. B.: Malignant lymphoma; clinico-pathologic survey of 618 cases. Amer. J. Path. **18**, 381 (1942).
11. BERMAN, L.: Malignant lymphomas; their classification and relation to leukemia. Blood **8**, 195 (1953).
12. WARREN, S., PICENA, J. P.: Reticulum cell sarcoma of lymph nodes. Amer. J. Path. **17**, 385 (1941).
13. JACOBS, D. S.: Primary gastric malignant lymphoma and pseudolymphoma. Amer. J. clin. Path. **40**, 379 (1963).
14. FARIS, F. D., SALTZSTEIN, S. L.: Gastric lymphoid hyperplasia: A term confused with lymphosarcoma. Cancer **17**, 207 (1964).
15. SALTZSTEIN, S. L.: Pulmonary malignant lymphomas and pseudolymphomas; classification, therapy and prognosis. Cancer **16**, 928 (1963).
16. KAPLAN, H.: Role of intensive radiotherapy in the management of Hodgkin's disease. Cancer **19**, 356 (1966).
17. CALLENDER, G. R.: Tumors and tumor-like conditions of the lymphocyte, the myelocyte, the erythrocyte and the reticulum cells. Amer. J. Path. **10**, 443 (1934).
18. GALL, E. A., MORRISON, H. R., SCOTT, A. T.: The follicular type of malignant lymphoma: a survey of 63 cases. Ann. intern. Med. **14**, 2073 (1941).
19. — RAPPAPORT, H.: Seminar on diseases of lymph nodes and spleen. In: Proceedings of 23rd Seminar, American Society of Clinical Pathology, 1958. Ed.: J. R. MCDONALD.
20. BRAUNSTEIN, H., GALL, E. A.: The cytologic and histochemical features of malignant lymphoma. In: Progress in Hematology, Vol. 3. Ed.: L. M. TOCANTINS. New York: Grune & Stratton 1962, p. 137.
21. DORFMAN, R. F.: Enzyme histochemistry of normal, hyperplastic and neoplastic lymphoreticular tissues. In: The Lymphoreticular Tumours in Africa. Ed.: F. C. ROULET. Basel-New York: S. Karger 1964, p. 304.
22. RAPPAPORT, H.: Tumors of Hematopoietic System. Armed Forces Institute of Pathology, Washington, D. C., 1966.
23. LUKES, R. J.: The Pathologic Picture of the Malignant Lymphomas, Reprinted from Proceedings of the International Conference on Leukemia-Lymphoma. Lea & Febiger 1968.
24. PETERS, M. V.: A study of survivals in Hodgkin's disease treated radiologically. Amer. J. Roentgenol. **63**, 299 (1950).
25. LUKES, R. J., CRAVER, L. L., HALL, T. C., RAPPAPORT, H., RUBIN, P.: Hodgkin's disease, report of Nomenclature Committee. Cancer Res. **26**, 1311 (1966).
26. HANSON, T. A. S.: Histologic classification and survival in Hodgkin's disease. Cancer **17**, 1595 (1964).
27. FRANSSILA, K. O., KALIMA, T. V., VOUTILAINEN, A.: Histologic classification of Hodgkin's disease. Cancer **20**, 1594 (1967).
28. KELLER, A. R., KAPLAN, H. S., LUKES, R. J., RAPPAPORT, H.: Correlation of histopathology with other prognostic indicators in Hodgkin's disease. Cancer **22**, 487—499 (1968).
29. BLOCK, J. B., EDGECOMB, J., EISEN, A., VAN SCOTT, E. J.: Mycosis fungoides; natural history and aspects of its relationship to other malignant lymphomas. Amer. J. Med. **34**, 228 (1963).

Discussion

The Relationship between Lymphocytic Leukemias and Lymphomas*

William W. Sheehan

With 3 Figures

In any discussion of hematopoietic neoplasms, it is customary to distinguish between diseases which present as localized tumors, the malignant lymphomas, and those which present as systemic diseases, the leukemias. The necessity for such a distinction arises from considerations of certain unique features of the hematopoietic system. The blood-forming organs which make up the hematopoietic system constitute only a portion of a larger system, the reticular tissue, which is widely distributed throughout the entire body. This tissue derives its name from the primitive reticular cell, an ubiquitous, undifferentiated and pluripotent cell, from which all of the stromal and hematopoietic tissues of the body are derived [1]. The resultant widespread anatomic distribution of hematopoietic precursor cells gives rise to two unique features of hematopoietic neoplasms: 1) the fact that primary hematopoietic neoplasms may arise virtually anywhere in the body, and 2) that many hematopoietic neoplasms appear to be systemic at the time of their clinical inception.

Dr. Lukes has confined his discussion primarily to the malignant lymphomas and has presented a classification of these tumors which is based on the distinction of various cytologic features of the proliferating cells. I intend to discuss the systemic proliferative diseases of lymphoid origin, paying particular attention to those features which point out the relationships and differences between these neoplasms and the localized tumors of corresponding cytologic type. In addition, I would like to review current terminology used in the classification of these disorders.

The distinction between localized and systemic neoplasms is usually clear-cut. In most instances, a malignant lymphoma presents with enlargement of a single lymph node or anatomically related group of lymph nodes. Less frequently it may arise as a mass lesion in a nonlymphoid organ, such as the gastrointestinal tract. It is rare for a lymphoma to be first detected in the liver or spleen. Recent studies, employing extensive staging procedures, have demonstrated that initial extension of the disease tends to follow lymphatic pathways involving contiguous lymph node

* Supported by Training Grant CA 05183 from The National Cancer Institute, NIH, USPHS.

groups [2]. Involvement of the spleen or liver is an indication of advanced disease, and when present, there is a tendency to the formation of masses or multiple nodules. Bone marrow involvement is also a late occurrence and tends to be focal. As in other malignant tumors, vascular invasion may occur, usually in advanced cases. When it occurs, follow up studies have demonstrated a poor prognosis. Anemia and thrombocytopenia are uncommon until late in the course of the disease. Circulating cells in the peripheral blood are rarely observed early in the disease, although they may appear in large numbers in the terminal phases of the disease.

The systemic diseases present with an entirely different picture. Lymph node enlargment may or may not be prominent, but when present, tends to be symmetrical and widespread. The liver and spleen are frequently enlarged at the time of diagnosis,

Table 1. *Terms that have been applied to leukemias of lymphocytic origin*

Chronic lymphocytic leukemia
Small cell and large cell varieties have been described
Subacute lymphocytic leukemia
Lymphosarcoma cell leukemia
Acute and chronic varieties have been described
Notched cell leukemia
Acute lymphocytic leukemia
Acute lymphoblastic leukemia
Stem-cell leukemia
Undifferentiated leukemia

or become enlarged soon thereafter. In these organs, the cellular proliferation tends to be evenly distributed, rather than nodular. The bone marrow is usually diffusely involved by the cellular proliferation, and anemia and thrombocytopenia become apparent early in the disease. Characteristically, large numbers of the proliferating cells are found in the peripheral blood at the time of diagnosis.

Up to this point, use of the term leukemia has been deliberately avoided. The lack of precise definition and usage of this term has led to a number of misunderstandings. Some observers have used the term to designate all disorders in which abnormal cells are demonstrable in the peripheral blood. As a result, the occurrence of circulating, abnormal cells late in the course of otherwise typical malignant lymphomas has led some observers to talk about the "transformation" of malignant lymphoma into leukemia. We feel that it is more logical to simply consider this occurrence as a late phase of the disease, or the natural evolution of the disease. Rather than apply the term "leukemia" in such cases, we simply add the term "leukemic" to the proper cytologic designation of the established malignant lymphoma. An example of this would be malignant lymphoma, poorly differentiated lymphocytic type, leukemic. Thus, for purpose of this discussion, the term leukemia will be applied only to those diseases which are systemic at onset, according to the above-mentioned distributional criteria, and which demonstrate appreciable numbers of the proliferating cells in the peripheral blood.

With this in mind, let us now turn to a consideration of the criteria for the cytologic classification of the systemic diseases of lymphoid origin. Table 1 lists a number of terms that have been applied to the various lymphocytic leukemias. This by no means exhausts the number of terms that are to be found in the literature, and it is unlikely that any one observer uses all of these terms. Nonetheless, it does serve to focus our attention on two key points: 1) that although most texts describe only two kinds of lymphocytic leukemia, acute and chronic, many observers have encountered difficulties in assigning all cases into these two categories; and 2) that the very variety of intermediate terms that have been used suggests that a spectrum of cytologic differentiation has been observed in these cases.

From this list of terms, we have selected only four to include in the center column of Table 2, which depicts what presently appears to be the most practical working

Table 2. *Classification of the systemic proliferative diseases and tumors of lymphoid origin* [a]

Predominant component cell	Systemic proliferative diseases (tumor formation may occur)	Initially localized tumors (systemic involvement occurs frequently)
Primitive reticular cell		Malignant lymphoma (M. L.), undifferentiated
Undifferentiated hematopoietic cell	Undifferentiated (stem-cell) leukemia	
Lymphoblast	Acute lymphoblastic leukemia	
Poorly differentiated lymphocyte	Lymphosarcoma cell leukemia	M. L., poorly differentiated lymphocytic
Differentiated lymphocyte	Chronic lymphocytic leukemia	M. L., well differentiated lymphocytic
	Macroglobulinemia	

[a] Modified from RAPPAPORT, H.: Tumors of the hematopoietic system [1].

classification of the systemic neoplasms of lymphoid origin. They are listed in parallel with the malignant lymphomas of similar cytologic composition. This table is slightly modified from Table 1 of RAPPAPORT's "Tumors of the Hematopoietic System" [1]. I shall discuss each of these terms in some detail.

The term stem-cell leukemia implies that there is a cytologic variant of leukemia composed of cells which fail to demonstrate any degree of differentiation beyond that of the undifferentiated hematopoietic cell. In practice, this term is applied to cases in which the observer is unable to distinguish differentiation. This is usually done solely on the basis of the appearance of the cells in Romanowsky-stained preparations. However, HAYHOE has shown that histochemical techniques (specifically, Sudan Black B, peroxidase, leukocyte alkaline phosphatase and the periodic acid-Schiff reaction) will differentiate between lymphocytic leukemias and those of myeloid or monocytic origin [3]. In applying each of these histochemical tests to a large number of cases of acute leukemia, he was able to assign all of the cases to either lymphocytic or myeolid or monocytic categories and thus eliminate the undifferentiated category. Thus, although the theoretical existence of a true stem-cell

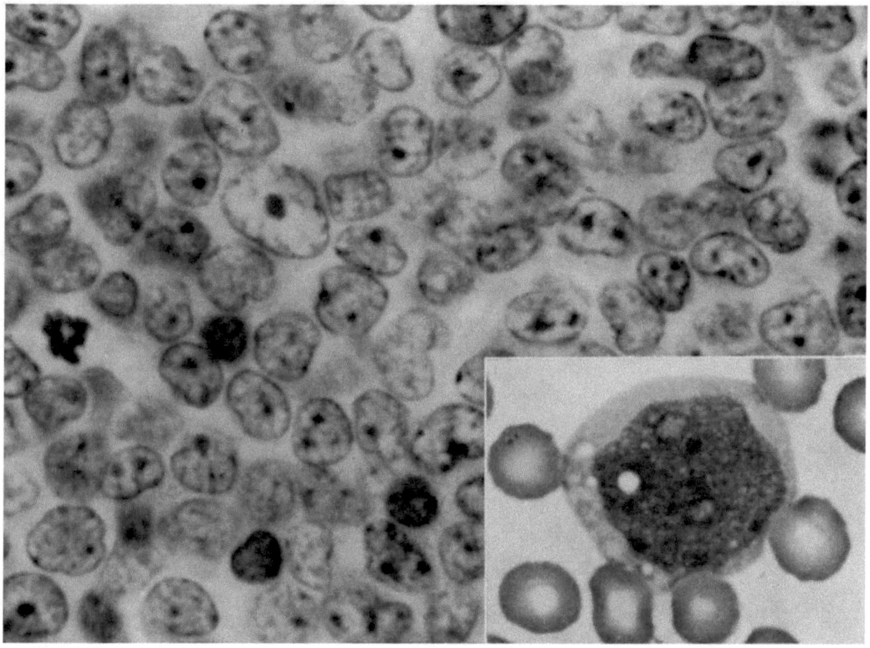

Fig. 1. Acute lymphoblastic leukemia. In routine H & E sections of lymph nodes the cells are large, yet smaller than histiocytes (upper, left). The nuclear chromatin is finely dispersed throughout the nucleus rather than coarsely clumped. Nucleoli are prominent, but not enlarged. Mitoses are frequent. Similar features are noted in Romanowsky-stained preparations (insert). Both ×1000

leukemia cannot be excluded at the present time, it is probably very rare if it occurs at all. However, since most laboratories are not equipped to carry out such studies on a routine basis, it is likely that this category will continue to be used. For this reason only, the term is retained.

We use the term acute lymphoblastic leukemia to designate those systemic disorders characterized by a proliferation of immature cells, at least some of which demonstrate features indicating some degree of lymphocytic differentiation. In typical cases, Romanowsky-stained preparations show the majority of the cells to be large cells with a relatively thin rim of blue cytoplasm. The cells have large nuclei with a delicate chromatin pattern. One or more large, pale-staining nucleoli is usually present (Fig. 1). The absence of specific granules or Auer rods, and the presence of occasional cells in which the nuclear chromatin shows a tendency to coarse clumping, permit identification of the cells as lymphoblasts. Where nuclear differentiation is absent or equivocal, the absence of Sudanophilia and peroxidase activity with a neutrophile alkaline phosphatase score above 40 and a PAS reaction which shows no diffuse staining, but which may show coarse granules in some of the cells, permits identification of the cells as lymphoblasts.

In optimally fixed H & E stained sections, the cells of acute lymphoblastic leukemia are characteristic, yet not distinguishable from the more immature examples

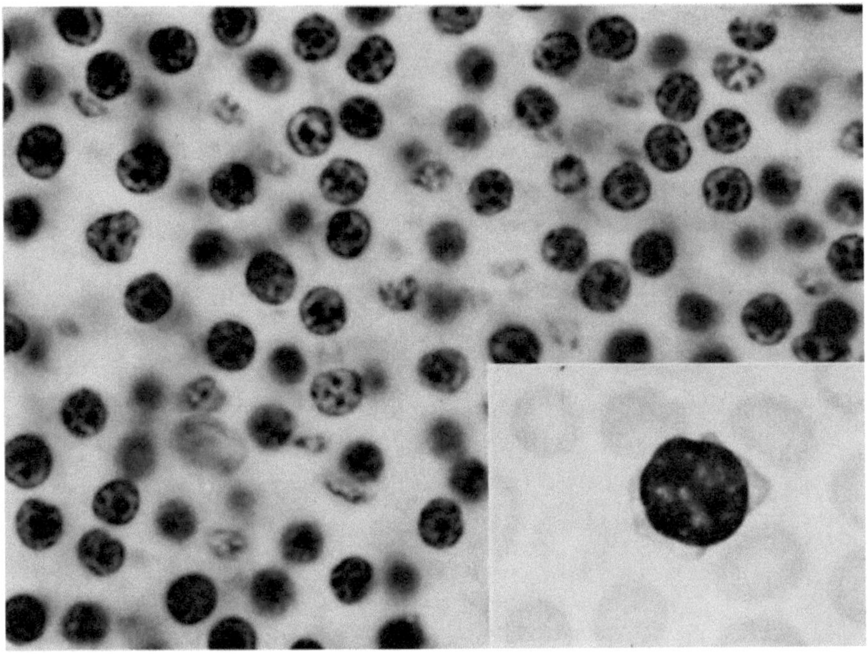

Fig. 2. Chronic lymphocytic leukemia. In routine sections of lymph nodes the cells are small, round and regular. The nuclear chromatin is coarsely clumped in both H & E and Romanowsky-stained preparations. Nucleoli can only occasionally be distinguished from chromatin clumps. Both ×1000

of malignant lymphoma, poorly differentiated lymphocytic type. The small amount of cytoplasm is usually difficult to distinguish. The nuclear chromatin is finely divided and evenly dispersed throughout the nucleus which contains one or more distinct, but not enlarged nucleoli. Although the nuclei are large compared to other cells of the lymphocytic series, they are not as large as the nuclei of histiocytes or endothelial cells present in the sections (Fig. 1). This feature clearly distinguishes them from the cells of undifferentiated malignant lymphoma, in which the nuclei are invariably as large or larger than those of histiocytes present in the tumor.

This distinction is confirmed in Romanowsky preparations. When the cells from imprints of the Burkitt's tumor (a variant of malignant lymphoma, undifferentiated) have been compared to the cells of acute lymphoblastic leukemia, differences in the cytology and in histochemical reactions have been noted and recently published by the World Health Organization [4].

At the opposite end of the spectrum is chronic lymphocytic leukemia which demonstrates all of the above-mentioned distributional features which characterize the systemic diseases. The peripheral blood regularly shows a marked lymphocytosis. Although there is a considerable range of cell size that may be observed from case to case and even within a given case, the characteristic coarse clumping of the nuclear chromatin in the majority of the proliferating cells is the reliable diagnostic feature. This is true both in Romanowsky-stained smears and in H & E stained sections (Fig. 2).

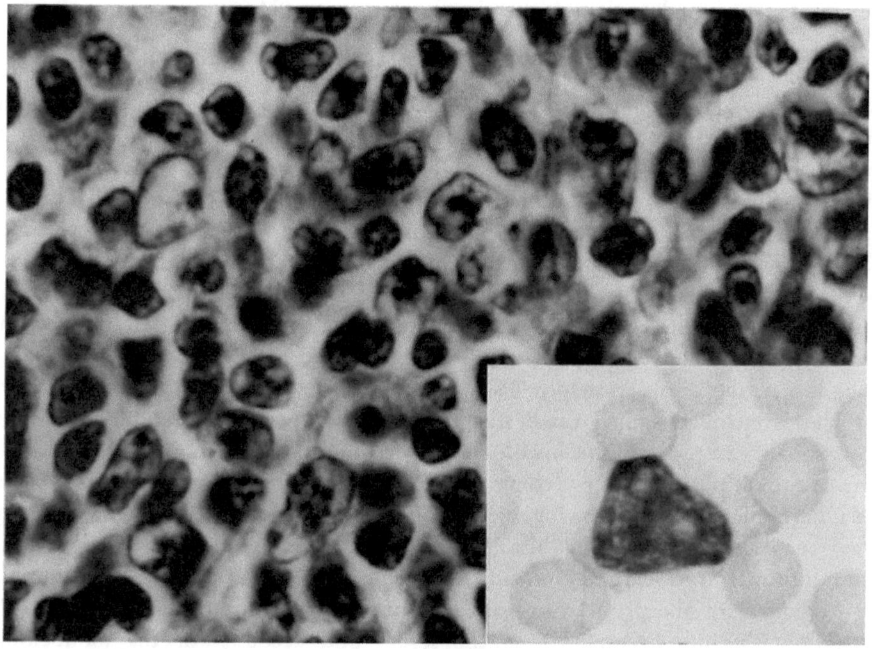

Fig. 3. Lymphosarcoma cell leukemia. In routine sections of lymph nodes the cells are larger than mature lymphocytes yet smaller than histiocytes (upper, left) and are less uniform. The nuclei are angulated and indented and show moderate clumping of chromatin. Cells observed in Romanowsky-stained peripheral blood smears contain nuclei with large pale nucleoli surrounded by dense rims of chromatin. Both ×1000

A significant number of cases do occur, however, in which the circulating cells show nuclear features which are intermediate between those of chronic lymphocytic leukemia and acute lymphoblastic leukemia. In such cells, the chromatin is less coarsely clumped than that of well-differentiated lymphocytes, yet not as finely divided as that of lymphoblasts. A striking feature of such cells is the presence, in a significant proportion of the cells, of a single, large, pale blue nucleolus surrounded by a dense rim of chromatin (Fig. 3).

These characteristic cells were first described by ISAACS in 1937. He called them lymphosarcoma cells since those which he observed appeared in the peripheral blood in the terminal phases of lymphosarcoma. He entitled his report "Lymphosarcoma Cell Leukemia" [5]. It has been estimated that as many as 20 per cent of cases of malignant lymphoma of the poorly differentiated lymphocytic type will have abnormal circulating cells in the peripheral blood in the terminal phases of the disease. We frequently see such cases and refer to them as malignant lymphoma, poorly differentiated lymphocytic type, leukemic, rather than introduce the term leukemia, which we feel implies a more fundamental change.

An entirely different situation exists, however, when one encounters a patient whose illness develops suddenly, shows the typical distributional features of systemic diseases, and in whom one finds morphologically identical cells in large numbers in the peripheral blood at the time of his presentation. One of ISAAC's original cases, for example, presented with a leukemic blood picture (94,000 per cu. mm.) which was persistent over a period of seven years. In recent years, the term lymphosarcoma cell leukemia has been applied to these kinds of cases, the systemic proliferative disease of lymphocytes of intermediate degree of differentiation. Such cases are the cytologic counterpart of the localized tumor, malignant lymphoma, poorly differentiated lymphocytic type.

In the past, most of these cases have been included with those called chronic lymphocytic leukemia. Justification for introducing this category is not yet well established. However, a recent report has shown that when these cases are separated from chronic lymphocytic leukemia, a small but statistically significant difference in median survival is demonstrable [6]. No studies in which therapy differed depending upon this distinction have been reported.

The last of the disorders which I shall discuss is WALDENSTRÖM's macroglobulinemia. This is included among the systemic proliferative disorders on the basis of its distributional features and the histologic pattern of involvement in such organs as the liver and spleen. It differs from the other systemic disorders in three respects: 1) Peripheral blood involvement is uncommon. 2) Although involvement of the bone marrow may be extensive, the histologic pattern is frequently that of numerous nodular infiltrates rather than the diffuse involvement which is typical in lymphocytic leukemias. 3) The proliferating cells produce electrophoretically identical IgM macroglobulins which accumulate in the serum and account for the monoclonal macroglobulin spike which is characteristic of this disease.

On a cytologic basis, WALDENSTRÖM's macroglobulinemia is a systemic proliferation, predominantly composed of well-differentiated, mature-appearing lymphocytes. The abnormal protein production is reflected by the fact that a variable number of the cells demonstrate the characteristic cytoplasmic features of plasma cells while retaining the nuclear features of lymphocytes. These plasmacytoid-lymphocytes are recognizable in Romanowsky-stained preparations as well as in routine H & E sections. The high carbohydrate content of the macroglobulin results in a strongly positive reaction with the periodic acid-Schiff stain. The occasional presence of PAS positive intranuclear inclusions is a characteristic, but not invariable, finding.

In summary, hematopoietic neoplasms are divided into two main categories: localized tumors and systemic proliferative diseases. This distinction is based upon the patterns of infiltration and distribution throughout the body, rather than upon the presence or absence of the proliferating cells in blood or bone marrow. The systemic proliferative diseases of lymphoid origin are subclassified on a cytologic basis. In addition to chronic lymphocytic and acute lymphoblastic leukemia, an intermediate category, lymphosarcoma cell leukemia and a usually non-leukemic disorder, WALDENSTRÖM's macroglobulinemia, are included. The terms undifferentiated or stem-cell leukemia are retained to designate those leukemias whose origins are uncertain on the basis of the technique used.

References

1. RAPPAPORT, H.: Tumors of the hematopoietic system. In: Atlas of Tumor Pathology, section III, Fascicle 8. Armed Forces Institute of Pathology, Washington, D. C., 1966, p. 13.
2. ROSENBERG, S. A., KAPLAN, H. S.: Evidence for an orderly progression in the spread of Hodgkin's disease. Cancer Res. **26** PART 1, 1225 (1966).

3. HAYHOE, F. G. J.: Clinical and cytological recognition and differentiation of the leukemias. In: Proceedings of the International Conference on Leukemia-Lymphoma. Ed.: C. J. D. ZARAFONETIS. Philadelphia: Lea & Febiger 1968, p. 307.

4. World Health Organization: Histopathological definition of Burkitt's Tumor. Eds.: C. BERARD, G. T. O'CONOR, L. B. THOMAS, and H. TORLONI. Bull. Wld. Hlth. Org. **40**, 601 (1969).

5. ISAACS, R.: Lymphosarcoma cell leukemia. Ann. intern. Med. **11**, 657 (1937).

6. ZACHARSKI, L. R., LINMAN, J. W.: Chronic lymphocytic leukemia versus chronic lymphosarcoma cell leukemia. Amer. J. Med. **47**, 75 (1969).

The Clinical Evaluation and Staging of Patients with Malignant Lymphoma

SAUL A. ROSENBERG [1]

With 1 Figure

Introduction

During the past decade there have been significant changes in our attitude toward patients with malignant lymphoma, especially those with Hodgkin's disease. There has been a gradually increasing optimism in the aggressive approach to such patients based upon improvement in our therapeutic modalities and the projected curative results now possible. In parallel with these developments has been a much greater interest and skill in the clinical evaluation and study of the untreated patient with malignant lymphoma. Logical therapeutic decisions cannot be made without an accurate assessment of the extent of disease in these patients: to identify those patients who may benefit from aggressive radiotherapeutic approaches and similarly to identify those who should be approached primarily with chemotherapy. Clinical investigations of therapeutic programs have provided significant information in the untreated patients relating to their extent of disease, patterns of disease presentation, and the value of various diagnostic techniques for identifying the sites of malignant lymphoma. These data have important implications as to the value of current and proposed staging systems.

The wide acceptance and utilization of the modern histopathologic classification of Hodgkin's disease [1, 2] and the therapeutic results which are correlated with the clinical stage of this disease have provided stimuli for obtaining valuable information which is improving our understanding of Hodgkin's disease. Though the other malignant lymphomas are equally important, there is much less satisfactory information available of the value of histopathologic classifications [3], diagnostic techniques, patterns of disease, and the reliability and significance of clinical staging systems.

---

[1] From the Departments of Medicine and Radiology, Stanford University School of Medicine. Data reported herein obtained from studies in collaboration with HENRY S. KAPLAN, M. D., supported, in part, by USPHS Grant CA 05838.

Clinical Evaluation

Though modern diagnostic techniques, primariliy radiological, are of great assistance in evaluating the patient with malignant lymphoma [4], a careful history and physical examination remains a most important diagnostic approach. In obtaining a history from an untreated patient, attention must be directed to the presence or absence of the characteristic systemic symptoms of lymphoma. Though occurring more commonly in patients with Hodgkin's disease, unexplained fever, excessive sweating especially at night, and generalized pruritus are commonly found in patients with advanced disease. These symptoms carry important prognostic considerations, especially the presence of fever and night sweats [5]. Often, these symptoms are severe and are unquestionable. However, there are patients with more subtle systemic symptoms: a very low grade fever which would not be identified without temperature recording, minimal sweating perhaps just of the neck, the upper thorax or the head, and localized pruritus. In addition, fatigue, anorexia, and weight loss may be complaints of patients with malignant lymphoma. These more subtle or non-specific symptoms may be correlated to prognosis but they have not been evaluated with sufficient accuracy to be sure.

The presence of pain should be ascertained as it relates to possible retroperitoneal adenopathy and foci of bone involvement. Unusual cardiorespiratory symptoms which may indicate serious involvement of mediastinal airway or vascular structures are of prime importance. Rarely, a patient will present with neurological symptoms as a result of local peripheral nerve compression or, more seriously, spinal cord compression by epidural masses and even more rarely, with meningeal or intracranial disease. Swelling of the ankles or upper extremities may indicate local venous or lymphatic obstruction by enlarged lymph nodes.

The physical examination must be done with great care to identify abnormal lymph nodes in the peripheral lymph node bearing areas. Careful palpation of the occipital, pre-auricular, cervical, supraclavicular, infraclavicular, axillary, brachial, epitrochlear, pectoral, iliac, inguinal, femoral, and popliteal areas must be done. In certain areas, especially in younger people, palpable lymph nodes are quite common. However, their size, consistency, mobility, and location should be carefully described by an experienced observer. When equivocal lymphadenopathy is found in an area which would sufficiently change the stage of disease so as to alter the therapeutic approach, biopsy of these nodes is necessary. Two areas which are very commonly involved and require special attention and skill are the medial supraclavicular areas bilaterally and the apex of each axilla. These examinations cannot be done superficially but must be done carefully with deep palpation and, if possible, by several observers. Waldeyer's ring must be evaluated by an experienced examiner. In the abdomen, careful determination of hepatic size, enlargement of the spleen and of abdominal masses must be noted. Especially in the non-Hodgkin's group, involvement of mesenteric nodes or bowel by lymphoma has important therapeutic implications. If movable masses are found in the abdomen, the examination should be repeated on subsequent days for their persistence. The patient should be evaluated with punch tenderness over the entire spine and iliac wings. If tenderness is found, then special attention radiologically should be directed toward the areas of suspicion.

Involvement of the skin especially in patients of the non-Hodgkin's group may be difficult to determine, since non-specific cutaneous manifestations are occasionally seen. When in doubt, biopsy of skin lesions may be necessary.

Radiological procedures are essential for the initial evaluation of patients with malignant lymphoma. The routine chest X-ray should be supplemented with whole lung tomography. The data of Davidson [4] provide strong evidence that supplementary information is derived from this procedure in a majority of patients. Mediastinal and hilar lymph nodes are common in Hodgkin's disease and, to a lesser extent, in the non-Hodgkin's group. Identification of pulmonary parenchymal nodules or infiltration is of importance in selecting the proper therapeutic program. The presence of pleural fluid should be carefully determined and frequently lateral decubiti views may be indicated. A routine skeletal survey does not frequently provide diagnostic information in the untreated patient. However, attention should be directed to the vertebrae and pelvis on the available chest and abdominal films. For any patients with skeletal pain or bone tenderness more detailed radiological studies and bone scans are indicated. Routine investigations of the stomach, small bowel, and colon, are usually not worthwhile in untreated patients with Hodgkin's disease. In the non-Hodgkin's group, however, they are always indicated, since involvement of these viscera is more frequent [6].

The retroperitoneal space is frequently involved with malignant lymphoma and can best be evaluated with bilateral lower extremity lymphography. This study is essential in the initial evaluation of all patients with malignant lymphoma as supported by the data of Lee and others [4, 7]. The lymphogram may be supplemented in selected cases with an inferior venacavagram, especially for evaluation of the region above the second lumbar vertebra which usually is not evaluated on the lymphogram. An intravenous pyelogram is desirable, especially in those patients with extensive abdominal disease to ascertain the position and patency of the ureters and to identify the kidneys in relation to proposed radiotherapeutic fields.

The bone marrow must be carefully examined in all patients with non-Hodgkin's lymphoma and those with advanced Hodgkin's disease. Though a bone marrow aspirate may identify abnormal lymphoid cells in the non-Hodgkin's group, it is almost always negative in those with Hodgkin's disease [8, 9]. Therefore, a bone marrow biopsy with either the Westerman-Jensen needle or open surgical type is an important initial step before deciding upon the cinical stage and therapeutic program for these patients. In our experience at Stanford bone marrow involvement has not been identified in untreated patients with clinical Stage I or II Hodgkin's disease. The setting of patients with bone marrow involvement in Hodgkin's disease is usually of those with widespread lymph node disease frequently with systemic symptoms, anemia, and an elevated serum alkaline phosphatase. However, these are not always present and occasional examples of patients with no abnormalities other than widespread lymph node disease have been seen [8].

The laboratory evaluation of patients with malignant lymphoma should include the routine studies of a complete blood count, sedimentation rate, attention to white cell morphology, and a serum alkaline phosphatase. As will be emphasized, the liver function tests are not sufficiently reliable, though a 45 minute BSP retention, LDH and transaminase levels are usually obtained. Parameters of hemolysis are desirable in selected patients. All patients when first seen should have a serum protein electrophoretic pattern and those in the non-Hodgkin's group should have an immunoelectrophoresis as well.

The determination of cutaneous anergy of the delayed hypersensitivity type is desirable and of interest in patients with Hodgkin's disease but cannot yet be used for prognostic or staging purposes.

Laparotomy and Splenectomy

In recent years we have resorted to exploratory laparotomy and splenectomy in selected patients who have had equivocal evidence of Hodgkin's disease below the diaphragm. This experience, analyzed by GLATSTEIN [10] demonstrated that approximately half of the patients with clinically enlarged spleens did not have histologic involvement of that organ, and conversely, approximately one in three spleens which were normal in size, contained demonstrable foci of Hodgkin's disease.

In these selected patients, we demonstrated the inability to identify patients with involvement of the liver when using the usual liver funcion tests, hepatic size, hepatic scan, or needle biopsy, as shown in Table 1. False positive clinical evaluations

Table 1. *Hodgkin's disease (selected series). Clinical evaluation of liver involvement at laparotomy*

	Without systemic symptoms		With systemic symptoms	
Clinical evaluation	+	—	+	—
Positive at laparotomy	5	2	8	6
Negative at laparotomy	3	25	5	8
% positive	23%		48%	

8/21 patients with liver involvement had a negative needle biopsy.

were found in eight of twenty-one patients within the limitations of the diagnostic accuracy of hepatic exploration and biopsy. Six of fourteen patients with systemic symptoms had demonstrable hepatic Hodgkin's disease without any clinical suspicion, pre-operatively. There was a high degree of correlation of hepatic and splenic involvement. Liver involvement was not found in the absence of splenic involvement, and the larger the size of the involved spleen the greater the incidence of hepatic disease.

These results have stimulated our group and others to resort to exploratory laparotomy and splenectomy routinely in the evaluation and staging of the untreated patient with Hodgkin's disease. An analysis of fifty consecutive untreated patients has been reported by GLATSTEIN [11] and extended our earlier observations.

The results of 100 consecutive, untreated patients are tabulated in Table 2. Liver involvement is much less frequent in the unselected group, but has not occurred in the absence of involvement of the spleen. Half of the patients with enlarged spleens did not have involvement of that organ when examined histologically. Seven examples of involvement of the lymph nodes in the hilum of the spleen have been observed, occasionally as the only site of disease below the diaphragm. There has been only one example of mesenteric lymph node involvement.

Of 57 lymphograms reported as negative, two were shown to have para-aortic lymph node involvement. Of 23 reported as positive, 17 were confirmed. Of 20 reported as equivocal, three were positive and 17 negative.

It is our conclusion that an accurate assessment of Hodgkin's disease below the diaphragm cannot be made without exploratory laparotomy and splenectomy.

Table 2. *Results of laparotomy in 100 consecutive untreated patients with Hodgkin's disease*

Site	Preoperative assessment	A Systemic symptoms absent	B Systemic symptoms present	Total
Liver	Clinically positive	0 / 4 [a]	1 / 11	1 / 15
	Clinically negative	1 / 53	1 / 32	2 / 85
Spleen	Clinically positive	2 / 6	6 / 10	8 / 16
	Clinically negative	11 / 51	9 / 33	20 / 84
Abdominal nodes	Positive lymphangiogram	8 / 11 (1)	10 / 12	18 / 23 (1)
	Negative lymphangiogram	5 / 33 (4)	2 / 24 (1)	7 / 57 (5)
	Equivocal lymphangiogram	3 / 13 (1)	1 / 7	4 / 20 (1)

[a] No. with HD / No. examined.
( ) Patients with ⊕ splenic hilar nodes, but ⊖ para-aortic node biopsy.

Patterns of Disease

The improved accuracy in assessing sites of involvement in patients with Hodgkin's disease who have not been treated has provided a considerable insight into the nature of this disease. It is quite clear that Hodgkin's disease in the untreated patient is not randomly distributed throughout the lymphoid tissues of the body. There are patterns of involvement which support the concept of an orderly progression of this disease, probably via lymphatic channels. There is a correlation between involvement of the right neck and the mediastinum (Table 3) and the left neck and

Table 3. *Hodgkin's disease. Correlation of cervical and mediastinal involvement*

	Right neck only	Left neck only	Both sides
Mediastinum involved	12 (86%)	17 (50%)	37 (66%)
Mediastinum uninvolved	2	17	19
Total	14	34	56

abdominal sites (Table 4). The association of involvement of the spleen with involvement of the liver has been confirmed in a retrospective analysis of the experience at Stanford by KAPLAN. Of 37 patients with hepatic involvement, all but two had concurrent or prior involvement of the spleen. Even the two exceptions were so poorly documented as to be questionable. Of great significance is the observation that in 56 patients with clinical involvement of the spleen 63% had concurrent or subsequent involvement of the liver. Spleen involvement in Hodgkin's disease can no longer be considered as if it were "merely a lymph node", but identifies a group of patients at high risk for having or subsequently developing involvement of the liver.

Table 4. *Hodgkin's disease. Correlation of cervical and abdominal involvement*

	Right neck only	Left neck only	Both sides
Abdomen involved	1 (7%)	17 (50%)	29 (52%)
Abdomen uninvolved	13	17	27
Total	14	34	56

Table 5 demonstrates the correlation of abdominal and mediastinal disease in patients with supraclavicular or infraclavicular Hodgkin's disease. These patterns of disease suggest that the upper abdomen is contiguous to the low neck probably via the thoracic duct, not as an exception, but in the majority of patients and involvement of the mediastinum is not associated with an increased frequency of identifiable abdominal disease. This by-passing of the mediastinum is noted in all histologic sub-groups (Table 6).

Table 5. *Hodgkin's disease. Correlation of mediastinal and abdominal involvement. 114 untreated patients staged with laparotomy*

	Mediastinum Involved	Uninvolved
Abdomen involved	21 (30%)	29 (64%)
Abdomen uninvolved	48	16
Total	69	45

The concept of an orderly progression of Hodgkin's disease, based upon patterns of disease in the untreated patient [12] can now be extended. KAPLAN analyzed 340 patients for contiguity of involvement. Table 7 demonstrates the very high degree of contiguity observed, ranging from 88% to 100% for various sites [13].

Similar studies of the non-Hodgkin's group are in progress and hopefully applying the newer histopathologic classification [3], routine laparotomy and bone marrow

Table 6. *Hodgkin's disease. Correlation of mediastinal and abdominal involvement. 114 patients staged with laparotomy*

	Lymphocyte predominance		Nodular sclerosis		Mixed cellularity		Lymphocyte depletion		Total	
Mediastinum	+	—	+	—	+	—	+	—	+	—
Abdomen +	0	8 (57%)	16 (26%)	9 (60%)	5 (62.5%)	11 (73%)	0	1	21 (30%)	29 (64%)
Abdomen —	0	6	45	6	3	4	0	0	48	16
Total	0	14	61	15	8	15	0	1	69	45

Table 7. *Hodgkin's disease. Contiguity of lymphatic sites of involvement in 340 untreated cases* [13]

Site	Total No. instances involved	Sole site involved	Additional sites involved	Anatomic relationship to other sites Non-contiguous	Contiguous	% Contiguous
1. Right axillary nodes	78	5	73	8	65	89
2. Left axillary nodes	90	3	87	3	84	97
3. Right cervical-supraclav. nodes	199	12	187	1	186	99
4. Left cervical-supraclav. nodes	241	23	218	6	212	97
5. Mediastinal nodes	211	5	206	1	205	99.5
6. Hilar nodes	39	0	39	0	39	100
7. Para-aortic nodes	114	1	113	1	112	99
8. Iliac, inguinal, femoral nodes	54	5	49	1	48	98
9. Spleen	44	0	44	5	39	88

studies, we may be able to identify which groups of patients of the non-Hodgkin's type may have predictable patterns of involvement. Unfortunately, this data is not yet available to us.

Staging Classification

There has been considerable change in the staging classifications of Hodgkin's disease in the last several decades. The initial classification of Craver modified by Peters was changed at the Paris and Rye conferences in 1965 and 1966 as a result of the increased utilization of lymphography. It seemed clear at that time that patients with widespread lymph node involvement should not be combined with those with hepatic, bone marrow, and pulmonary disease in that their therapeutic

Table 8. *Hodgkin's disease. Definition of clinical stages. Recommended at the Rye conference* [14]

Stage I	Disease limited to one anatomic region [a] (I_1) or to two contiguous anatomic regions (I_2) on the same side of the diaphragm.
Stage II	Disease in more than two anatomic regions or in two non-contiguous regions on the same side of the diaphragm.
Stage III	Disease on both sides of the diaphragm, but not extending beyond the involvement of lymph nodes, spleen, and/or Waldeyer's ring.
Stage IV	Involvement of the bone marrow, lung parenchyma, pleura, liver, bone, skin, kidneys, gastrointestinal tract, or any tissue or organ in addition to lymph nodes, spleen, or Waldeyer's ring.

All stages will be subclassified as "A" or "B" to indicate the absence or presence, respectively, of systemic symptoms. The following documented symptoms, otherwise unexplained, are significant: (a) fever; (b) night sweats; and (c) pruritus.

[a] See Fig. 1.

Table 9. *Hodgkin's disease. Stanford modification of the Rye staging system*

Stage I	Involvement of a single lymphoid region.
Stage II_n	Involvement of two or more lymphoid regions, but limited to one side of the diaphragm. A subscript $-_n$, indicates the number of regions involved.
Stage III	Involvement of lymph nodes above and below the diaphragm, and/or Waldeyer's ring, and/or the spleen. A subscript $-_s$ (III_s) indicates involvement of the spleen.
Stage IV	Involvement of extranodal sites such as the lung, liver, bone marrow, bone, skin, and/or other viscera in addition to lymph nodes and/or Waldeyer's ring, and/or the spleen. If the extranodal involvement is limited, and in contiguity with lymphoid involvement, the designation IV_1 shall be used.

All patients will be sub-classified A or B to indicate the absence or presence, respectively, of documented unexplained fever, night sweats, or generalized pruritus.

approach and prognoses were widely divergent. The Rye classification [14] has been widely adopted and remains the most valuable classification to date (Table 8 and Fig. 1). However, the classification only has important validity and utility if the diagnostic work-up has been complete. If, for example, lymphography is not used in the evaluation of patients, then staging so derived will have little comparative meaning to series which utilize this diagnostic approach. Similarly, the use of exploratory laparotomy and splenectomy will significantly change the accuracy of the identified groups. Any staging system to be of value for comparative purposes must employ the same diagnostic methods.

The Rye staging classification for Hodgkin's disease is deficient in several respects and should be modified (Table 9).

There has been reluctance in practice to group together in Stage I, patients who have only one lymphoid region involved and those with two contiguous regions despite their similar prognosis. Since this has not stood the test of utilization, it is suggested, that Stage I be limited to those patients who have only one lymphoid region. The Stage II group remains a broad one and it is suggested that subscripts indicating the number of lymphoid regions involved be used. It seems clear from the data presented that involvement of the spleen does not carry the same implication as if it were a lymph node. A future classification should take into account this special significance of splenic involvement as it relates to subsequent hepatic disease and probably connotes poorer prognostic consequences. The data from Stanford [5] and from Musshoff [15] suggest strongly that involvement of non-lymphoid structures which

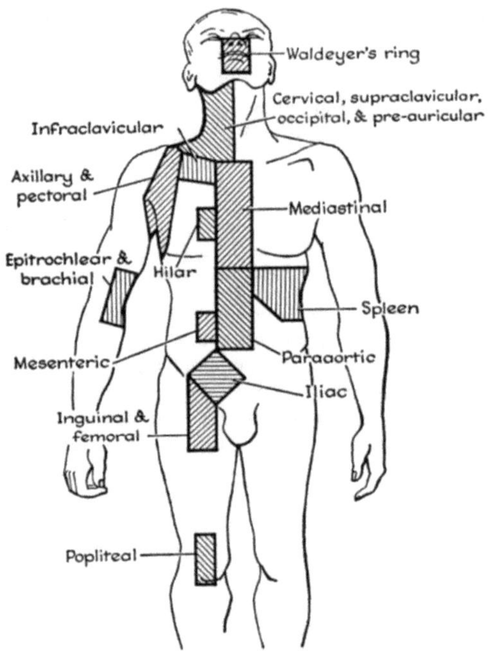

Fig. 1. Schematic representation of the regional areas used in the staging of Hodgkin's disease

are contiguous to involved lymphoid tissue, probably by direct extension, do not indicate a poor prognosis. For example, direct involvement of the lung, presumably from mediastinal or hilar lymph nodes to a limited extent which may still allow radiotherapy to be delivered is still associated with a good prognosis. Other examples of such localized extra nodal involvement are the sternum, clavicle, vertebra, pericardium, pleura and localized subcutaneous and skin involvement from underlying lymph node masses. These localized extra nodal sites should be identified as a more favorable group since in Musshoff's series their survival and curability are identical to patients with Stage II disease. For Hodgkin's disease it is also important to document the prognostic significance of generalized pruritus. The present staging classification implies the same unfavorable prognosis of this symptom as with fever and sweating. Many experienced clinicians question this association and studies are under way to document its importance.

There are a number of major differences between the non-Hodgkin's lymphoma group and those with Hodgkin's disease as it relates to staging and prognosis. We must await the results of clinical studies, and correlations with the newer histopathologic classifications before having confidence in proposed staging systems. However, it is quite clear that the non-Hodgkin's group frequently presents or is associated with extra nodal involvement early in the course of disease [6, 16]. Some of these settings are most favorable and it is proposed that Stage I should include involvement of an isolated extra nodal site. Stage II, in addition to including patients with two or more lymphoid regions, should include patients with an apparent primary extra nodal lesion and involvement of the local draining lymph node region. At this time, we still designate widespread extra-nodal disease as Stage IV. However, it is quite clear that patients with involvement of the bone marrow by nodular or well differentiated lymphocytic lymphoma may still have a good prognosis.

Summary

The therapeutic program cannot be outlined for the untreated patient with malignant lymphoma until he has undergone an exhaustive investigation and carefully assigned a staging designation. There has been a gradual evolution of the diagnostic studies required to detect disease which now include routine bi-pedal lymphography, bone marrow biopsy, whole chest tomography and exploratory laparotomy with splenectomy. These detailed studies have provided new information on the patterns of disease especially relating in Hodgkin's disease, involvement of the low neck and the upper abdomen, and involvement of the spleen with that of the liver. Because of these observations and the relatively favorable prognosis of certain extranodal sites in Hodgkin's disease, changes of the Rye staging classification are required. A tentative proposal modifying the Rye staging system is presented.

References

1. Lukes, R. J., Butler, J. J., Hicks, E. B.: Natural history of Hodgkin's disease as related to its pathologic picture. Cancer **19**, 317 (1966).
2. — Report of the nomenclature committee. Cancer Res. **26**, 1311 (1966).
3. Rappaport, H.: Tumors of the hematopoietic system. In: Atlas of Tumor Pathology, Section III, Fascicle 8. Armed Forces Institute of Pathology, Washington, D. C., 1966.
4. Davidson, J. W., Clarke, E. A.: Influence of modern radiological techniques on clinical staging of malignant lymphoma. Canad. Med. Ass. J. **99**, 1196 (1968).
5. Keller, A. R., Kaplan, H. S., Lukes, R. J., Rappaport, H.: Correlations of histopathology with other prognostic indicators in Hodgkin's disease. Cancer **22**, 487 (1968).
6. Rosenberg, S. A., Diamond, H. D., Jaslowitz, B., Craver, L. F.: Lymphosarcoma: a review of 1269 cases. Medicine **40**, 31 (1961).
7. Lee, B. J.: Correlation between lymphangiography and clinical status of patients with lymphoma. Cancer Chemother. Rep. **52**, 205 (1968).
8. Rosenberg, S. A.: Contribution of lymphangiography to our understanding of lymphoma. Cancer Chemother. Rep. **52**, 213 (1968).
9. Grann, V., Pool, J. L., Mayer, K.: Comparative study of bone marrow aspiration and biopsy in patients with neoplastic disease. Cancer **19**, 1898 (1966).
10. Glatstein, E., Guernsey, J. M., Rosenberg, S. A., Kaplan, H. S.: The value of laparotomy and splenectomy in the staging of Hodgkin's disease. Cancer **24**, 709 (1969).

11. GLATSTEIN, E., TRUEBLOOD, H. W., ENRIGHT, L. P., ROSENBERG, S. A., KAPLAN, H. S.: Surgical staging of abdominal involvement in unselected patients with Hodgkin's disease. Radiology, in print.
12. ROSENBERG, S. A., KAPLAN, H. S.: Evidence for an orderly progression in the spread of Hodgkin's disease. Cancer Res. **26**, 1225 (1966).
13. KAPLAN, H. S.: On the natural history, treatment, and prognosis of Hodgkin's disease. Lecture before the Harvey Society of New York, March 1969. In press.
14. ROSENBERG, S. A.: Report of the committee on the staging of Hodgkin's disease. Cancer Res. **26**, 1310 (1966).
15. MUSSHOFF, K., RENEMANN, H., BOUTIS, L., AFKHAM, J.: Die extranoduläre Lymphogranulomatose (Hodgkin's disease). Diagnose, Therapie und Prognose bei zwei unterschiedlichen Formen des Organbefalls. Ein Beitrag zur Stadieneinteilung der Lymphogranulomatose. Fortschr. Röntgenstr. **109**, 776 (1968).
16. BANFI., A., BONADONNA., G., CARNEVALI, G., FOSSATI-BELLANI, F.: Malignant lymphomas: Further studies on their preferential sites of involvement and possible mode of spread. Lymphology **2**, 130 (1969).

Discussion

The Staging of Lymphoma

LAWRENCE W. ALLEN, STEPHEN B. STRUM, JOHN E. ULTMANN, and HENRY RAPPAPORT [1]

The data presented by Dr. ROSENBERG suggest that exploratory laparotomy may play a significant role in the staging of lymphoma. One year ago, aware of their findings in selected patients, we began to perform diagnostic laparotomy and splenectomy in all patients under 65 with Hodgkin's disease apparently confined to lymph nodes, and more recently in patients with other lymphomas, admitted to the Argonne Cancer Research Hospital for staging and treatment. The following summarizes our results in the first 21 patients with Hodgkin's disease and compares our findings with those of the Stanford group.

Preliminary studies include a careful history, physical examination, complete blood counts, a battery of liver function tests, including bromsulphalein retention, alkaline phosphatase, transaminases, and serum protein electrophoresis, liver and spleen scan employing radioactive technetium and liver biopsy if indicated, chest x-rays with lung tomograms if hilar adenopathy is found, and bone films with bone scan and biopsy if indicated, inferior vena cavagram, azygogram, and bilateral lower extremity lymphogram. Then if Stage IV disease, that is, visceral involvement has not been proven, laparotomy and splenectomy are performed.

The laparotomy is done by a surgical team experienced in this procedure. After careful inspection and palpation of the abdominal contents, the surgeon takes biopsies from any suspicious areas of the liver, a large wedge from the left lobe, and a deep needle biopsy of each lobe. Multiple lymph nodes are then removed from any lymph node groups which are suspicious from cavagraphy, lymphography, inspection or palpation, and lymph nodes are routinely biopsied from the para-aortic, iliac, and mesenteric chains and the porta hepatis. Following this the spleen is removed along with splenic hilar lymph nodes. Metal clips are placed at the sites from which lymph nodes were removed, at the most lateral margins of disease, at the splenic pedicle, and along the splenic artery. At the close of the procedure, a core bone biopsy is

---

[1] From the Departments of Medicine and Pathology of the Pritzker School of Medicine of the University of Chicago and the Argonne Cancer Research Hospital (operated by the University of Chicago for the United States Atomic Energy Commission), Chicago, Illinois 60637

Supported in part by United States Public Health Service Grant CA-5183 and the Hematology General Research Fund.

taken from the iliac crest. Post-operatively, an abdominal x-ray verifies that the lymph nodes in question have been removed.

Twenty-one patients, ten male, eleven female, ages 8—45 with apparent Stage I, II, or III Hodgkin's disease have had laparotomies performed specifically for staging, from January 1, 1969 to December 31, 1969. Of the 21, 18 have had splenectomy. There were no deaths. There was no morbidity except for one patient who, four days postoperatively, had acute gastrointestinal bleeding due to a reactivation of peptic gastritis.

Eleven patients have had normal or equivocal contrast studies to evaluate retroperitoneal lymphadenopathy. Two of these patients, both with normal studies, had

Table 1. *Laparotomy and splenectomy in staging of Hodgkin's disease*

Clinical findings		Lymph node		Spleen		Liver	
		+	—	+	—	+	—
IVC/LAG							
Normal or equivocal	(11)	2	9				
Abnormal	(6)	2	4				
Not done	(2)	0	2				
Spleen palpation/scan							
Not felt and neg. scan	(13)			3	10		
Splenomegaly and/or pos. scan	(5)			3	2		
Liver function tests							
Normal	(13)					0	13
Abnormal	(8)					0	8

IVC = Inferior venacavagram; LAG = Lymphangiogram; + = Biopsy diagnostic of Hodgkin's disease; — = Biopsy negative for Hodgkin's disease.

Hodgkin's disease in lymph nodes on biopsy (Table 1). Six patients had abnormal studies indicating abdominal disease. However, in only two of these six patients did biopsy confirm this disease. In two patients for whom no studies were available, lymph node biopsies were negative. Histologic findings in lymph nodes which appeared abnormal on lymphangiogram but did not contain Hodgkin's disease, included reactive hyperplasia and lipoid granulomata or granulomatous lymphadenitis.

Eighteen patients have had splenectomy during their staging procedure (Table 1). In 13 of these, the spleen was not palpable and the spleen scan was considered normal. Of these 13, 3 had splenic disease. Five patients had either a palpable spleen, an abnormal scan, or both; of these 5, 3 had splenic involvement. In only 2 of the 6 cases with splenic involvement did the surgeon suspect this at the time of laparotomy. In all cases, the splenic involvement was obvious by gross examination after serial 3 mm sections were made. Thus, of the 18 patients who had splenectomy 6, or 33 per cent, had splenic Hodgkin's disease. Several case studies illustrate the clinical presentations of Hodgkin's disease in the spleen. The first patient had fever, night sweats, generalized adenopathy, and a markedly abnormal inferior venacavagram. The spleen was neither palpable nor abnormal by scan. The spleen, however, was in fact the largest of those involved with Hodgkin's disease, weighed 290 gms, and contained multiple nodules. The next patient was asymptomatic, had a large iliac lymph node, and the spleen, though not palpable, appeared slightly large by scan. This was in fact the smallest involved spleen, weighed only 78 gms, and also contained multiple nodules. The next patient was asymptomatic and had only a large left supraclavicular lymph node, a normal lymphangiogram and a clinically negative spleen. This spleen, weighing 110 gms, nonetheless, had a single nodule of Hodgkin's disease less than 5 mm in diameter and is representative of the three patients who had single splenic nodules.

Twenty-one patients have had multiple liver biopsies. Although 8 of the group had at least 1 abnormal liver function test, we have not found definite liver involvement by Hodgkin's disease in a single patient. Six showed portal lymphocytic infiltrates which varied from mild to severe.

Core bone biopsies in 21 patients did not reveal a single instance of Hodgkin's disease.

Staging was advanced because of laparotomy in 3 of 12 patients, thought to be Stage I or II prelaparotomy, by the finding of unsuspected Hodgkin's disease in the spleen or abdominal lymph nodes.

On the other hand, 6 of 9 patients suspected of having Stage III disease by virtue of either lymph node or splenic involvement were found at laparotomy to have no evidence of abdominal involvement. Thus, 9 of the 21 had a change in their staging as a result of laparotomy and splenectomy.

How do these results compare with those reported by Dr. ROSENBERG? Although our numbers are relatively small, the similarities are great. There was no significant morbidity in either series. Clinically suspected disease has been refuted by this procedure and a disturbingly high incidence of clinically occult disease, especially in the spleen has been detected. The higher correlation with lymphography findings in the Stanford series may be related, in part, to differing radiographic criteria for lymph node abnormality but the lesson learned is the same, namely, that lymphography is not an infallible diagnostic tool.

The relatively high incidence of hepatic involvement associated with splenic involvement as reported by GLATSTEIN, GUERNSEY, ROSENBERG, and KAPLAN [1] in the first series of laparotomies in selected patients with Hodgkin's disease is not confirmed by their subsequent finding of a low incidence of hepatic involvement in unselected patients. The absence of definite hepatic involvement in our series of unselected patients now closely resembles the data reported by Dr. ROSENBERG.

Thus we see that lymphangiography, although it remains very useful in planning radiation ports and follow-up of abdominal lymph nodes, may have limited value as a staging procedure because it may falsely suggest that abdominal disease is present, and, more importantly, may fail to reveal significant abdominal disease.

Laparotomy and splenectomy are useful in the management of apparently localized lymphoma because it will help define the natural history of the disease, assist in definitive staging, potentially remove a major site of disease, help accomplish accurate port design by the careful mapping of disease activity and judicious placement of silver clips, and prevent radiation injury to vital organs such as the left kidney, pleura, lung, and diaphragm. Moreover, it may improve follow-up because of the permanency of silver clips compared to the finite life-span of lymphogram dye. There is now reason to believe that it may improve the tolerance for radiation therapy. It remains to be proven that it will increase the tolerance for drug therapy.

We have emphasized the value of performing diagnostic laparotomy and splenectomy in the staging of lymphoma. It is also important to stress the manner in which the node biopsies are obtained and evaluated. First, the largest node should be included in the biopsy, not just the most accessible one. The reason for this is that the more superficial lymph node may reveal only reactive hyperplasia, while the larger, less accessible, contiguous lymph node may show gross involvement with lymphoma. Secondly, STRUM and RAPPAPORT [2] have emphasized that a lymph node which appears benign on routine section may show small areas of involvement with lymphoma when a careful search is made by the technique of semi-serial section of the node. They presented six cases of Hodgkin's disease in which lymph node biopsy sections showed minute foci of Hodgkin's disease despite the fact that these nodes generally had a preserved nodal architecture and a cellular composition that in most cases was not suggestive of disease. One of these cases was that of a 26-year-old woman with a left supraclavicular lymph node showing nodular sclerosing type of Hodgkin's disease, who was asymptomatic, had an otherwise normal physical examination and routine staging procedures, but at diagnostic laparotomy was found to have a single splenic nodule of Hodgkin's disease. Routine sections of the multiple lymph nodes removed showed only reactive hyperplasia, but following semi-serial section, a minute focus of disease was found in one lymph node. Failure to detect either the splenic nodule or the lymph node focus might have led to inadequate radiation therapy.

Based on the findings of the Stanford group and the firm support lent by our own results and by others, we believe the time is right to consider diagnostic laparotomy and splenectomy as a critical step in the evaluation of malignant lymphoma especially in Hodgkin's disease where Stage IV disease cannot be proven and the patient is being approached with curative intent. This should be done at large treatment centers where interested and experienced internists, surgeons, pathologists, and radiation therapists cooperate in the care and study of patients with lymphoma.

References

1. GLATSTEIN., E., GUERNSEY, J. M., ROSENBERG, S. A., KAPLAN, H. S.: The value of laparotomy and splenectomy in the staging of Hodgkin's disease. Cancer **24**, 709—718 (1969).
2. STRUM, S. B., RAPPAPORT, H.: The significance of focal involvement of lymph nodes for the diagnosis and staging of Hodgkin's disease. Cancer **25**, 1314—1319 (1970).

An Empirical Cellular Approach to the Improvement of Cancer Chemotherapy [1]

W. R. Bruce and H. Lin

With 1 Figure

Over the past two years successful strategies have been developed for effectively dealing with a small number of experimental tumors in mice. These strategies have been arrived at rather empirically on the basis of a cellular approach to the tumor. The logical extension of these methods to other experimental tumors would seem to be only a matter of time. However, of more importance, it should be possible to use the approach, with appropriate modification, to optimize the treatment of human tumors. In effect we are suggesting that it may be possible that human tumors can be effectively treated with chemotherapeutic agents we now possess and that significantly improved results will follow the use of appropriate drugs at appropriate dosages, combinations, and correct timing. But what are the appropriate drugs, the appropriate dosages, and the proper combinations, and what is the correct timing?

The approach that has been used with the experimental tumors differs from the usual one in which the effectiveness of treatments is evaluated by tumor regression alone. Rather, the effects of the drugs on the survival of individual tumor cells have been measured. The effects of combinations and of timing of the drugs were then determined, and finally a treatment strategy was formulated. A schematic presentation of this treatment strategy is shown in Fig. 1.

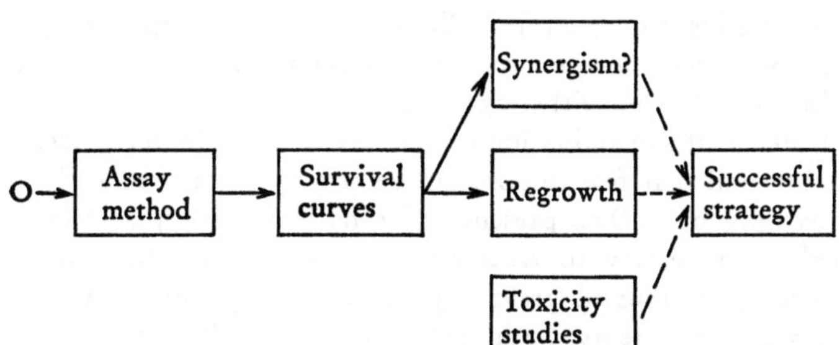

Fig. 1. Schematic presentation of treatment strategy

[1] Reprinted by permission of Cancer Res. 29, 2308—2310 (1969).

The first step is the development of an assay system for the malignant stem cells of the tumor in question. By the term "malignant stem cells" we mean those problem cells within the tumor which can continue to proliferate and whose continued multiplication leads to the death of the animal. We must be able to count these cells so that we can determine the effects of our treatment at a cellular level. Several methods for determining the number of cells with proliferative capacity within a tumor are known. Certainly there is room for improving and simplifying these methods, but one method has proven particularly useful and can probably be used more extensively. This is the endpoint dilution assay system originally described by HEWITT and independently developed by SKIPPER. This method provides a measure of the number of tumor cells which, on transplantation into other animals, can proliferate and kill the recipient. With such a method for counting the number of malignant cells, it is possible to look quantitatively at the effects of drug schedules.

The second step is the measurement of the survival of tumor cells after different dosages of drugs. Since survival is, of course, a function of both the dose rate and the duration of exposure to a drug, we have found it convenient to think in terms of dose-survival curves (when the animal is exposed to the drug over a constant period of time) and time-survival curves (when the animal is exposed to a constant dosage rate of the drug). The survival curves in both cases are typically exponential in shape over several decades, but at lower survival values there is usually a change in the slope corresponding to a fraction of the population that is less sensitive to the drug in question. The reason for the resistance may be genotypic or it may be phenotypic—a consequence of difference in the penetration of the drug to different portions of the tumor or to differences in the sensitivities of cells in different parts of the generations or growth cycles. In either case it is clearly advantageous to use the doses and the exposure times corresponding to the steepest portion of the survival curve, and it is inefficient to use a drug at doses corresponding to the latter portion of the survival curves where there is little tumor destruction for each increment of the dose given.

The third step in the approach is to look for synergism in the action of the agents. This as necessary since almost certainly no single agent will be able to deal effectively with most of our tumors. Most of the survival curves show the presence of resistant cell populations. Combinations of agents which kill cells on the basis of different mechanisms reduce the possibility that cells with genotypic and phenotypic resistance appear. It is not necessary to understand the mechanism of the resistance before testing for synergism. Combinations of drugs, each given at their most effective doses, may be used together to determine whether the combination kills more malignant cells than either agent alone.

The fourth step is the examination of the recovery of the tumor cell population. We will probably find that few tumors can be effectively treated with combinations of agents given only once. The presence of cells in phenotypically resistant states will likely make it necessary to treat and re-treat. Information on the regrowth kinetics of the tumor is thus of great importance in determining what time should be allowed between treatments. Such information will allow treatment before the tumor regrows extensively and before the effects of the treatment are lost.

Our present chemotherapeutic agents have a limited degree of selectivity on tumor cells, and thus we must examine a fifth area in which more data are needed. This is drug toxicity. While we have information on the toxicity of most agents

Table 1

Tumors	Assay method	Survival curves	Synergism	Regrowth	Successful strategy	References
L1210 leukemia	+	+	+	+	+	[5, 14, 16, 19]
AKR lymphoma, transplanted	+	+	+	+	+	[3, 4, 17]
Carcinoma 755	+	+	+	+	+	[11]
AKR lymphoma, spontaneous	+	+	+	+	–	[12; SKIPPER et al. (personal communication)]
Fortner plasmacytoma (hamster)	+	+	–	+	+	[6]
Sarcoma (albino, C3H)	+	r [a]	–	–	–	[7]
Lymphoblastic leukemia (CBA)	+	r	–	–	–	[8]
P-388 lymphocytic leukemia	+	r	–	–	–	[2]
LSA ascites tumor (C57BL)	+	r	–	–	–	[15]
Rhabdomyosarcoma (WAG rat)	+	r	–	–	–	[13]
Mammary carcinoma (C3H)	+	r	–	–	–	[10]
KHT sarcoma (C3H)	+	r	–	–	–	[10; HILL and BUSCH (personal communication)]
Squamous carcinoma (WHT/Ht)	+	r	–	–	–	[9]
Osteosarcoma (C57 X CBA) F_1	+	r (+)	–	+	–	[18]
Plasma cell tumor Adj. PC-5	+	+	–	–	–	[1]
Spontaneous solid tumors in experimental animals	–	–	–	–	–	
Human tumors	–	–	–	–	–	

Current status of Cancer Chemother. Res. [a] r, radiation survival curve only.

given in a single schedule, we do not have systematic information on the effects of combinations of agents or on the effects of repeated doses of combined drug schedules. This information is necessary for the definition of workable drug schedules and can be obtained before the survival curves for all tumors are obtained.

It is not possible to define *a priori* a schedule which may be effective in treating a given tumor even when we have all the information outlined above. However, it is possible to state four general principles. First, drugs should be employed which produce a substantial reduction in the survival of the malignant cells. Second, doses of these drugs should be used that correspond to the steepest portion of the survival curves in order to achieve the maximum degree of malignant cell reduction for the minimum drug exposure. Third, the drugs should be used in combinations that show demonstrable synergism. Fourth, the combinations should be given repeatedly before the tumor has grown substantially, but after the animal has recovered from previous treatment.

The current status of cancer chemotherapy research from the point of view of the flow diagram (Fig. 1) is summarized in Table 1. Several tumors have been studied in detail with respect to assay methods, survival curves, synergism, and tumor recovery, and successful strategies have been developed. Other tumors are in the process of investigation. Many assay systems for transplanted tumors have been developed, but few have been used to examine the effects of chemotherapeutic agents. No asssays have yet been developed either for examining the survival of tumor cells in solid spontaneous tumors in animals or for systemically examining survival of malignant cells in human tumors.

We feel that, in light of previous success with the approach given in Fig. 1, we are warranted in making the following recommendations:

a) The available assay methods for transplanted solid experimental tumors in animals should be exploited to determine the effects of chemotherapeutic agents on the survival of malignant cells within solid tumors. Optimum methods for treating these tumors should be developed.

b) Methods for assaying malignant cells of spontaneous solid tumors in animals should be developed to determine whether the sensitivities of these cells are similar to those of the transplanted experimental tumors. Strategies for treating these tumors should be developed.

c) Methods for assaying for malignant stem cells from certain of the human tumors should be developed. Such technics will allow us both to investigate the action of drugs on these tumors while they are in the patient and to compare the results with the studies in the experimental animals.

The approach which we recommend differs considerably from the current approaches of cancer chemotherapy research. It does not depend on elucidating biochemical pathways or on explaining cell survival curves. It may not lead to any new insights into the mechanism of action of the agents. We feel, however, that this empirical cellular approach will quickly tell us whether we now have chemotherapeutic agents which are capable of effectively treating human tumors and what the optimum drugs, combinations, and timings are.

Summary

A critical step in developing a successful strategy for dealing with experimental tumours is the development of assay methods for the malignant stem cells of the tumour. When such an assay is available, it is possible to determine the effect of dosages, combinations and timing of drugs on this important tumour population. It would appear that the development of assays for stem cells in human tumours should receive a high priority.

References

1. BERGSAGEL, D. E., VALERIOTE, F. A.: Growth characteristics of a mouse plasma cell tumor. Cancer Res. **28**, 2187—2196 (1968).
2. BERRY, R. J., ANDREWS, J. R.: Quantitatives Studies of radiation effects on cell reproductive capacity in a mammalian transplantable tumor system *in vivo*. Ann. N. Y. Acad. Sci. **95**, 1001—1008 (1961).

3. Bruce, W. R., Meeker, B. E., Powers, W. E., Valeriote, F. A.: Comparison of the dose and time-survival curves for normal hematopoietic and lymphoma colony-forming cells exposed to vinblastine, vincristine, arabinosyl cytosine and amethopterin. J. Nat. Cancer Inst. **42,** 1015—1023 (1969).
4. Bruce, W. R., Van Der Gaag, H. A.: Quantitative assay for the number of murine lymphoma cells capable of proliferating *in vivo*. Nature **199,** 79—80 (1963).
5. Goldin, A., Venditti, J. M., Humphreys, S. R., Mantel, N.: Quantitative evaluation of chemotherapeutic agents against advanced leukemia in mice. J. Nat. Cancer Inst. **21,** 495—511, 1958.
6. Griswold, D. P., Jr., Schabel, F. M., Jr., Wilcox, W. S., Simpson-Herren, L., Skipper, H. E.: Success and failure in the treatment of solid tumors. I. Effect of cyclophosphamide on primary and metastatic plasmacytoma in the hamster. Cancer Chemother. Rep. **52,** 345—387 (1968).
7. Hewitt, H. B.: Studies of the quantitative transplantation of mouse sarcoma. Brit. J. Cancer **7,** 367—383 (1953).
8. Hewitt, H. B.: Studies of the dissemination and quantitative transplantation of a lymphocytic leukemia of CBA mice. Brit. J. Cancer **12,** 378—401 (1958).
9. — Chan, D. P. S., Blake, E. R.: Survival curves for clonogenic cells of a murine keratinizing squamous carcinoma irradiated *in vivo* or under hypoxic conditions. Int. J. Radiat. Biol. **12,** 535—549 (1967).
10. Kallman, R. F., Silini, G., Van Putten, L. M.: Factors influencing the quantitative estimation of the *in vivo* survival of cells from solid tumors. J. Nat. Cancer Inst. **39,** 539—549 (1967).
11. Laster, W. R., Jr., Mayo, J. G., Simpson-Herren, L., Griswold, D. P., Jr., Lloyd, H. H., Schabel, F. M., Skipper, H. E.: Success and failure in the treatment of solid tumors. II. Kinetic parameters and "cell cure" of moderately advanced carcinoma 755. Cancer Chemother. Rep. **53,** 169—188 (1969).
12. Lin, H., Milley, G. I. A., Bruce, W. R.: Effects of cyclophosphamide (CY), 1,3-bis-(2-chloroethyl)-1-nitrosourea (BCNU), vinblastine (VLB) and cytosine arabinoside (Ara-C) on lymphoma cells from the spontaneous lymphoma of AKR mice. Proc. Amer. Ass. Cancer Res. **10,** 51 (1969).
13. Reinhold, H. S.: Quantitative evaluation of the radiosensitivity of cells of a transplantable rhabdomyosarcoma in the rat. Europ. J. Cancer **2,** 33—42 (1966).
14. Schabel, F. M.: *In vivo* Leukemic cell kill kinetics and "curability" in experimental system. In: The Proliferation and Spread of Neoplastic cells, 21st Annual Symposium on Fundamental Cancer Research, Houston, Texas, 1967. Baltimore: Williams & Wilkins Co 1968, pp. 379—408.
15. Silini, G., Maruyama, Y.: Studies of the LSA ascites lymphoma of C57 BL mice. I. Transplantation characteristics and radiosensitivity of cells during serial passages. J. Nat. Cancer Inst. **35,** 841—849 (1965).
16. Skipper, H. E., Schabel, F. M., Jr., Wilcox, W. S.: Experimental evaluation of potential anticancer agents. XIII. On the criteria and kinetics associated with "curability" of experimental leukemia. Cancer Chemother. Rep. **35,** 1—111 (1964).
17. Valeriote, F. A., Bruce, W. R., Meeker, B. E.: Synergistic action of cyclophosphamide and 1,3-bis(2-chloroethyl)-1-nitrosourea on a transplanted murine lymphoma. J. Nat. Cancer Inst. **40,** 935—944 (1968).
18. Van Putten, L. M.: Oxygenation and cell kinetics after irradiation in a transplantable osteosarcoma. In: Effects of Radiation on Cellular Proliferation and Differentiation, Proceeding Series of a Symposium held in Monaco, April, 1968. Vienne: International Atomic Energy Agency 1968, pp. 493—505.
19. Wodinsky, I., Swiniarski, J., Kensler, C. J.: Spleen colony studies of leukemia L 1210. I. Growth kinetics of lymphocytic L 1210 cells *in vivo* as determined by spleen colony assay. Cancer Chemother. Rep. **51,** 415—421 (1967).

Radiation Therapy with Curative Intent in the Malignant Lymphomas

HENRY S. KAPLAN

A. Introduction

The fundamental concepts underlying the definitive treatment of Hodgkin's disease and the other malignant lymphomas with radiotherapy are not new; they were defined more than forty years ago by the late Swiss radiotherapist, RENÉ GILBERT [1] and effectively applied by Dr. VERA PETERS [2, 3] and others during the kilovoltage era of radiotherapy. However, the advent of modern megavoltage apparatus has freed the radiotherapist of the severe technical limitations formerly imposed by his equipment and made it possible to implement fully the ideas advocated by GILBERT. These technical advances, coupled with the great improvements in the accuracy of diagnostic evaluation and staging described above by my colleague, Dr. SAUL ROSENBERG [4], have now brought about a veritable revolution in the clinical management and prognosis of these once-dreaded neoplasms [5].

B. Technical Considerations

The principal technical factors which determine the efficacy of radiation therapy for the malignant lymphomas are: the total radiation dose per field; the size, shape, and number of treatment fields; and the beam energy.

1. *Dose.* Any given site of involvement can be permanently eradicated with a high degree of reliability with doses of 3,500 to 4,500 rads delivered in three and a half to five weeks. Apparently complete disappearance of enlarged lymph nodes also occurs after substantially smaller doses, but such responses are likely to be transient, and recurrences are common [6]. Since re-irradiation of recurrences is likely to be poorly tolerated by the normal tissues, it is imperative to use optimal dose levels for all involved sites during the first course of treatment.

2. *Fields.* When multiple chains of lymph nodes must be irradiated, it is highly undesirable to use multiple small treatment fields because of the risk of overlapping of fields resulting in excessive normal tissue doses, or of excessive gaps between fields, leading to underdosage to diseased nodes. It is therefore essential to use a long treatment distance to permit multiple lymph node chains to be encompassed within as few fields as possible. Each large field must be carefully shaped to the contours of

the lymph node chains by the use of lead shields to provide maximal protection to such vital structures as the lungs, heart, liver, kidneys, and spinal cord. A gap is always left between adjacent fields at the skin surface; its width must be carefully calculated to permit perfect abutment of the adjacent fields at the midplane of the body. It is usually possible to encompass all of the relevant lymph nodes in just two sets of matched anterior and posterior opposed fields: the "mantle" field, covering the cervical, supraclavicular, infraclavicular, axillary, hilar and mediastinal nodes down to the level of the diaphragm [7]; and the "inverted Y", covering the splenic pedicle, celiac, paraaortic, iliac, inguinal and femoral nodes [8]. When the lymphoid tissues of Waldeyer's ring are to be treated, as in the non-Hodgkin's lymphomas, and in the presence of high cervical adenopathy in Hodgkin's disease, opposing lateral fields are delineated to include the nasopharynx, base of tongue, posterior pharyngeal wall, and tonsillar region. Extended-field, "total lymphoid" radiotherapy is technically demanding and potentially extremely hazardous, and should not be attempted by radiologists who do not devote their entire time to radiation therapy.

3. *Beam Energy.* The dual requirement for relatively high doses and very large fields dictates the use of megavoltage radiation beams generated by linear accelerators, multikilocurie cobalt-60 teletherapy units, or betatrons. Comparable doses of 200 Kv X-rays would elicit intolerably severe skin reactions over such large fields. Since the first course of radiation therapy offers the best chance for cure, it is of particular importance to use megavoltage beams from the beginning.

C. Acute Morbidity of Radiation Therapy

Dryness and soreness of the throat and dysphagia often occur during treatment of the "mantle" field, and may occasionally be severe enough to warrant brief interruption of treatment or a decrease in the daily dose rate. Nausea, vomiting, and/or diarrhea may occur during treatment of the retroperitoneal and pelvic nodes, but are usually easily controlled with medication. Leukopenia and/or thrombocytopenia typically reach the nadir during treatment of the last field and may then fall low enough to interrupt treatment for a week or two. Temporary alopecia may be expected in the occipital regions on either side of the midline after treatment of the "mantle" field.

D. Late Complications of Radiation Therapy

Hypothyroidism has been documented in about 5 to 10% of our patients, and has responded readily to treatment. Radiation pneumonitis occurs in about 10% of cases within three to six months after treatment to a "mantle" field, but is seldom severe. It is usually manifested by a hacking, nonproductive cough, mild to moderate dyspnea on exertion, and accentuation of radiographic markings in the paramediastinal lung zones corresponding to the treatment field contours. These signs and symptoms persist for a few months and then gradually disappear, leaving little or no residual symptomatic impairment, though careful physiologic measurements continue to disclose evidence of restrictive pulmonary disease.

Radiation pericarditis [9] has occurred in about 7% of our cases after treatment to the "mantle" field, but is usually almost asymptomatic and manifested primarily by the development of cardiomegaly. Other diagnostic procedures then reveal the presence of fluid in the pericardial sac, and a friction rub may be heard. The typical course is benign; prompt and complete resolution occurs with bedrest and the use of mild diuretics in the great majority of cases. However, occasional cases may progress to chronic constrictive pericarditis, necessitating surgical pericardiectomy for relief.

A more common but less serious complication is the Lhermitte syndrome, in which numbness, tingling, or "electric" sensations are experienced in the arms, legs, and/or lower back, and characteristically elicited or aggravated by sharp forward flexion of the head. There is never any associated motor dysfunction. These symptoms disappear gradually over a period of several months. Transverse myelitis is much more serious, but fortunately quite rare; it can usually be traced to technical errors, such as the use of an inadequate gap between the "mantle" and "inverted Y" fields.

Isolated instances of myelogenous leukemia have been reported in patients surviving several years after radiotherapy for Hodgkin's disease [10], but conclusive proof that such leukemias are indeed radiation-induced has not yet been presented. Other major hematologic complications have been surprisingly rare [11].

E. Indications for Selection of Treatment in Previously Untreated Cases

Stages I A and II A: Radiation therapy with curative intent is the treatment of choice. It has not yet been established whether total lymphoid radiotherapy yields significantly better results than local high-dose radiotherapy confined to the site(s) of involvement.

Stages I B, II B, and III A: Total lymphoid radiation therapy with curative intent is the treatment of choice.

Stage III B: Total lymphoid radiotherapy and multiple-drug combination chemotherapy [12] have each yielded results superior to those of single-drug chemotherapy or palliative radiotherapy. Sequential treatment with total lymphoid radiotherapy followed by combination chemotherapy, now under clinical investigation, may well prove to be the treatment of choice [13].

Stages IV A and IV B: Chemotherapy is usually indicated; the highly effective but more hazardous multiple-drug combinations should be reserved for relatively young and otherwise healthy patients. Palliative radiotherapy is indicated whenever symptoms or signs of *local* nature are a prominent clinical feature.

F. Indications for Treatment of Relapse in Previously Treated Patients

When Stage I or II disease previously treated with local radiotherapy later relapses in sites other than those already irradiated, a complete diagnostic study to exclude Stage IV sites of involvement should be performed again. If the extent of the relapsing disease is limited to Stage II or III, radiotherapy to potentially curative dose levels should be given to all previously untreated lymphoid regions. When the site of relapse is in a previously heavily irradiated region, re-irradiation is likely to be so hazardous as to make chemotherapy the treatment of choice; exceptions should be made only after consultation with an experienced radiation therapist. Documented extralymphatic site(s) of relapse, unless strictly localized, constitute an indication for chemotherapy.

G. Prognosis

Intensive, wide-field megavoltage radiotherapy has drastically altered the prognosis of Hodgkin's disease. Carefully staged and optimally treated cases may be expected to exhibit relapse-free survival rates at five years of 85 to 90% in Stages I and II, 70% in Stage III A, 40 to 50% in Stage III B, and an overall five-year survival for all stages of 65 to 70% [11]. Since at least 95% of all primary relapses occur during the first five years, relapse-free survival for this interval or longer may be considered tantamount to cure [14]. Thus, the classical view that the malignant lymphomas are inevitably fatal is no longer tenable; instead, the physician who adopts an aggressive approach to early diagnosis, followed by prompt referral to highly qualified radiotherapists and/or chemotherapists for careful staging and treatment, can expect to be rewarded by the long-term disease-free survival of the majority of his patients.

Summary

With the advent of modern supervoltage radiotherapy apparatus, the treatment of Hodgkin's disease and the other malignant lymphomas with high-dose, large-field radiotherapy has become technically feasible. Concurrently, other advances in histopathological classification, clinical staging, and new techniques of diagnostic evaluation have developed over the years. Each of these areas is explored in this article, which also includes a brief review of possible complications of radiotherapy, follow-up care, and indications of relapse and the need for retreatment. The desirability of early diagnosis and prompt referral of the lymphoma patient to qualified radiotherapists and/or chemotherapists is emphasized, since an overall five-year survival rate of 65 to 70 per cent or more is attainable with optimal care.

References

1. Gilbert, R.: Radiotherapy in Hodgkin's disease (malignant granulomatosis). Amer. J. Roentgenol. **41**, 198 (1939).
2. Peters, M. V.: A study of survivals in Hodgkin's disease treated radiologically. Amer. J. Roentgenol. **63**, 299 (1950).
3. — Middlemiss, K. C. H.: A study of Hodgkin's disease treated by irradiation. Amer. J. Roentgenol. **79**, 114 (1958).
4. Rosenberg, S. A.: The clinical evaluation and staging of patients with malignant lymphoma. This volume, page 32.
5. Kaplan, H. S.: Clinical evaluation and radiotherapeutic management of Hodgkin's disease and the malignant lymphomas. New Engl. J. Med. **278**, 892 (1968).

6. KAPLAN, H. S.: Evidence for a tumoricidal dose level in the radiotherapy of Hodgkin's disease. Cancer Res. **26**, 1221 (1966).
7. PAGE, V., GARDNER, A., KARZMARK, C. J.: Physical and dosimetric aspects of the radiotherapy of malignant lymphomas. I. The mantle technique. Radiology **96**, 609 (1970).
8. — — — II. The inverted Y technique. Radiology **96**, 619 (1970).
9. STEWART, J. R., COHN, K. E., FAJARDO, L. F., HANCOCK, E. W., KAPLAN, H. S.: Radiation-induced heart disease: a study of twenty-five patients. Radiology **89**, 302 (1967).
10. EZDINLI, E. Z., SOKAL, J. E., AUNGST, C. W., KIM, U., SANDBERG, A. A.: Myeloid leukemia in Hodgkin's disease: chromosomal abnormalities. Ann. intern. Med. **71**, 1097 (1969).
11. KAPLAN, H. S.: On the natural history, treatment, and prognosis of Hodgkin's disease. Harvey Lect. **1968—1969** (in press).
12. DEVITA, V. T., SERPICK, A., CARBONE, P. P.: Combination chemotherapy of advanced Hodgkin's disease: the NCl program. Proc. Amer. Ass. Cancer Res. **10**, 19 (1969).
13. BULL, J. M., DEKIEWIET, J. W. C., ROSENBERG, S. A., KAPLAN, H. S.: Cyclic chemotherapy (MOPP) combined with extended-field radiotherapy for Hodgkin's disease. Clin. Res. **18**, 189 (1970) (abst.).
14. KAPLAN, H. S.: Prognostic significance of the relapse-free interval after radiotherapy in Hodgkin's disease. Cancer **22**, 1131 (1968).

Discussion

The Curative Radiotherapy of Lymphomas

Ralph E. Johnson

With 5 Figures

An increasing enthusiasm in the radiotherapy of lymphomas has resulted from recognition that many adequately irradiated patients have subsequently remained free of disease for extended periods of time. Appreciation of this has understandably led to progressively more radical attempts to improve results. But radiotherapeutic efforts have been hampered by the fact that even for patients with apparently localized Hodgkin's disease or malignant lymphoma, the disease process is frequently more disseminated than apparent from diagnostic evaluation. This is evidenced by several reports, including our earlier description [1] of the unreliability of the lymphogram in demonstrating occult involvement of retroperitoneal nodes. The recent experience described by Dr. Rosenberg at Stanford with the biopsy at laparotomy of lymphographically normal-appearing retroperitoneal lymph nodes similarly highlights the propensity for subclinical spread throughout the lymphatic system. This latter is the basis for so-called "prophylactic" irradiation of clinically uninvolved regions. The experience of Peters [2] suggesting the efficacy of prophylactic therapy in early Hodgkin's disease has generated considerable interest and I will briefly summarize our experience in this regard.

Between 1965 and 1969, a prospective trial was performed by the Radiation Branch of the National Cancer Institute. Employing the clinical evaluation outlined in Table 1, a total of 136 patients with previously untreated Hodgkin's disease were classified as Stage I or Stage II (Table 2). Most of these patients were then randomly assigned to either extended field (EF) or total nodal irradiation (TNI) as illustrated in Figure 1. EF therapy consisted of irradiating the involved plus anatomically adjacent lymph nodes. TNI consisted of the prophylactic irradiation of all major lymph nodes areas above and below the diaphragm, including the spleen. The randomization to EF versus TNI therapy was stratified for clinical extent of disease (i. e. Stage I versus Stage II), presence or absence of constitutional symptoms, and histopathological classification.

Several aspects of this clinical trial may be commented upon at this time. The first relates to the accuracy of the clinical staging evaluation in terms of investigating the possible presence of extranodal dissemination [3]. Of the 96 patients with Stage

Table 1. *Pretreatment diagnostic evaluation of Hodgkin's disease*

1. Careful history (with documentation of constitutional symptoms) and physical examination.
2. Complete blood count and bone marrow biopsy.
3. PA and lateral chest radiographs with whole chest tomography in the presence of hilar or mediastinal lymphadenopathy.
4. Metastatic bone survey with a radiostrontium bone scan in the presence of bone pain, elevated serum alkaline phosphatase, or suspicious radiographic findings on the metastatic series.
5. Bipedal lymphography and intravenous pyelography.
6. Liver function studies including BSP clearance and alkaline phosphatase (liver biopsy if tests abnormal).
7. Renal function tests including urinanalysis.
8. Other tests as deemed indicated on individual patients including the selective use of thoracotomy and laparotomy for equivocal clinical findings.

Table 2. *Clinical staging of Hodgkin's disease*

Stage [a]	Clinical extent of involvement
I	Disease limited to a single group of lymph nodes.
II	Disease limited to two or more lymph node areas on the same side of the diaphragm.
III	Disease involving areas on both sides of the diaphragm but confined to lymph and the spleen.

[a] Each clinical stage is subdivided according to the absence (A) or presence (B) of pruritus, night sweats, or otherwise unexplained fever.

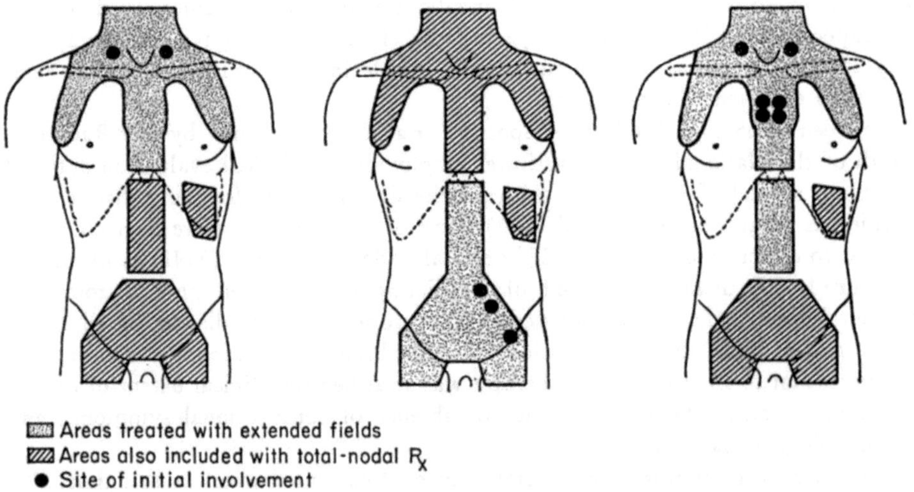

Fig. 1. Examples illustrating the randomization of Stage I—II Hodgkin's disease patients to extended field versus total nodal irradiation

I A—II A Hodgkin's disease, 14 have relapsed to date. Four of these initial 14 relapses have involved extension of disease to extranodal sites (one each in liver, bone, bone marrow, and pericardium). The remaining 10 relapses consisted of extension of disease to anatomically non-adjacent lymph nodes which were untreated in patients receiving EF therapy.

Among the 40 patients with Stage I B—II B disease, there have been 16 relapses to date. Four of these 16 had extranodal involvement detectable at the time of relapse in the absence of simultaneous active disease in previously untreated lymph nodes (two in bone and one each in liver and lung). An additional two patients had demonstrable bone involvement concurrent with relapse of disease in non-irradiated lymph nodes. Thus the diagnostic error in evaluating occult extranodal dissemination has been several fold higher for those patients with (15%) as compared to those without (4%) constitutional symptoms. And the most frequent site of clinically unrecognized occult extranodal involvement has been bone.

This experience relates directly to the potential usefulness of exploratory laparotomy in evaluating the suitability of Hodgkin's disease patients for curative radiotherapy. Since the retroperitoneal lymph nodes and spleen can be prophylactically irradiated not only with minimal difficulty but also with therapeutic effectiveness as will be described, the principal advantage of routine laparotomy pertains to the detection of occult liver involvement not discernible with more conventional techniques. Certainly the diagnostic yield from routine laparotomy for the 96 Stage I A—II A patients would have been negligible since only a single patient has developed extension to the liver. Even for the 40 Stage I B—II B patients, the solitary case of extension to liver at the time of initial relapse indicates the relative accuracy of our diagnostic evaluation in terms of detecting occult liver involvement in patients with clinically early stage Hodgkin's disease. I should comment, however, that we have routinely subjected those selected patients with abnormal liver function tests to surgical biopsy and thereby restaged several patients on the basis of liver biopsy.

The randomized comparison of TNI and EF therapy has demonstrated a measurable decrease in the relapse rate with more comprehensive prophylactic treatment (Fig. 2). As mentioned, this has primarily resulted from a reduced frequency of relapse in lymph node sites anatomically non-adjacent to the area(s) of primary involvement. However, a definite advantage for TNI compared to EF therapy has been observed only for those patients with histology other than nodular sclerosis. Improved disease-free rates have not been obtained with TNI for Stage I—II A patients with nodular sclerosis histology, this group having fared remarkably well with both EF and TNI therapy. A reliable estimate cannot be made for Stage I B to II B patients because of the relatively low frequency of nodular sclerosis histology in patients with this clinical staging.

Sufficient time has now elapsed for the difference in relapse rates between TNI and EF therapy to become reflected in the overall survival rates. As shown in Fig. 3, the 5-year survival rate for combined histology in the Stage I A—II A patients exceeds 95% for the preferred radiotherapy techniques as based on histology. Similarly for the Stage I B—II B group (Fig. 4), the better survival following TNI is a consequence of the lower relapse rate as compared to EF therapy.

During the course of this study, we have also treated a number of patients with Stage III Hodgkin's disease. For patients with clinical evidence of Hodgkin's disease

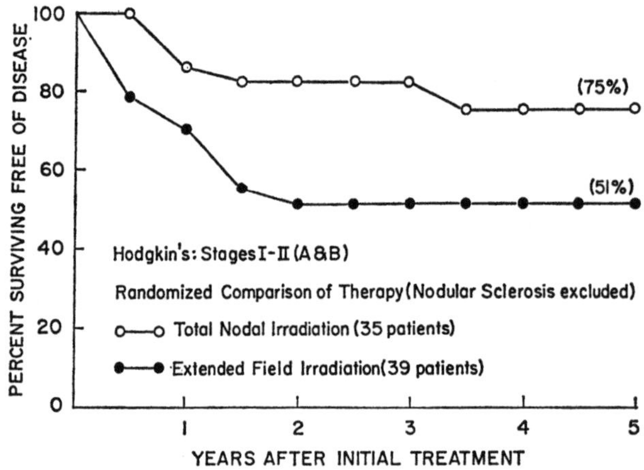

Fig. 2. Comparison of relapse rates for Stage I—II Hodgkin's disease patients randomly assigned to extended field versus total nodal irradiation. No difference in disease free survival has been observed for the two treatment techniques for patients with nodular sclerosis histology and the latter are not included in this analysis (life table method)

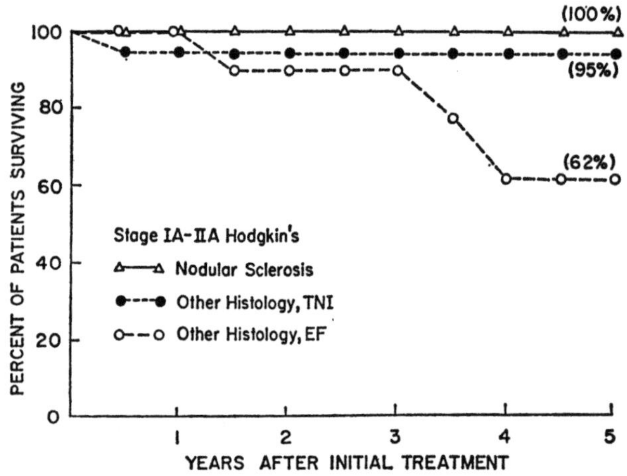

Fig. 3. Survival of Stage IA—IIA Hodgkin's disease patients treated with extended field versus total nodal irradiation by random assignment

both above and below the diaphragm, radiotherapy was at best considered unorthodox treatment if not unjustified by many oncologists a few years ago. Even today, a number of radiologists are scarcely enthusiastic about aggressive radiotherapy of Stage III patients. Our experience has indicated that whereas the results for Stage III B have been less than satisfactory because of the high rate of relapse in extranodal sites, the results for Stage III A have been very encouraging. For the 19 Stage III A patients treated between 1964 and 1969, the 5-year free of disease rate (life table analysis) is 75%, demonstrating that radical radiotherapy should now be viewed as the indicated treatment for this subgroup.

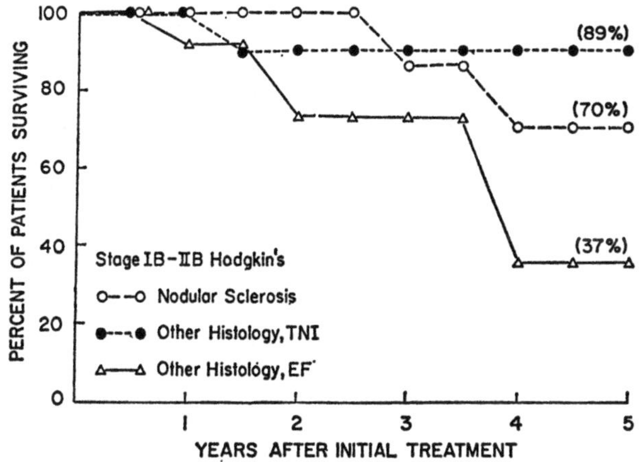

Fig. 4. Survival of Stage IB—IIB Hodgkin's disease patients treated with extended field versus total nodal irradiation by random assignment

With respect to the management of lymphosarcoma, it has likewise been demonstrated that a substantial proportion of patients with clinically localized disease are amenable to cure with radiotherapy. Compared to Hodgkin's disease, however, relatively little attention has been directed toward aggressive radiotherapy for patients with more generalized lymphosarcoma. Currently, patients with generalized lymph node involvement by lymphosarcoma are almost uniformly treated palliatively either with chemotherapy or limited radiotherapy.

Concurrent with the clinical trials on Hodgkin's disease, we began to investigate the treatment approaches summarized in Table 3 for lymphosarcoma patients having generalized lymph node involvement (Stage III). The preliminary results of this investigation [4] are summarized in Fig. 5. Of particular encouragement has been the 40% 5-year survival continuously free of disease for these 16 patients. Although this pilot study involved a limited number of patients, thus not permitting definitive conclusions, the survival has been so remarkably good that a larger scale investigation of these techniques has been undertaken.

In summary, the era of negativism toward patients with Hodgkin's disease and other lymphomas has clearly ended. Investigation of aggressive radiotherapy has demonstrated that considerable optimism is justified and the immediate needs are twofold. The first is for increased dissemination of current information as to the

Table 3. *Treatment techniques for patients with generalized lymph node involvement by lymphosarcoma (stage III)*

Treatment A:	Sequential irradiation of all major lymph node areas (total nodal irradiation) above and below the diaphragm with a tumor dose of 2000 rads delivered in 2—3 weeks.
Treatment B:	Total body irradiation (10 rads thrice weekly to a dose of 100—150 rads) followed by total nodal irradiation as above after a rest interval to permit bone marrow recovery.

results achievable with present therapeutic methods and in this regard, symposia such as this serve an important function. The obvious and immediate byproduct of more adequately informing the general medical community is that referring physicians will inevitably become more critical in terms of demanding appropriate treatment of their patients.

The second need is for the radiotherapy community to gain the necessary experience with newer methods used in the treatment of Hodgkin's disease and the malignant lymphomas. It is unfortunate that the techniques yielding these improved

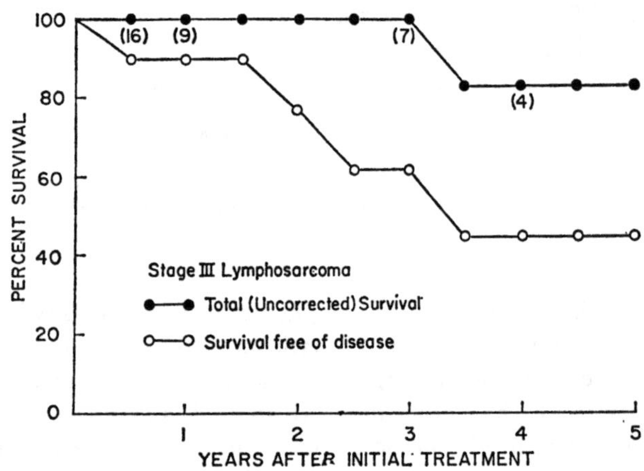

Fig. 5. Overall survival and survival continuously free of disease (life table analysis) for 16 consecutive patients with previously untreated Stage III lymphosarcoma

results are relatively complex and contain multiple opportunities for rather subtle and yet critical errors. To this end, periodic workshops devoted to indepth consideration of the constantly evolving technical aspects of radiotherapy are rather urgently required. For only with such targeted efforts at continuing education can the dramatically improved prognosis for Hodgkin's disease and the malignant lymphomas be translated into a reality for the majority of patients newly diagnosed in the future.

References

1. JOHNSON, R. E., COOK, P. L.: Hodgkin's disease: the negative lymphogram in guiding radiotherapy. Amer. J. Roentgenol. **102**, 883 (1968).
2. PETERS, M. V.: Prophylactic treatment of adjacent areas in Hodgkin's disease. Cancer Res. **26**, 1232 (1966).
3. JOHNSON, R. E., THOMAS, L. B., CHRETIEN, P.: Correlation between clinico-histologic staging and extranodal relapse in Hodgkin's disease. Cancer **25**, 1071 (1970).
4. — O'CONOR, G. T., LEVIN, D.: Primary management of advanced lymphosarcoma with radiotherapy. Cancer **25**, 787 (1970).

Discussion

Reasons for Failure of the Curative Radiotherapeutic Management of Patients with Lymphomas

MELVIN L. GRIEM

With 2 Figures

The reasons for failure in the management of lymphomas by radiotherapy with curative intent might be outlined as follows: (1) The dose of radiation therapy in a given time period is insufficient to produce complete tumor cell depopulation. (2) The radiation therapist does not have sufficient knowledge of the extent of disease to adequately cover all of the disease sites by ionizing radiation. (3) There are possibilities of technical errors with inappropriate beam direction, improper dosimetry or improper treatment planning. (4) The tolerance of the normal tissue to ionizing radiation has been excessive resulting in either severe morbidity or mortality.

Dr. KAPLAN has already pointed out the importance of giving an adequate dose of ionizing radiation in a given time period and that when this dose is given the probability of recurrent disease at the treated site can be reduced to a minimum of well below 5%. Similar data have been presented by a number of other workers including Dr. RALPH SCOTT who worked with the patient material available at the University of Chicago. Since 1937 adequate dosimetry and very careful treatment time was carried out by Dr. ANNA HAMANN. Dr. SCOTT set up very specific criteria for analysis of 75 patients of over 300 who had the diagnosis of Hodgkin's disease in the period 1937 through 1960. He required that there be histological confirmation of disease, that prior to radiation therapy and in subsequent four year periods following radiation therapy, no chemotherapy was administered and that follow-up could be conducted for the period of four years or to death and autopsy to indicate the control of the disease in the treated site. He accumulated the data on over 75 patients and constructed two graphs relating the time of overall treatment in days to the dose of radiation considered the minimum tissue dose delivered to the tumor. Fig. 1 demonstrates this data all of which was done with 250 KV equipment. This figure represents those patients in whom no recurrence was found in the four year period and who were considered successfully treated. The heavy line represents the least squares fit of the data and the fine line represents the 95% confidence limit.

Fig. 2 represents those patients in whom the treatment was considered a failure. A heavy line and the fine lines from the previous graph have been repeated on this graph. Note that no failure is found above the 95% confidence line. If one considers this data and the data presented by Dr. Kaplan and corrections are made for the different quality of radiation used, then the data presented by Dr. Kaplan and this data are consistent. We believe that by delivering 4,000 rads in a time period of four weeks as a minimum tumor dose, the probability of recurrence in the treated area should be well below 5%.

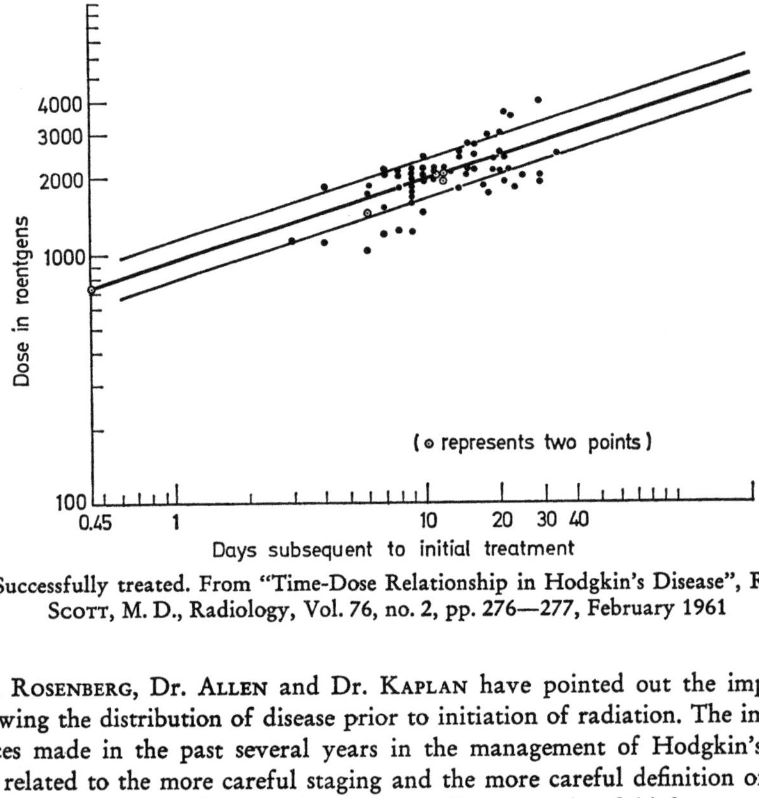

Fig. 1. Successfully treated. From "Time-Dose Relationship in Hodgkin's Disease", Ralph M. Scott, M. D., Radiology, Vol. 76, no. 2, pp. 276—277, February 1961

Dr. Rosenberg, Dr. Allen and Dr. Kaplan have pointed out the importance of knowing the distribution of disease prior to initiation of radiation. The important advances made in the past several years in the management of Hodgkin's disease can be related to the more careful staging and the more careful definition of disease prior to initiation of radiation therapy. A small rectangular field for treatment of lymph node chains is no longer considered the best approach to treatment of this malignancy and the radiation therapist has been challenged to design radiation fields to conform to the extent of known disease and possible extensions of that disease. In the more advanced stages of Hodgkin's disease, there is no question that the radical radiation therapy including the majority of the lymph node groups in the body has yielded excellent results.

Dr. Kaplan has pointed out the need for careful treatment planning. There should be no reason for a geographic misalignment of the treatment fields in relation to the patient and the tumor. Techniques are currently available with simulators of radiation therapy equipment to properly align the treatment fields to the patient. Likewise, the radiological physicist is well equipped to provide the radiation therapist with accurate knowledge concerning the dose a particular area of the body is receiving. There is no reason for a geographic miss nor is there any reason for improper dosimetry. Recently, we have added one additional feature to the treatment, that is, the use of a confirmatory film which is placed under the patient each time to indicate where the treatment was given and monitor the accuracy of the daily therapy set up. This film recently was developed by two manufacturers, Eastman Kodak and Dupont. It responds to an exposure of between 150 and 300 rads and indicates the fields in relation to the patient for each treatment. Small deviations from the ideal are immediately corrected by this monitoring method.

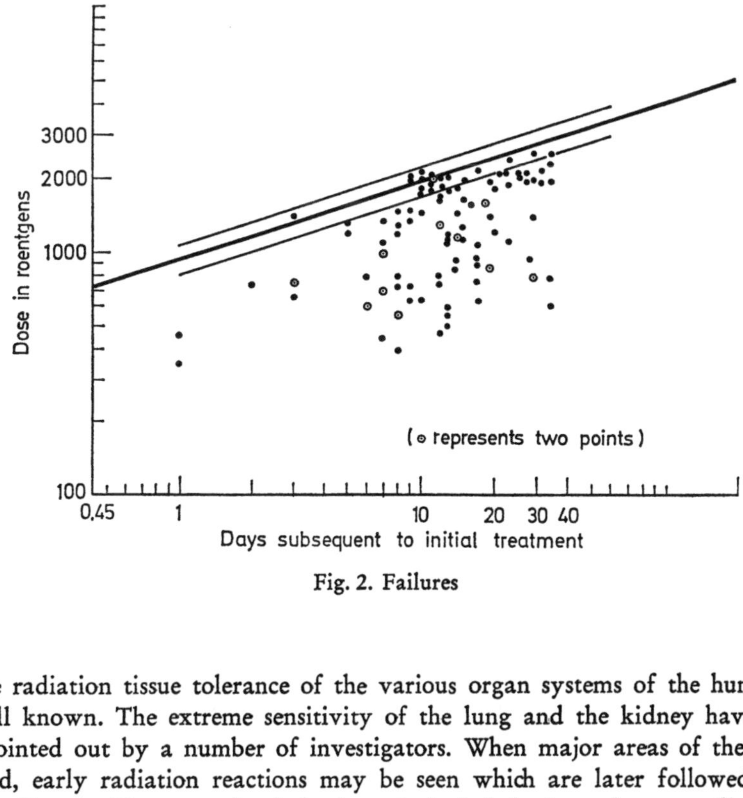

Fig. 2. Failures

The radiation tissue tolerance of the various organ systems of the human body are well known. The extreme sensitivity of the lung and the kidney have already been pointed out by a number of investigators. When major areas of the lung are included, early radiation reactions may be seen which are later followed by pulmonary fibrosis. If too much of the lung is included, the pulmonary fibrosis may be sufficient to result in pulmonary insufficiency with associated morbidity and mortality. The kidney is extremely sensitive to radiation and should be avoided or the dose should be reduced when one considers major areas of kidney mass. Radiation nephritis is a well known entity which results in anemia, kidney failure, malignant hypertension and death in severe cases. Dr. Kaplan has pointed out the sensitivity of the heart and liver to radiation and has documented the complications of intensive radiation to the heart and liver. Although these two organs are less sensitive than the lung and kidney, complications from radiation of the heart and liver can be decreased or avoided by proper treatment planning. Radiation injury of the spinal cord is also a problem. Here again proper treatment planning generally can avoid major complications from radiation myelitis and now only occasional problems are seen which suggest irreversible injury of the spinal cord. The bowel is also a sensitive organ, but does not present the problems that have been mentioned. The bone marrow may also be depressed by radiation therapy, however by proper treatment planning and spacing of treatment, bone marrow depression can be minimized and radiation therapy with curative intent can usually be accomplished.

Failure of radiation therapy to cure lymphomas represents the modern challenge to the well trained physician who specializes in radiation therapy. However, radiation therapy with curative intent should be possible in a very high percentage of patients by minimizing these reasons for failure.

Extracorporeal Irradiation of Blood in the Treatment of Chronic Lymphocytic Leukemia[1]

EUGENE P. CRONKITE

With 4 Figures

The technique of extracorporeal irradiation of the blood (ECIB) was devised in 1921 by HEYMANS [1]. The history of the development of the procedure has been reviewed elsewhere [2].

My interest in further development of this technique arose from the fact that the lymphocytes are radiosensitive and that if it were possible to kill these in an extracorporeal shunt by irradiation, one should be able to deplete the body of lymphocytes and thus be able to study the feedback loops that control restoration of the lymphocyte mass to normal. The technique would be analogous to bleeding to study erythropoiesis. In a series of publications we perfected the technique [3—7]. The original studies were performed in a cumbersome manner utilizing an x-ray machine necessitating about 30 meters of Tygon tubing as an extracorporeal shunt. A more compact gamma irradiator was developed in order to bring the animals closer to the source and minimize the volume of blood in the extracorporeal shunt [8].

The technique has become exceptionally useful in studying lymphopoiesis and various aspects of allografting and humoral immunity [9—11]. Pre- and post-skin grafting treatment with ECIB prolongs the acceptance of unrelated skin grafts [9, 10]. ECIB prior to primary immunization with tetanus toxoid substantially reduces the primary response [11]. There is no effect upon secondary responses. From application of extracorporeal irradiation of the lymph (ECIL) it has been established that there is an obligatory anatomic pathway for transport of antigenic information from the graft through afferent lymphatics into the regional lymph nodes. After the well known transformation and proliferation of lymphocytes which takes about 5 days, activated lymphocytes, committed to attack the allograft are released through the efferent lymphatics exclusively, enter the blood, transporting cell bound antibody, proceed to the graft and affect its rejection [12].

In Fig. 1 the relationships of the blood to organs in which lymphocytes are being produced or stored is shown. The lymphocyte is truly ubiquitous. From the work of HARRIS and KUGLER [13] and OSMOND and EVERETT [14], lymphocytes are

[1] Research supported by the U. S. Atomic Energy Commission.

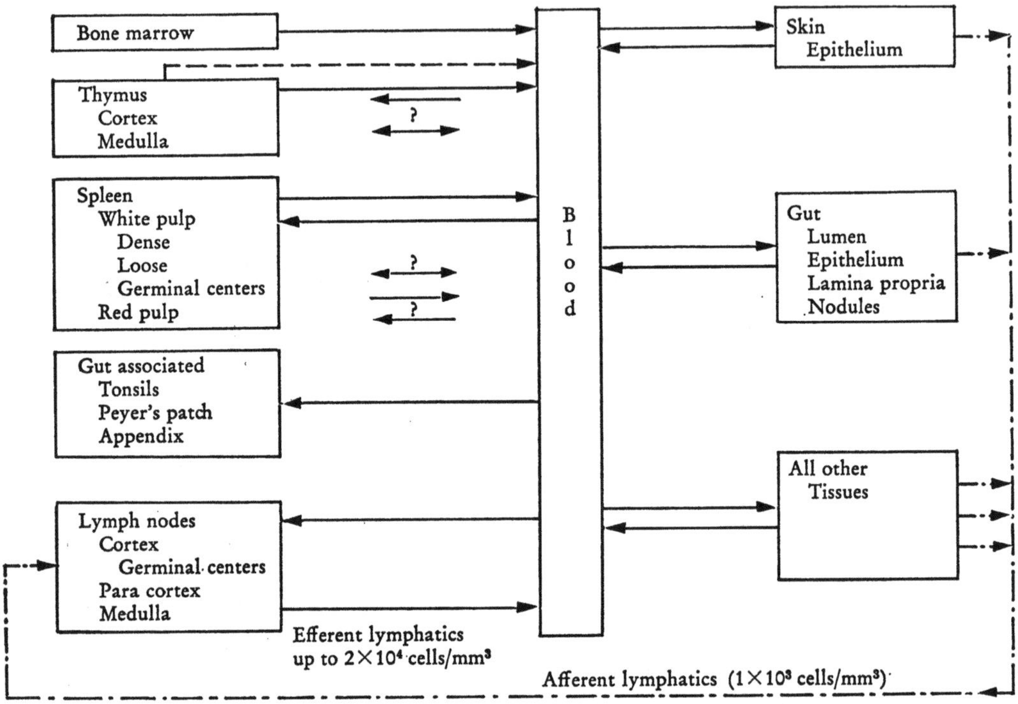

Fig. 1. Schematic compartmentation of relationships of the blood lymphocytes to lymphoreticular tissues

clearly produced in the bone marrow and seem to be contributed to the blood. The reverse exchange of lymphocytes migrating to the bone marrow is less impressive [13—15]. In a large series of studies by several investigators the migration of lymphocytes out of the thymus into the blood via the vein and thymic lymphatics is well established [16—19]. From the studies of Goldschneider and McGregor [19] and Ford [20], the recycling of lymphocytes through specific anatomical areas of the white pulp of the spleen has been clearly shown. From the work of Gowans and Knight [21], the apparent one-way migration of lymphocytes from blood to the gut-associated lymphoid tissues is established along with the migration of cells into the lumen [22]. A single prolonged 48-hour continuous extracorporeal irradiation of the blood has shown that one can deplete predominantly the paracortical region of the lymph nodes, the cuff of small lymphocytes surrounding germinal centers in the spleen and the dense and loose white pulp surrounding the malpighian bodies. There is no influence upon the germinal centers [6, 23]. From the preceeding and other studies [2, 24] it has been shown that there is an easily mobilizable pool of lymphocytes that predominantly involves the so-called thymic dependent areas [25] of the lymph nodes and spleen and a relatively tightly fixed pool of lymphocytes that apparently is largely located in the outer cortex of the lymph node and the medullary regions [23]. The size of these pools has been estimated [2, 24].

After it was clearly established in model systems that one could significantly deplete tissues and that there was relatively little harm from extracorporeal irradiation

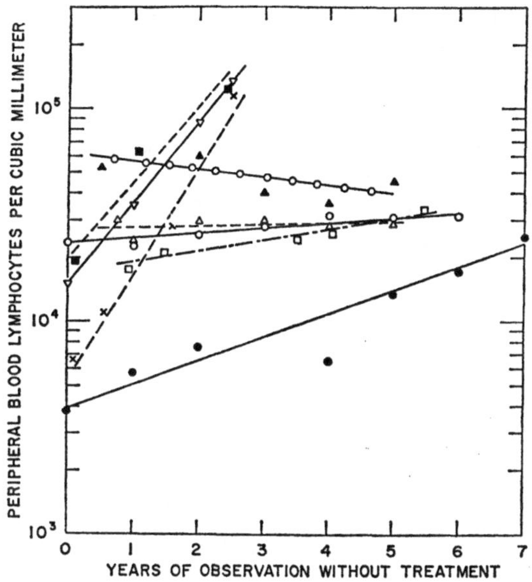

Fig. 2. Examples of the great variation in rate of increase of blood counts in untreated chronic lymphocytic leukemia

of the blood, we commenced studies on bovine chronic lymphocytic leukemia [9]. It was possible to decrease the concentration of leukemic cells in peripheral blood and there was an apparent improvement in the welfare of the animals since they commenced eating again and some gained weight.

Thereafter we and others commenced the study and treatment of various types of human leukemia [26—30]. Since it was shown in the calf that prolonged ECIB would produce striking hemolysis [31] studies were undertaken on the radiosensitivity of the human red cell [32]. It was established that doses of radiation *in vitro* to the normal human red cell up to 35,000 rads did not substantially decrease its life span. A computer program was also worked out for given flow rates, transit dose, blood volume and shunt volumes to estimate how long it would take during treatment for a substantial fraction of the patient's red cells to accumulate 35,000 rads [32]. In the course of treating acute myeloblastic leukemia, chronic granulocytic leukemia and chronic lymphocytic leukemia, even though hemorrhagic manifestations and changes in the platelet count were not observed, ascribable to ECIB, we studied the radiation sensitivity of human platelets [33] with doses *in vitro* up to 75,000 r chromium-labeled autotransfused platelets did not have a reduced survival time. In 5 individuals undergoing treatment for chronic lymphocytic leukemia the chromium labeled survival time was determined prior to the commencement of ECIB and during ECIB. There was no difference in the apparent survival time.

We have studied intensively various aspects of chronic lymphocytic leukemia. As pointed out by Dameshek [34], chronic lymphocytic leukemia has a highly variable course. In our studies [30] shown in Fig. 2, the highly variable change in lymphocyte count is shown in a series of 8 patients studied without treatment over a period of 7 years. One patient is now in her 10th year with a slowly, continually, exponentially rising lymphocyte count with bone marrow invasion but no detectable lymphadenopathy and normal size spleen.

Utilizing labeling of leukemic cells *in vitro* with ^{3}H cytidine followed by autotransfusion, we have attempted to determine the behavior and the pool size of leukemic cells into which labeled cells would be diluted [35, 36]. The readily accessible compartment of leukemic lymphocytes in which the autotransfused tritiated cytidine labeled cells has varied from 0.33 to 4.6×10^{11} cells per patient. A typical example of the response to extracorporeal irradiation of the blood is shown in Fig. 3.

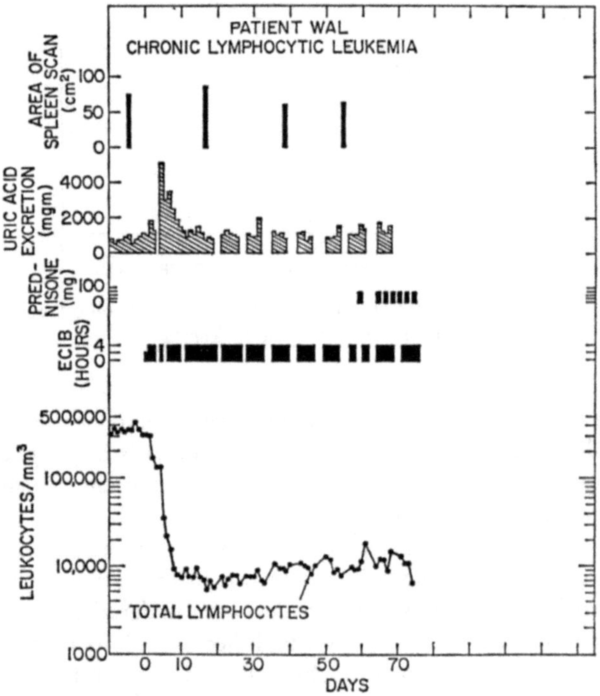

Fig. 3. An example of the effect of ECIB on the blood count, uric acid excretion and splenic size

This patient had very extensive lymphadenopathy and marked splenomegaly with an infiltrated marrow. Note the striking exponential decrease in the concentration of cells in the peripheral blood followed by a plateau despite the continued ECIB. Also note the marked increase in uric acid excretion and the initial increase in the splenic size followed by diminution. There was also a modest decrease in the size of some lymph nodes. In Fig. 4 is shown the variability in the exponential decrease of the lymphocyte count of the blood during ECIB. In other studies [37] the relation of the rate of decrease in cells in the peripheral blood to the apparent turnover rate of RNA in the autotransfused cells was studied. There appeared to be a correlation insomuch as the cells with the longer apparent turnover time of RNA were in individuals in whom there was a very striking rapid decrease in the concentration of lymphocytes during ECIB.

The relapse following cessation of treatment has also been highly variable. Some patients increased exponentially with doubling time of a few days and others remained stable for months followed by an exponential rise of varying slopes.

In conclusion we feel that ECIB has been beneficial in some individuals who had become refractory to chemotherapy. A similar view is shared by STORB et al. [27]. Several individuals have been treated who have never received previous chemotherapy. The response has been highly variable and in some individuals very encouraging and others very discouraging. It is possible that an effective management of some cases of chronic lymphocytic leukemia would involve intermittent ECIB,

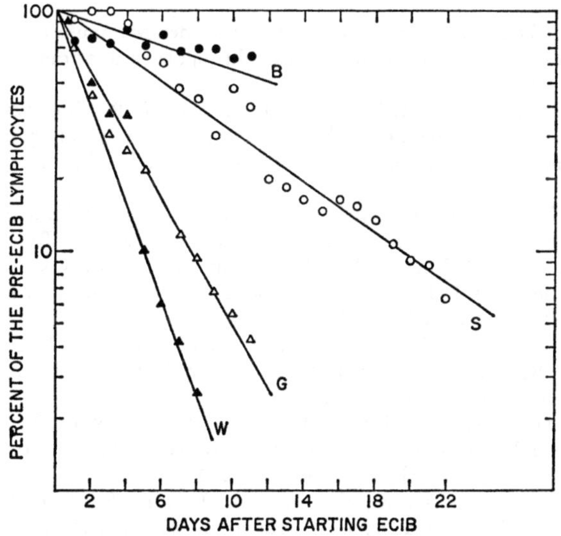

Fig. 4. Examples of the wide range in response to ECIB showing the exponential decrease in lymphocyte counts with different slopes

perhaps at intervals of several months in an endeavor to keep the blood and the readily accessible pool of lymphocytes cleaned out and hopefully avoid organomegaly and other complications of an expanding mass due to accumulation of immunologically incompetent cells [34]. The hypothesis assumes that normal lymphocytes will maintain themselves if not squeezed out by the accumulation of the incompetent cells.

Summary

ECIB produces a lymphopenia and depletion of those portions of the lymphopoietic system termed "thymic dependent" and to a lesser extent the outer cortex and medulla of lymph nodes and the red pulp of the spleen. The preceding was predictable on the basis of what was known about the traffic pattern of lymphocytes through the blood, lymphoid organs and lymphatics. If chronic lymphocytic leukemia (CLL) lymphocytes have similar pathways, a depletion should also be produced by ECIB and might have some therapeutic value. Several patients with CLL have been treated. The lymphocyte count has been decreased to varying degrees in all patients. The diminution in spleen size and lymph nodes has been variable. Patients relapse at widely different rates with blood lymphocyte doubling times of a few days to a stable low count for many months followed by exponential increases with varying slopes. In common with others, we feel that ECIB has a place in treating CLL refractory to chemotherapy and it may be useful in initial therapy of CLL since it has no widespread known harmful effects as is the case with alkylating agents.

References

1. Heymans, J. F.: Iso, Hyper et Hypo-thermisation des Mammifères par calorification et frigorification du sang de la circulation carotid-jugulaire anastomosée. Arch. int. Pharmacodyn. **25**, 1 (1921).
2. Cronkite, E. P., Chanana, A. D., Joel, D. D., Rai, K. R., Schiffer, L. M.: Influence of extracorporeal irradiation of the blood and lymph on lymphopoiesis and immunity. IAEA Symposium on the Effect of Radiation on Cellular Proliferation and Differentiation, Monaco, April 1—5, 1968.
3. — Jansen, C. R., Mather, G., Adamik, E., Sipe, C. R.: The induction of a prolonged lymphopenia by extracorporeal irradiation of the blood. Radiat. Res. **16**, 586 (1961).
4. — — Mather, G. C., Nielsen, N. O., Usenik, E. O., Adamik, E. A., Sipe, C. R.: Studies on lymphocytes I. Lymphopenia produced by prolonged extracorporeal irradiation of the blood. Blood **20**, 203 (1962).
5. Jansen, C. R., Cronkite, E. P., Mather, G. C., Nielsen, N. O., Rai, K. R., Adamik, E. A., Sipe, C. R..: Studies on lymphocytes II. Production of lymphocytosis by intravenous heparin in calves. Blood **20**, 443 (1962).
6. Cottier, H., Cronkite, E. P., Jansen, C. R., Rai, K. R., Singer, S., Sipe, C. R.: Studies on lymphocytes III. Effects of extracorporeal irradiation of the circulating blood upon the lymphoreticular organs in the calf. Blood **24**, 241 (1964).
7. Cronkite, E. P., Jansen, C. R., Cottier, H., Rai, K. R., Sipe, C. R.: Lymphocyte production measured by extracorporeal irradiation, cannulation and labeling techniques. Ann. N. Y. Acad. Sci. **113**, 566 (1964).
8. Kuhl, O. A., Ripperger, W., Huszagh, D. W., Cronkite, E. P.: Cobalt-60 irradiator for extracorporeal blood irradiation. Nucleonics **22**, 79 (1964).
9. Cronkite, E. P., Chanana, A. D., Schnappauf, Hp.: Extracorporeal irradiation of blood and lymph in animals: Its effect on homografts and on lymphoma. New Engl. J. Med. **272**, 456 (1965).
10. Chanana, A. D., Brecher, G., Cronkite, E. P., Joel, D. D., Schnappauf, Hp.: The influence of extracorporeal irradiation of the blood and lymph on skin homograft rejection. Radiat. Res. **27**, 330 (1966).
11. Stoner, R. D., Cottier, H., Sipe, C. R., Chanana, A. D., Joel, D. D., Cronkite, E. P.: The effects of ECIB and ECIL on tetanus antitoxin responses in calves. Radiat. Res. **37**, 539 (1969).
12. Chanana, A. D.: Studies on lymphocytes XII. The role of immunologically committed lymphocytes in rejecting skin grafts. Transplantation **7**, 459 (1969).
13. Harris, P. F., Kugler, J. H.: An investigation of lymphocyte production in guinea pig bone marrow. Acta haemat. **33**, 351—369 (1965).
14. Osmond, D. G., Everett, N. B.: Radioautographic studies of bone marrow lymphocytes *in vivo* and in diffusion chamber cultures. Blood **23**, 1—17 (1964).
15. Keiser, G., Cottier, H., Odartchenko, N., Bond, V. P.: Autoradiographic study on the origin and fate of small lymphoid cells in the dog bone marrow: Effect of femoral artery clamping during *in vivo* availability of H^3-thymidine. Blood **24**, 254 (1964).
16. Metcalf, D.: The nature and regulation of lymphopoiesis in the normal and neoplastic thymus. In: The Thymus. Ed.: G. E. W. Wolstenholme and Ruth Porter. Boston: Little, Brown and Company 1966, p. 242.

17. Iorio, R. J., Chanana, A. D., Cronkite, E. P., Joel, D. D.: Studies on lymphocytes XVI: Distribution of bovine thymic lymphocytes in the spleen and lymph nodes. Cell and Tissue Kinetics **3** (2), 161—173 (1970).
18. Murray, R., Woods, P.: Studies on the fate of lymphocytes. III. The migration and metamorphosis of *in situ* labeled thymic lymphocytes. Anat. Rec. **150**, 113 (1964).
19. Goldschneider, I., McGregor, D. D.: Migration of lymphocytes and thymocytes in the rat. I. The route of migration from blood to spleen and lymph nodes. J. exp. Med. **127**, 155 (1968).
20. Ford, W. L.: The kinetics of lymphocytes recirculation within the rat spleen. Cell and Tissue Kinetics **2**, 171 (1969).
21. Gowans, J. L., Knight, E. J.: The route of recirculation of lymphocytes in the rat. Proc. roy. Soc. B **159**, 257—282 (1964).
22. Kotani, M., Yamashita, A., Rai, F., Seiki, K., Horii, I.: Reutilization of DNA breakdown products from lymphocytes in lumen of intestine. Blood **29**, 616 (1967).
23. Ruchti, C., Cottier, H., Cronkite, E. P., Jansen, C. R., Rai, K. R.: Studies on lymphocytes. XVII. Differential lymphocyte depletion in lymphoreticular organs of the calf during continuous extracorporeal x-irradiation of the circulating blood. Cell and Tissue Kinetics, in press (1970).
24. Schnappauf, Hp., Schnappauf, U.: Drainage des Ductus thoracicus und Größe der „leicht mobilisierbaren" Lymphocyten bei Kälbern, Schafen und Hunden. Blut **XVI**, 209—220 (1968).
25. Parrott, D. M. V., De Sousa, M. A. B., East, J.: Thymus dependent areas in the lymphoid organs of neonatally thymectomized mice. J. exp. Med. **123**, 191 (1966 a).
26. Thomas, E. D., Epstein, R. P., Eschbach, J. W., Jr., Frager, D., Buckner, C. D., Marsaglia, G.: Treatment of leukemia by extracorporeal irradiation. New Engl. J. Med. **273**, 6 (1965).
27. Storb, R., Epstein, R. B., Buckner, C. D., Thomas, E. D.: Treatment of chronic lymphocytic leukemia by extracorporeal irradiation. Blood **31**, 490 (1968).
28. Schiffer, L. M., Atkins, H. L., Chanana, A. D., Cronkite, E. P., Greenberg, M. L., Stryckmans, P. A.: Extracorporeal irradiation of blood (ECIB) in man. II. Treatment of acute myelocytic leukemia. Blood **1**, 17 (1968).
29. Schiffer, L. M., Chanana, A. D., Cronkite, E. P., Greenberg, M. L., Joel, D. D., Schnappauf, Hp., Stryckmans, P. A.: Extracorporal irradiation of the blood. Seminars in Hematology **3**, 154 (1966).
30. Schiffer, L. M.: Kinetics of chronic lymphocytic leukemia. Ser. Haemat. **1**, 3 (1968).
31. Schnappauf, Hp., Joel, D. D., Chanana, A. D., DiGiacomo, R., Cronkite, E. P.: The influence of *in vitro* irradiation of blood on red cell survival after auto and homo transfusion of cells labeled with Iron-59 or Chromium-51. Radiat. Res. **25**, 646 (1965).
32. Schiffer, L. M., Atkins, H. L., Chanana, A. D., Cronkite, E. P., Greenberg, M. L., Johnson, H. A., Robertson, J. S., Stryckmans, P. A.: Extracorporeal irradiation of the blood in humans: Effects upon erythrocyte survival. Blood **27**, 831 (1966).
33. Greenberg, M. L., Chanana, A. D., Cronkite, E. P., Schiffer, L. M., Stryckmans, P. A.: Extracorporeal irradiation of blood in man: Radiation resistance of circulating platelets. Radiat. Res. **35**, 147—154 (1968).
34. Dameshek, W.: Chronic lymphocytic leukemia — accumulative disease of immunologically incompetent lymphocytes. Blood **29**, 566 (1967).
35. Fliedner, T. M.: Experimental studies on PHA-stimulated lymphocytes and autotransfusion of ^{3}H-cytidine labelled lymphocytes in chronic lymphocytic leukaemia. Reprint from: The Lymphocyte in Immunology and Haemopoiesis, Symposium held in Bristol, Edward Arnold (Publ.) Ltd., April, 1966.
36. Stryckmans, P. A., Chanana, A. D., Cronkite, E. P., Greenberg, M. L., Schiffer, L. M.: Studies on lymphocytes. IX. The survival of autotransfused labeled lymphocytes in chronic lymphocytic leukemia. Europ. J. Cancer **4**, 241—246 (1968).
37. — — — — — Studies on lymphocytes. X. Influence of extracorporeal irradiation of the blood on lymphocytes in chronic lymphocytic leukemia: apparent correlation with RNA turnover. Radiat. Res. **37**, 118 (1969).

Some Biochemical and Pharmacologic Considerations of Agents in the Management of Acute Leukemia[1]

ALAN C. SARTORELLI

With 1 Figure

The successful induction by chemotherapeutic agents of complete remission of disease in the therapy of acute leukemia necessarily requires a selective toxic action by the antileukemic agent(s) employed on neoplastic cells as compared to the most sensitive of the tissues of the host. That preferential kill of malignant cells by drugs can be attained has been amply demonstrated in both experimental systems [1] and in patients with a variety of neoplastic diseases [2—4].

Some Factors Contributing to Selective Toxicity

The selective toxicity of certain carcinolytic agents to leukemic cells appears to derive from at least two factors. The first is that a larger portion of the leukemic cell population as compared to normal cell types of the host is in the proliferative state and that individuals in the S-phase of the cell cycle are those most sensitive to the chemotherapeutic agents that are currently available for the treatment of the leukemias. The second factor in the successful achievement of preferential kill of leukemic cells is the presence of biochemical differences between tumor cells and normal tissues of the host that are of sufficient magnitude to allow chemical exploitation. At present, the most significant example of such a metabolic difference that has resulted in therapeutic advantage is provided by the extreme sensitivity of acute lymphoblastic leukemia to L-asparaginase [5, 6], the differential sensitivity being due to a limited capacity of leukemic cells to fabricate sufficient L-asparagine thereby being dependent upon an external supply of this amino acid. Normal tissues presumably possess levels of asparagine synthetase sufficient to provide enough asparagine to meet the metabolic demands of growth and function in these tissues, and are therefore relatively insensitive to the influence of L-asparaginase [7—10]. Other biochemical differences between malignant cells and those of the host appear

[1] Support was provided by Grant CA-02817 from the National Cancer Institute, USPHS and Grant T-23 from the American Cancer Society.

to exist; conceivably therapeutic advantage of these quantitative differences could be attained in man. For example, SILBER et al. [11] reported that leukemic cells of man incorporate methionine into RNA at a rate that greatly exceeded that of normal leukocytes; the increased incorporation presumably is indicative of enhanced methylation of various species of RNA of neoplastic cells. The findings imply that methylation of RNA is inherently important to the proliferation and survival of leukemic cells and encourages the search for agents that interfere with these metabolic events.

MOORE and LEPAGE [12] have shown that the glutamine antimetabolites azaserine (O-diazoacetyl-L-serine) and diazonorleucine (6-diazo-5-oxo-L-norleucine), agents that cause potent blockade of purine nucleotide biosynthesis *de novo*, are selectively toxic to transplanted neoplastic cells. The concentration of each of these agents required to cause at least 90% inhibition of the formation of purine nucleotides in mouse spleen, the most sensitive of the normal tissues examined, was approximately 2.5-fold greater than was needed to accomplish a comparable degree of blockade of this pathway in the Ehrlich carcinoma. Although the precise biochemical basis for this selective toxicity is unknown, it appears reasonable to relate the phenomenon to the findings that the levels of glutamine are lower than normal in animal tumors [13, 14] and in the plasma of tumor-bearing animals [14]. A competitive relationship exists between azaserine or diazonorleucine and glutamine at the level of phosphoribosylformylglycineamidine synthetase, the target enzyme of the purine nucleotide biosynthetic pathway for these inhibitors; however, in the absence of substrate (glutamine) the enzyme is covalently bound by the antimetabolites resulting in long-lived blockade of the formation of purine nucleotides [15]. The report that plasma glutamine levels were generally lower than normal in patients with acute myeloblastic and lymphoblastic leukemias, as well as in patients with other neoplasms [16], implies that the low availability of glutamine will render phosphoribosylformylglycineamidine synthetase vulnerable to azaserine and diazonorleucine and encourages a further evaluation of the utility of these agents in malignant disease, particularly in combination with preformed purine analogs with which they synergize [17, 18].

An understanding of the metabolic basis for the sensitivity and resistance of normal tissues to antileukemic agents is important to the proper scheduling of dosage, and may result in means to overcome certain types of toxicity. One of the best understood actions at the molecular level is that of the guanine analog, 6-thioguanine, a compound well tolerated by the gastrointestinal tract, but extremely toxic to bone marrow. 6-Thioguanine is deaminated to an inactive form by guanine deaminase; the absence of this enzyme would be expected to result in toxicity to both tumor and normal cells which are unable to catabolize this agent. Essential to sensitivity, however, is the necessity for conversion of this purine analog to the nucleotide form. The importance of these factors for tissue sensitivity to 6-thioguanine was shown in experiments by MARCHESI and SARTORELLI [19]; these studies demonstrated that while rabbit bone marrow was essentially void of guanine deaminase activity, it was very efficient at converting 6-thioguanine to its active inhibitory nucleotide form. In contrast, the intestinal mucosa possessed an active guanine deaminase, thereby catabolizing a large fraction of the 6-thioguanine to which this tissue became exposed. Additionally contributing to the relative lack of toxicity of 6-thioguanine to intestinal mucosa was the presence of a nucleotide-forming system less active than that of the bone marrow. Although bone marrow tissue is quite sensitive to 6-thioguanine the relatively non-toxic effects of this compound on the intestinal mucosa suggests that it should be strongly considered as a replacement for 6-mercaptopurine in the treatment of acute leukemia.

Pharmacologic Factors

It is important to recognize that the relationship between dose and response is described by an extremely steep line, both for host toxicity and tumor susceptibility, and that the therapeutic indices of most known antileukemic agents are extremely

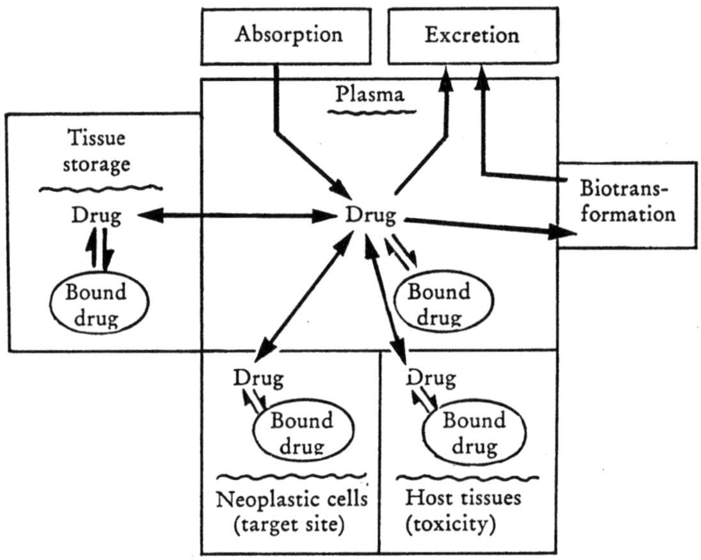

Fig. 1

low. Thus, for optimum therapeutic efficacy it is essential that (a) the quantity of chemotherapeutic agent to which a leukemic patient is exposed be sufficient to attain a critical concentration of the active form of the drug at the target site within the leukemic cells, and (b) that the affected metabolic process essential to cell survival be maintained for a period sufficient to result in the death of the malignant cells. Additional drug serves only to produce toxicity to the host. Because of the extremely low therapeutic differential between normal and leukemic cells, it would seem imperative to tailor the dose and frequency of administration of a carcinostatic agent(s) to accomplish the maintenance of critical drug-induced metabolic alterations within neoplastic cells. The accomplishment of such an approach depends upon a knowledge of the active form of the drug and the biochemical lesions associated with its mechanism of action. These parameters are strongly influenced by a number of pharmacological factors, summarized in Fig. 1; they include the route of drug administration, the extent and rate of absorption through a number of membranes, the degree of structural modification by the processes of biotransformation, the route and rate of excretion, and the tissue and cellular localization and degree of binding of the agent.

The importance of the route of administration was demonstrated by HENDERSON [20] in an experimental tumor system using 6-mercaptopurine. The concentration of this agent required for 50% inhibition of tumor growth varied greatly with the site or form of the neoplasm and with the route of drug administration. The variation was due in part to the quantity of 6-mercaptopurine to which the neoplastic cells were directly exposed, as well as the amount of the active nucleotide form of this agent that was synthesized by the malignant cells; therefore, regardless of the route of drug administration the maximum concentration of 6-mercaptopurine ribonucleotide present in neoplastic cells at the concentration required for 50% inhibition of growth was the same. Of importance was the finding that the maximum intracellular concentration of the active nucleotide form of the drug at the 50% growth-inhibitory concentration differed for tumors growing at different sites within the host, indicating that the sensitivity of biochemical events that governs the degree of responsiveness of tumors to chemotherapeutic agents is dependent upon the environment of the neoplastic cells. Thus, it is conceivable, for example, that leukemic cells present in the central nervous system may have a different sensitivity than their counterparts in other body compartments.

Following absorption, a chemotherapeutic agent may be either distributed uniformly throughout body water or it may preferentially orient itself in certain tissues of the host. In the plasma compartment the drug may exist in a free state or be bound to plasma proteins. Methotrexate provides an example of a compound that is bound to plasma proteins with about 50% of the drug present in the plasma, and approximately 90% of the related antifolate dichloromethotrexate, being bound to albumin [21, 22]; such binding in theory limits the effective blood concentration of these drugs. Commonly used weak organic acids such as salicylates displace methotrexate from its plasma albumin binding sites, a factor conceivably of importance to the attainment of a proper therapeutic blood level of this agent in patients receiving certain additional drugs.

Tissue storage is a factor that has received little attention in the selection of optimum conditions for utilization of antineoplastic agents. One of the classic examples of this phenomenon in pharmacology is the attainment of relatively high concentrations of ultrashort acting barbiturates such as hexobarbital and thiopental in depot fat. Such orientation of the therapeutic agent can result both in undesired termination of the action of a drug by decreasing its concentration in the plasma, as well as prolonging its toxic actions by relatively slow release from this tissue storage site.

Biotransformation may serve to either inactivate or activate an antileukemic agent with respect to both toxicity and antitumor activity. The role of drug metabolism in the action of the folic acid antagonists was investigated by OLIVERIO and LOO [23], who demonstrated that dichloromethotrexate undergoes oxidative change both in man and in experimental animals; the oxidation product was identified as 7-hydroxydichloromethotrexate [24]. The metabolic conversion of dichloromethotrexate to the 7-hydroxy derivative results in a compound that is only $^{1}/_{1000}$ as effective as the parent agent as an inhibitor of the "target enzyme" dihydrofolate reductase [25]. The enzyme responsible for the oxidative modification of dichloromethotrexate has been shown to be aldehyde oxidase [26]; the major site of detoxification is the liver, with enzyme also present in kidney and gastrointestinal mucosa [27]. Most mammalian species oxidize dichloromethotrexate to the 7-hydroxy derivative; however, the hydroxylation of methotrexate is considerably more species specific. Thus, the rabbit and guinea pig are considerably more resistant to the toxic effects of methotrexate than are either man or the rat or mouse [28]. The enzymatic basis for this difference is that the liver aldehyde oxidase of guinea pig and rabbit hydroxylates and inactivates the folate analogs at a rapid rate; whereas, in that of the mouse and rat as well as in that of man little metabolism of these drugs occurs [28, 29]. The consequences of the extensive biotransformation of dichloromethotrexate to the maintenance of effective plasma levels can be demonstrated using mice as the experimental model (BERTINO, J. R., SARTORELLI, A. C., IANNOTTI, A. T., BOOTH, B. A., and JOHNS, D. G.: Unpublished observations). When plasma levels of dichloromethotrexate and methotrexate are measured at various times after the intravenous administration of either agent, a considerably more rapid rate of loss of dichloromethotrexate occurs, presumably reflecting the greater susceptibility of this agent to the catabolic effects of the enzyme aldehyde oxidase. If a similar situation were to obtain in man, dichloromethotrexate would possess distinct advantage over methotrexate for the treatment of meningeal leukemia by intrathecal administration. High doses of dichloromethotrexate could be employed, since drug leaving the central nervous system would not be expected to induce significant systemic toxicity because of relatively rapid catabolism.

The drug-metabolizing enzyme system of the endoplasmic reticulum may be relevant to the action of some carcinostatic agents. Cyclophosphamide provides an illustration of an antileukemic agent that is activated by the microsomal enzyme system to a growth-inhibitory form [30]. Rodents have a comparatively active microsomal drug-metabolizing system, whereas such enzyme activity in man is generally considered to be low. Nevertheless, these enzymes are of considerable importance to the attainment of the maximum therapeutic potential of antileukemic agents that are either activated or destroyed by this system, and they may contribute to variability of patient response to drug action, since the activity of the microsomal enzymes is influenced by other drugs, diet, and age, as well as by several additional factors [31]. Commonly used drugs such as phenobarbital, phenylbutazone, chlorcyclizine, imipramine, and triparanol, as well as the chlorinated insecticides, induce an increase in the activity of drug-metabolizing enzymes, whereas certain agents such as chlorpromazine [32] and cortisol [33] first depress and then stimulate the activity of these enzymes of the endoplasmic reticulum.

Finally, the route and rate of excretion can influence the efficacy of antileukemic agents. A recent report [34] indicated that in patients with disseminated malignancy methotrexate was both filtered and actively secreted by the renal tubules. The simultaneous presence of weak organic acids such as salicylate and p-aminohippurate decreased the rate of clearance of methotrexate. These findings derive from the fact that methotrexate is a weak organic acid and thereby probably shares a renal tubular secretory pathway characteristic for organic anions. Thus, for this agent and perhaps for other antileukemic drugs, the excretion of the compound will be dependent in part upon the status of the patient with regard to other medication as well as the integrity of the excretory pathway; these factors will influence both toxicity and therapeutic efficacy.

Biochemical Considerations

The proper manipulation of pharmacologic factors is necessary to achieve the greatest degree of differential toxicity between leukemic cells and the most sensitive of the host tissues during the administration of chemotherapeutic agents. The absolute limits of the therapeutic gains achieved by such manipulation, however, would be expected to be dictated by the small metabolic differences between tumors and normal tissues that convey a degree of selective toxicity with certain chemotherapeutic agents. We have recently stressed the need to exploit presently known therapeutic differentials in an effort to achieve even greater selective toxicity to neoplastic cells, and we have described some experimental approaches that might lead to the development of more potent therapies for the treatment of malignant diseases [35]. It was suggested that the therapeutic potency of agents with known utility in the treatment of tumors in man, that is, drugs with some degree of differential toxicity to malignant and normal tissues, might be enhanced by further exploitation of knowledge concerning the metabolic lesions produced by these agents associated with cell death. These metabolic sites of vulnerability of tumor cells, which in some instances can be equated in part with differential toxicity, can conceivably be rendered more susceptible to drug action by either rational modification of the structure of an existing agent active at that site or by the use of drug combinations to achieve greater biochemical perturbation of a particular metabolic event. Structural modification of an effective antileukemic agent should be directed towards the development of a compound with greater affinity for the target site. BAKER [36] has described the concept of the development of site-directed antimetabolites with a function capable of alkylating either the active site of the enzyme (endo-alkylation) or some reactive group on the enzyme surface other than the catalytic center (exo-alkylation). The binding of inhibitors to the active site of enzymes from different sources that catalyze the same reaction should be expected to be reasonably similar, since few evolutionary or mutational changes within the catalytic site would be expected. However, in the transition from a normal cell to that of a malignant one, alterations might result in areas adjacent to the active center of the enzyme without loss of catalytic activity. Thus, small differences in regions proximate to the active site of a given target enzyme might well be exploitable. From a theoretical basis, it would appear advantageous to expose the tumor-bearing host to a concentration and frequency of administration of carcinolytic agent that is just sufficient to accomplish the degree and duration of blockade of a particular metabolic event, resulting in the eventual death of the leukemic cells. The more tightly a chemotherapeutic agent binds to its target site, the greater the probability that the affected cell will not survive. To successfully design a clinically useful irreversible inhibitor requires that (a) the drug-sensitive enzymic loci are precisely known, and (b) differences exist between the enzymes of leukemic cells of man and their counterparts in the most susceptible of host tissues. We are presently attempting such an approach with several α-(N)-heterocyclic carboxaldehyde thiosemicarbazones, compounds that exhibit antineoplastic potency against a relatively wide spectrum of transplanted rodent neoplasms [35] and spontaneous lymphomas in dogs [37]. These compounds are potent inhibitors of the enzyme ribonucleoside diphosphate reductase, which is of central importance to the replication of DNA, catalyzing the reduction of ribonucleotides to deoxyribonucleotide forms. The most promising members of this class of antineoplastic agents are 1-formylisoquinoline thiosemicarbazone [38, 39], its 4- and 5-hydroxy derivatives [40—42], and both 2-formyl-3-hydroxypyridine thiosemicarbazone and 2-formyl-5-hydroxypyridine thiosemicarbazone [41, 43—45]. Inhibition of the syntheses of RNA and protein is produced by relatively high concentrations of these agents; however, antineoplastic potency is correlated with, and therefore appears to be dependent upon, blockade of ribonucleoside diphosphate reductase and the resultant interference with the biosynthesis of DNA [46—50]. Studies on the mechanism of inhibition of ribonucleoside diphosphate reductase activity using an enzyme prepared from the Novikoff rat tumor suggested that 1-formylisoquinoline thiosemicarbazone and 2-formylpyridine thiosemicarbazone functioned to inhibit by a similar mechanism. The results were consistent with the concept that these derivatives interacted with the enzyme by coordination of the iron-charged protein at the site occupied by the required coupled reducing system. The systematic modification of these two thiosemicarbazones allowed a probe of the inhibitor binding site [47, 51]. The 3-, 4-, and 5-methyl derivatives of 2-formylpyridine thiosemicarbazone, 4- and 5-methyl-1-formylisoquinoline thiosemicarbazone, and 3-formylisoquinoline thiosemicarbazone were strong inhibitors of the enzyme, but 6-methyl-2-formylpyridine thiosemicarbazone, 3-methyl-1-formylisoquinoline thiosemicarbazone and 2-formylquinoline thiosemicarbazone were 5- to 20-fold less active. The results suggested that the enzyme had little bulk tolerance at the 3-position of 1-formylisoquinoline thiosemicarbazone and 6-position of 2-formylpyridine thiosemicarbazone, positions of equivalence with respect to orientation of these agents on the enzymatic site to which they bind. Thus, a group capable of alkylation of the enzyme could conceivably be substituted in positions 4 or 5 of these inhibitor molecules without apparent interference of inhibitor binding; we are currently engaged in an effort to design such an irreversible inhibitor.

Combination Chemotherapy

The use of combinations of agents to achieve additional gain in the therapy of leukemia can be based on biochemical, pharmacological, and toxicological knowledge. Drugs with differing toxicities to host tissues have been used successfully in admixture to intensify toxicity to the population of leukemic cells with considerably less damage to the host [52]. Of more pertinence to the subject matter of the present report are the approaches in which the selection of drugs for use in combination are based upon biochemical and pharmacologic considerations. As has been previously discussed [17, 18, 35], rational mixtures can be achieved by capitalizing on a knowledge of the mechanism of drug action and the metabolic parameters required to attain and sustain critical drug-induced lesions.

There are a number of barriers that any agent must surmount before an effective concentration at the "target site" can be achieved; these are chiefly a succession of membranes, such as the gastrointestinal tract, the membranes enclosing the blood and other body fluids, the membranes surrounding individual cells, and also those about the various intracellular structures. Selectivity of such membranes may well alter the susceptibility of a leukemic cell to a growth-inhibitory agent. A pertinent example of this phenomenon is shown by the report of KESSEL et al. [53] wherein the transport of methotrexate by transplantable murine neoplastic cell lines was a determinant of sensitivity; those tumors that effectively transported the folic acid antagonist were quite sensitive to this agent, whereas resistant cell lines poorly incorporated methotrexate. It is conceivable that the permeability of leukemic cells to a cytotoxic agent can be modified by the addition of a second agent. YAMADA and his co-workers [54, 55] have provided an experimental illustration of this phenomenon with the report that rodent hepatoma cells pretreated *in vitro* with Tween 80 had an increased sensitivity to nitrogen mustard N-oxide; enhanced sensitivity was correlated with greater uptake of the alkylating agent.

The greatest chance of success with combination therapy employing an agent to alter membrane permeability would appear to be in those instances in which the active compound is transported slowly and is bound intracellularly and, therefore, would not diffuse outward from cells with altered membranes. It remains to be seen whether such an approach can be employed successfully at the clinical level. It appears unlikely that means can be found by which drugs that alter membrane permeability might preferentially act upon leukemic cells; therefore, in such combination chemotherapy selectivity of action may well be dependent largely upon the active carcinostatic agent. A good candidate drug for attempted modification of transport appears to be methotrexate. The studies of HAKALA [56] and of GOLDMAN [57] indicate that the rate of uptake of the folic acid analog methotrexate, whose transport into neoplastic cells is a carrier-mediated process characterized by different uni-directional influx and efflux mechanisms, is elevated by substances such as dinitrophenol, azide, antimycin A, oligomycin, iodoacetate and anaerobiosis. Azide-induced increase in the rate of influx of methotrexate was associated with a rise in both the maximum transport velocity and the influx Michaelis constant. In addition, efflux of the antimetabolite was slowed by azide. Although it is unlikely that these toxic agents could find clinical utility in combination with methotrexate, their activity encourages the design of agents capable of depressing energy stores, which (a) have less toxicity to the host, and (b) may increase the intracellular concentration of the folic acid analog. Such compounds will be useful in combination with methotrexate against leukemic cells that have acquired resistance to this agent by virtue of an altered transport mechanism or a rise in the intracellular levels of the target enzyme dihydrofolate reductase. In the latter situation, difficulty derives from an inability to administer a quantity of drug large enough to attain intracellular concentrations capable of titrating a significant amount of the increased number of molecules of dihydrofolate reductase [58].

A knowledge of the mechanism of action of an antileukemic agent on occasion allows the addition of a second drug to provide an element of selective antineoplastic action by reducing the toxicity of the growth-inhibitory compound for normal tissue without significantly altering carcinostatic potency. The use of leucovorin (folinic acid) which supplies a precursor of the end-product of the inhibited enzyme dihydrofolate reductase, provides such an antidote to the action of methotrexate. With this combination the host, but not the tumor, is in some circumstances rescued from the lethal effects of the folic acid antimetabolite [59—63].

Increased antileukemic activity can theoretically be attained when one agent prevents the enzymatic destruction of an active compound or when the excretion of the carcinostatic agent is delayed. The tumor-inhibitory potency of 6-mercaptopurine and 6-chloropurine against adenocarcinoma 755 was enhanced by the simultaneous administration of 4-hydroxypyrazolo(3,4-d)pyrimidine (allopurinol); this agent is a potent inhibitor of xanthine oxidase, the enzyme converting the carcinostatic purine analogs to inactive products [64]. The combination of 6-mercaptopurine and allopurinol was compared by LEVIN et al. [65] to 6-mercaptopurine alone in the induction and maintenance of remission of acute leukemia in children. The median length of remission for the group treated with the combination was not significantly different from that of children treated with 6-mercaptopurine alone. Rather than eliminate such a drug mixture from clinical consideration, it should be stressed that the use of an agent that prevents the destruction of an active tumor-inhibitory compound should theoretically be efficacious only in those situations in which an insufficient concentration of the active drug is maintained in the environment of leukemic cells; this condition might be expected to occur with a drug that is rapidly excreted or catabolized or is slowly transported into neoplastic cells. The inability of allopurinol to increase the antileukemic activity of 6-mercaptopurine suggests that the achievement of a remission of this disease was not limited by the availability of the purine analog to the neoplastic cells.

Pharmacologic manipulation can be used to alter the intracellular conversion of a drug to its active antileukemic form. This type of mechanism is provided by the combination of 6-mercaptopurine and 6-methylmercaptopurine ribonucleoside, a mixture that causes synergistic inhibition of the growth of several transplanted murine neoplasms [66, 67]. Enhanced carcinostasis requires the initial conversion of 6-methylmercaptopurine ribonucleoside to its nucleotide form by the enzyme adenosine kinase; 6-methylmercaptopurine ribonucleotide is a potent inhibitor of phosphoribosylpyrophosphate amidotransferase [68] blockade of which causes an accumulation of phosphoribosylpyrophosphate. This metabolite is then utilized as a source of ribosephosphate for the conversion of 6-mercaptopurine to its active antileukemic nucleotide form [69]. The combination of 6-mercaptopurine and 6-methylmercaptopurine ribonucleoside has been employed in the treatment of patients with several forms of metastatic cancer [70]; the mixture was active against acute myelogenous leukemia; however, it is questionable that the response was superior to that obtained with 6-mercaptopurine alone. Cells of the bone marrow, and presumably malignant individuals derived therefrom, appear to be deficient in their capacity to carry out purine nucleotide biosynthesis *de novo* [71]; the implication is that, in leukemic cells derived from bone marrow, the target enzyme phosphoribosylpyrophosphate amidotransferase is not available for blockade by 6-methylmercaptopurine ribonucleotide, a requisite for effective functioning of this combination. Thus it would seem that additional trial of this mixture should be carried out in other malignant disease forms responsive to 6-mercaptopurine.

Drugs may also be selected for admixture on the basis of biochemical considerations. The use of the concepts of sequential [72], concurrent [73] and complementary inhibition has been discussed in recent reviews [18, 35]. Sequential inhibition relates to the utilization of two or more drugs in combination to inhibit different enzymes in a limited portion of a multi-enzyme sequence. The action of 6-thioguanine employed alone would appear to describe the phenomenon of sequential blockade. Thus, this agent might be considered to synergize with itself in that it produces multiple enzymatic blocks which should function to limit the synthesis of guanine nucleotides [74].

Complementary inhibition involves the use of two agents to interfere in neoplastic cells with the formation and function of certain polymeric structures. The selection of agents for such admixture is based upon the employment of a drug to create lesions at the level of macromolecular structures with a compound that interferes with synthesis and repair of the affected structure through blockade of enzymic reactions involved in the fabrication of precursor molecules. The experimental model that led to the development of this concept was based upon a directed metabolic attack at the level of RNA using combinations of actinomycin D and ribonuclease [75]. Actinomycin D was visualized to function to inhibit the biosynthesis of RNA; tumor cells, which theoretically survived the toxic action of this antibiotic, conceivably did so by conservation and utilization of preexisting RNA for metabolic function. Ribonuclease was employed in the combination to catabolize RNA molecules fabricated prior to administration of the actinomycin D. The employment of such a combination resulted in synergistic inhibition of transplanted tumors; however, it is clear that the envisioned mechanism of action represents an over-simplification. A variety of other factors are involved. For example, the status of a cell with respect to its growth cycle is important for the action of actinomycin D, with those individuals present in the G_1 phase being most sensitive to this agent [76]. This finding is probably a reflection of both the ability of this agent to interact with DNA, which is a measure of the availability of certain portions of the genome, and the functional capacity of the DNA-actinomycin D complex. These considerations may be in part responsible for the inhibition of the formation of ribosomal RNA that occurs at drug concentrations lower than those required to inhibit the synthesis of other kinds of RNA [77]. These findings stress that the magnitude and the number of lesions produced by a particular chemotherapeutic agent are dependent upon the concentration of the active form of the drug within the leukemic cell, as well as the receptivity of the target cell with respect to metabolic function.

An understanding of the role of cell cycle kinetics to cancer chemotherapy and the relatively widespread use of multiple mixtures of drugs have resulted in major advances in the management of acute leukemia. The use of biochemical and pharmacological principles has also led to some gains; however, the potential of these tools to cancer chemotherapy is virtually untapped. Knowledge of the biochemical mechanism of action of an effective chemotherapeutic agent and the pharmacologic factors influencing its action allows the utilization of this information to (a) tailor the magnitude and duration of therapy to the achievement of a particular metabolic event in neoplastic cells, (b) serve as a predictive test for cell sensitivity, and (c) design rational combination treatments. It would appear certain that additional gains in the treatment of acute leukemia would result from the widespread utilization of the principles of these scientific disciplines.

Summary

Selective toxicity of chemotherapeutic agents to leukemic cells appears to derive from (a) the fraction of neoplastic cells in the proliferative state relative to normal cell types and (b) the presence of biochemical differences between tumor cells and normal tissues of the host. Pharmacologic factors such as the route of drug administration, the extent and rate of absorption through a number of membranes, the degree of structural modification by the processes of biotransformation, the route and rate of excretion, and the tissue and cellular localization and degree of binding of the agent are important to the achievement of optimal therapeutic indices in the treatment of cancer. Biochemical approaches toward improving existing therapeutic differentials of known antineoplastic agents are also of significance and advances theoretically can be achieved by the systematic design of more effective inhibitors of enzymatic reactions which appear to be sites of vulnerability of neoplastic cells. Gains in therapeutic effectiveness can be attained through combination chemotherapy which utilizes both a knowledge of the mechanisms of drug action and the metabolic parameters required to attain and sustain critical drug-induced lesions.

References

1. BRUCE, R. W.: The action of chemotherapeutic agents at the cellular level and the effect of these agents on hematopoietic and lymphomatous tissue. Can. Cancer Conf. **7**, 53 (1967).
2. BURCHENAL, J. H.: Formyl discussion: long-term survival in Burkitt's tumor and in acute leukemia. Cancer Res. **27**, 2616 (1967).
3. FARBER, S., D'ANGIO, G., EVANS, A., MITUS, A.: Clinical studies of actinomycin D with special reference to Wilms' tumor in children. Ann. N.Y. Acad. Sci. **89**, 421 (1960).
4. ROSS, G. T., GOLDSTEIN, D. P., HERTZ, R., LIPSETT, M. B., ODELL, W. D.: Sequential use of methotrexate and actinomycin D in the treatment of metastatic choriocarcinoma and related trophoblastic diseases in women. Amer. J. Obstet. Gynec. **93**, 223 (1965).
5. HANDSCHUMACHER, R. E.: Mechanisms of control of tumor growth: asparaginase and asparaginase analogs. In: Exploitable Molecular Mechanisms and Neoplasia. Baltimore: Williams and Wilkins 1969, p. 565.
6. ADAMSON, R. H., FABRO, S.: Antitumor activity and other biologic properties of L-asparaginase (NSC-109 229)-A review. Cancer Chem. Rep. **52**, 617 (1968).
7. PATTERSON, M. K., JR., ORR, G.: L-asparaginase biosynthesis by nutritional variants of the Jensen sarcoma. Biochem. biophys. Res. Commun. **26**, 228 (1967).
8. BROOME, J. D., SCHWARTZ, J. H.: Differences in the production of L-asparaginase in asparaginase-sensitive and resistant lymphoma cells. Biochim. biophys. Acta (Amst.) **138**, 637 (1967).
9. HOROWITZ, B., MADRAS, B. K., MEISTER, A., OLD, L. J., BOYSE, E. A., STOCKERT, E.: Asparaginase synthetase activity of mouse leukemias. Science **160**, 533 (1968).
10. PRAGER, M. D., BACHYNSKY, N.: Asparagine synthetase in asparaginase resistant and susceptible mouse lymphomas. Biochem. biophys. Res. Commun. **31**, 43 (1968).
11. SILBER, R., BERMAN, E., GOLDSTEIN, B., STEIN, H., FARNHAM, G., BERTINO, J. R.: Methylation of nucleic acids in normal und leukemic leukocytes. Biochim. biophys. Acta (Amst.) **123**, 638 (1966).
12. MOORE, E. C., LEPAGE, G. A.: *In vivo* sensitivity of normal and neoplastic mouse tissues to azaserine. Cancer Res. **17**, 804 (1957).
13. ROBERTS, E., FRANKEL, S.: Free amino acids in normal and neoplastic tissues of mice as studied by paper chromatography. Cancer Res. **9**, 645 (1949).
14. — SIMONSEN, D. G.: Free amino acids and related substances in normal and neoplastic tissues. In: Amino Acids, Proteins and Cancer Biochemistry. Ed.: J. T. EDSALL. New York: Academic Press 1960, p. 121.
15. LEVENBERG, B., MELNICK., I., BUCHANAN, J. M.: Biosynthesis of the purines. XV. The effect of aza-L-serine and 6-diazo-5-oxo-L-norleucine on inosinic acid biosynthesis *de novo*. J. Biol. Chem. **225**, 163 (1957).

16. ROUSER, G.: Free or easily extractable amino acids in blood cells and body fluids. In: The Leukemias: Etiology, Pathophysiology and Treatment. New York: Academic Press 1957, p. 361.
17. VENDITTI, J. M., GOLDIN, A.: Drug synergism in antineoplastic chemotherapy. In: Advances in Chemotherapy, Vol. 1. Eds.: A. GOLDIN and F. HAWKING. New York: Academic Press 1964, p. 397.
18. SARTORELLI, A. C.: Approaches to the combination chemotherapy of transplantable neoplasms. In: Prog. Exptl. Tumor Res., Vol. 6. Ed.: F. HOMBURGER. Basel: S. Karger 1965, p. 228.
19. MARCHESI, S. L., SARTORELLI, A. C.: The biochemical basis for the differential sensitivity of intestinal mucosa and bone marrow to 6-thioguanine. Cancer Res. **23**, 1769 (1963).
20. HENDERSON, J. F.: Variation in selective toxicity: causes and consequences. Cancer Res. **29**, 2404 (1969).
21. HENDERSON, E. F., ADAMSON, R. H., OLIVERIO, V. T.: The metabolic fate of tritiated Methotrexate. II. Absorption and excretion in man. Cancer Res. **25**, 1018 (1965).
22. DIXON, R. L., HENDERSON, E. S., RALL, D. P.: Plasma protein binding of methotrexate and its displacement by various drugs. Fed. Proc. **24**, 454 (1965).
23. OLIVERIO, V. T., LOO, T. L.: Separation and isolation of metabolites of folic acid antagonists. Proc. Amer. Ass. Cancer Res. **3**, 140 (1960).
24. LOO, T. L., ADAMSON, R. H.: The metabolite of 3′,5′-dichloro-4-amino-4-deoxy-N^{10}-methylpteroylglutamic acid (dichloromethotrexate). J. Med. Chem. **8**, 513 (1965).
25. MISRA, D. K., ADAMSON, R. H., LOO, T. L., OLIVERIO, V. T.: Inhibition of dihydrofolate reductase by dichloromethotrexate and its metabolite. Life Sci. **2**, 407 (1963).
26. JOHNS, D. G., IANNOTTI, A. T., SARTORELLI, A. C., BOOTH, B. A., BERTINO, J. R.: The identity of rabbit-liver methotrexate oxidase. Biochim. biophys. Acta (Amst.) **105**, 380 (1965).
27. LOO, T. L., ADAMSON, R. H.: The enzymic oxidation of certain folic acid antagonists. Biochem. Pharmacol. **11**, 170 (1962).
28. JOHNS, D. G., IANNOTTI, A. T., SARTORELLI, A. C., BERTINO, J. R.: The relative toxicities of methotrexate and aminopterin. Biochem. Pharmacol. **15**, 555 (1966).
29. HENDERSON, E. S., ADAMSON, R. H., DENHAM, C., OLIVERIO, V. T.: The metabolic fate of tritiated methotrexate. I. Absorption, excretion, and distribution in mice, rats, dogs and monkeys. Cancer Res. **25**, 1008 (1965).
30. HOHORST, H. J., ZIEMAN, A., BROCK, N.: Alkylating substances in serum and urine after injection of cyclophosphamide. Arzneimittel-Forsch. **15**, 432 (1965).
31. CONNEY, A. H., BURNS, J. J.: Factors influencing drug metabolism. Advanc. Pharmacol. **1**, 31 (1962).
32. RALL, D. P.: Pharmacologic aspects of selective chemotherapy of leukemia and Burkitt's tumor. Combination chemotherapy: advertent and inadvertent. Cancer Res. **27**, 2650 (1967).
33. TEPHLY, T. R., MANNERING, G. J.: Inhibition of drug metabolism by steroid hormones. Pharmacologist **6**, 186 (1964).
34. LIEGLER, D. G., HENDERSON, E. S., HAHN, M. A., OLIVERIO, V. T.: The effect of organic acids on renal clearance of methotrexate in man. Clin. Pharmacol. Ther. **10**, 849 (1969).
35. SARTORELLI, A. C.: Some approaches to the therapeutic exploitation of metabolic sites of vulnerability of neoplastic cells. Cancer Res. **29**, 2292 (1969).
36. BAKER, B. R.: Design of active-site-directed irreversible enzyme inhibitors. New York: John Wiley and Sons 1967.
37. CREASEY, W. A., AGRAWAL, K. C., STINSON, K. K., SARTORELLI, A. C.: Antineoplastic effects and metabolism of α-(N)-heterocyclic carboxaldehyde thiosemicarbazones in dogs and mice. Fed. Proc. **29**, 681 (1970).
38. FRENCH, F. A., BLANZ, E. J., JR.: The carcinostatic activity of α-(N)-heterocyclic carboxaldehyde thiosemicarbazones. I. Isoquinoline-1-carboxaldehyde thiosemicarbazone. Cancer Res. **25**, 1454 (1965).
39. — — The carcinostatic activity of thiosemicarbazones of formyl heteroaromatic compounds. III. Primary correlation. J. Med. Chem. **9**, 585 (1966).

40. Agrawal, K. C., Booth, B. A., Sartorelli, A. C.: Potential antitumor agents. I. A series of 5-substituted 1-formylisoquinoline thiosemicarbazones. J. Med. Chem. **11**, 700 (1968).
41. — Sartorelli, A. C.: Potential antitumor agents. III. Sodium salts of α-(N)-heterocyclic carboxaldehyde thiosemicarbazones. J. pharm. Sci. **57**, 1948 (1968).
42. — — Potential antitumor agents. IV. Synthesis of 4-substituted 1-formylisoquinoline thiosemicarbazones by rearrangement of 1-methylisoquinoline-N-oxide. Abstr. Amer. Chem. Soc. MEDI-39, Sept., 1968.
43. Blanz, E. J., Jr., French, F. A.: The carcinostatic activity of 5-hydroxy-2-formylpyridine thiosemicarbazone. Cancer Res. **28**, 2419 (1968).
44. French, F. A., Blanz, E. J., Jr.: The carcinostatic activity of α-(N)-heterocyclic carboxaldehyde thiosemicarbazones. II. 3-hydroxypyridine-2-carboxaldehyde thiosemicarbazone. Cancer Res. **26**, 1638 (1966).
45. — — Carcinostatic hydrazones: some design principles, data and correlations. In: Cancer Chemotherapy, Gann Monograph No. 2. Tokyo: Maruzen Co. 1967, p. 51.
46. Sartorelli, A. C.: Effect of chelating agents upon the synthesis of nucleic acids and protein: Inhibition of DNA synthesis by 1-formylisoquinoline thiosemicarbazone. Biochem. biophys. Res. Commun. **27**, 26 (1967).
47. — Agrawal, K. C., Booth, B. A., Moore, E. C.: Inhibition of ribonucleotide diphosphate reductase by substituted α-(N)-heterocyclic aldehyde thiosemicarbazones.. Fourth Internat. Congress Pharmacol. Basel: Schwabe 1969, p. 195.
48. — Booth, B. A.: Biochemical effects of some pyridine aldehyde thiosemicarbazones. Proc. Amer. Ass. Cancer Res. **9**, 61 (1968).
49. — — Moore, E. C.: Studies on the site of action of pyridine aldehyde thiosemicarbazones. Proc. Amer. Ass. Cancer Res. **10**, 76 (1969).
50. — Zedeck, M. S., Agrawal, K. C., Moore, E. C.: Correlation of inhibition of DNA synthesis and *in vitro* inhibition of ribonucleotide reductase by 1-formylisoquinoline thiosemicarbazone. Fed. Proc. **27**, 650 (1968).
51. Moore, E. C., Agrawal, K. C., Booth, B. A., Sartorelli, A. C.: Potential irreversible inhibitors of ribonucleotide reductase: substituted α-(N)-heterocyclic aldehyde thiosemicarbazones. Fed. Proc. **29**, 908 (1970).
52. Frei, E., III, Freireich, E. J.: Progress and perspectives in the chemotherapy of acute leukemia. In: Advances in Chemotherapy, Vol. 2. Eds.: A. Goldin, F. Hawking, and R. J. Schnitzer. New York: Academic Press 1965, p. 269.
53. Kessel, D., Hall, T. C., Roberts, D. W., Wodinsky, I.: Uptake as a determinant of methotrexate response in mouse leukemias. Science **150**, 752 (1965).
54. Yamada, T., Iwanami, Y.: The transport of nitrogen mustard N-oxide through cellular membrane and its cytological effects in rat ascites hepatoma. Gann **53**, 225 (1962).
55. — — Baba, T.: The transport of ^{14}C-labeled nitrogen mustard N-oxide through cellular membrane treated with tween 80 *in vitro*. Gann **54**, 171 (1963).
56. Hakala, M. T.: On the nature of permeability of sarcoma-180 cells to amethopterin *in vitro*. Biochim. biophys. Acta (Amst.) **102**, 210 (1965).
57. Goldman, I. D.: Transport energetics of the folic acid analogue, methotrexate, in L1210 leukemia cells. Enhanced accumulation by metabolic inhibitors. J. biol. Chem. **244**, 3779 (1969).
58. Sartorelli, A. C., Booth, B. A., Bertino, J. R.: Folate metabolism in methotrexate-sensitive and -resistant Ehrlich ascites cells. Arch. Biochem. **108**, 53 (1964).
59. Mead, J. A. R., Venditti, J. M., Schrecker, A. W., Goldin, A., Keresztesy, J. C.: The effect of reduced derivatives of folic acid on the toxicity and antileukemic effect of methotrexate in mice. Biochem. Pharmacol. **12**, 371 (1963).
60. Goldin, A., Venditti, J. M., Kline, I., Mantel, N.: Eradication of leukaemic cells (L1210) by methotrexate and methotrexate plus citrovorum factor. Nature (Lond.) **212**, 1548 (1966).
61. Sullivan, R. D., Miller, E., Sikes, M. P.: Antimetabolite-metabolite combination cancer chemotherapy. Effects of intra-arterial methotrexate-intramuscular citrovorum factor therapy in human cancer. Cancer **12**, 1248 (1959).

62. Lefkowitz, E., Papac, R. J., Bertino, J. R.: Studies of head and neck cancer. III. Toxicity of 24 hour infusions of methotrexate (NSC-740) and protection by leucovorin (NSC-3590) in patients with epidermoid carcinomas. Cancer Chem. Rep. **51**, 305 (1967).
63. Hryniuk, W. M., Bertino, J. R.: Treatment of leukemia with large doses of methotrexate and folinic acid: clinical-biochemical correlates. J. clin. Invest. **48**, 2140 (1969).
64. Elion, G. B., Callahan, S., Nathan, H., Bieber, S., Rundles, R. W., Hitchings, G. H.: Potentiation by inhibition of drug degradation: 6-substituted purines and xanthine oxidase. Biochem. Pharmacol. **12**, 85 (1963).
65. Levine, A. S., Sharp, H. L., Mitchell, J., Krivit, W., Nesbit, M. E.: Combination therapy with 6-mercaptopurine (NSC-755) and allopurinol (NSC-1390) during induction and maintenance of remission of acute leukemia in children. Cancer Chem. Rep. **53**, 53 (1969).
66. Schabel, F. M., Jr., Laster, W. R., Jr., Skipper, H. E.: Chemotherapy of leukemia L1210 by 6-mercaptopurine in combination with 6-methylthiopurine ribonucleoside. Cancer Chem. Rep. **51**, 111 (1967).
67. Wang, M. C., Simpson, A. I., Paterson, A. R. P.: Combinations of 6-mercaptopurine and 6-(methylmercapto)purine ribonucleoside in the chemotherapy of the Ehrlich ascites carcinoma. Cancer Chem. Rep. **51**, 101 (1967).
68. Hill, D. L., Bennett, L. L., Jr.: Purification and properties of 5-phosphoribosyl pyrophosphate amidotransferase from adenocarcinoma 755 cells. Biochemistry **8**, 122 (1969).
69. Paterson, A. R. P., Wang, M. C.: Stimulation of 6-mercaptopurine anabolism in tumor cells by prior treatment with 6-(methylmercapto)purine ribonucleoside. Fed. Proc. **27**, 759 (1968).
70. Bodey, G. P., Brodovsky, H. S., Isassi, A. A., Samuels, M. L., Freireich, E. J.: Studies of combination 6-mercaptopurine (NSC-755) and 6-methylmercaptopurine ribonucleoside (NSC-40 774) in patients with acute leukemia and metastatic cancer. Cancer Chem. Rep. **52**, 315 (1968).
71. Lajtha, L. G., Vane, J. R.: Dependence of bone marrow cells on the liver for purine supply. Nature (Lond.) **182**, 191 (1958).
72. Potter, V. R.: Sequential blocking of metabolic pathways *in vivo*. Proc. Soc. exp. Biol. (N. Y.) **76**, 41 (1951).
73. Elion, G. B., Singer, S., Hitchings, G. H.: Antagonists of nucleic acid derivatives. VIII. Synergism in combinations of biochemically related antimetabolites. J. biol. Chem. **208**, 477 (1954).
74. Miech, R. P., Parks, R. E., Jr., Anderson, J. H., Jr., Sartorelli, A. C.: An hypothesis on the mechanism of action of 6-thioguanine. Biochem. Pharmacol. **16**, 2221 (1967).
75. Sartorelli, A. C.: Combination chemotherapy with actinomycin D and ribonuclease: an example of complementary inhibition. Nature (Lond.) **203**, 877 (1964).
76. Elkind, M. M., Kano, E., Sutton-Gibert, H.: Cell killing by actinomycin D in relation to the growth cycle of Chinese hamster cells. J. Cell Biol. **42**, 366 (1969).
77. Perry, R. P.: Selective effects of actinomycin D on the intracellular distribution of RNA synthesis in tissue culture cells. Exp. Cell. Res. **29**, 400 (1963).

Consideration of the Cell Cycle in Chemotherapy of Acute Leukemia[1]

BAYARD CLARKSON, AKIO TODO, MAKOTO OGAWA, TIMOTHY GEE, and JERROLD FRIED

With 12 Figures

There is now convincing evidence that it is possible to regularly cure certain experimental leukemias by using chemotherapeutic schedules specifically designed to exploit known information about the kinetic behavior of the leukemic cells, whereas other treatment schedules employing the same or higher total doses of the same drugs fail to effect any cures [1—9]. Much greater difficulty is encountered in treating spontaneous animal leukemias and human leukemia effectively, and the present paper is concerned with what we believe are the main reasons for these different results. To help focus attention on some of the critical points, two representative studies in patients with acute leukemia will be described for illustrative purposes, and general conclusions drawn from these studies in the context of previous information.

Methods

The patients were given continuous intravenous infusions of ^{3}H-thymidine (^{3}H-TdR; Sp.Ac. 6 C/mM) at a constant rate of 3 or 4 mc/24 hours, and samples of blood and marrow were taken periodically for autoradiographs [10]. The latter were processed as previously described [10, 11] and exposed for 12 to 20 weeks as noted. The background radioactivity was less than 1 grain per cell; cells containing 4 or more grains over the nucleus were registered as labeled. Flash ^{3}H-TdR labeling indexes (LI) were determined by 30 minutes incubation of marrow or blood samples with isotope (1 μc/ml) *in vitro*. The generation time (T_G) of leukemic and other cells was estimated by the median grain count (MGC) halving method [10—13]. T_G was

[1] From the Divisions of Chemotherapy Research, and Biophysics, Sloan-Kettering Institute for Cancer Research, and Department of Medicine, Memorial Hospital for Cancer and Allied Diseases, New York, N. Y. — This investigation was supported in part by research grants CA-05826 and CA-08748 from the National Cancer Institute, United States Public Health Service, the American Cancer Society, T-538A, The John C. McCarroll Memorial Fund, Hearst Foundation Fund, United Leukemia Fund, and the Junior Committee of the Society of Memorial Sloan-Kettering Cancer Center.

also computed using the geometric mean in place of the median as the former often has certain practical and theoretical advantages [14]. Identification of cell types and measurement of nuclear areas were performed as previously described [10, 13]. The concentration of hydroxyurea was assayed by Dr. F. S. Philips in PCA filtrates of whole blood samples, using a modification [15] of Nery's colorimetric method [16].

Results

First Case — Acute Lymphoblastic Leukemia

J. T. was a 26-year old man whose disease was diagnosed in March 1967. In June, a remission was induced with prednisone and methotrexate, but marrow relapse occurred in December despite maintenance therapy with methotrexate. At the time of admission to Memorial Hospital in March 1968, he had had no treatment for several weeks; his course while in the hospital is shown in Fig. 1. There were no physical signs of disease, and although the marrow was filled with leukemic cells, he was asymptomatic and the hemoglobin and platelet values remained almost normal during the ^{3}H-TdR infusion.

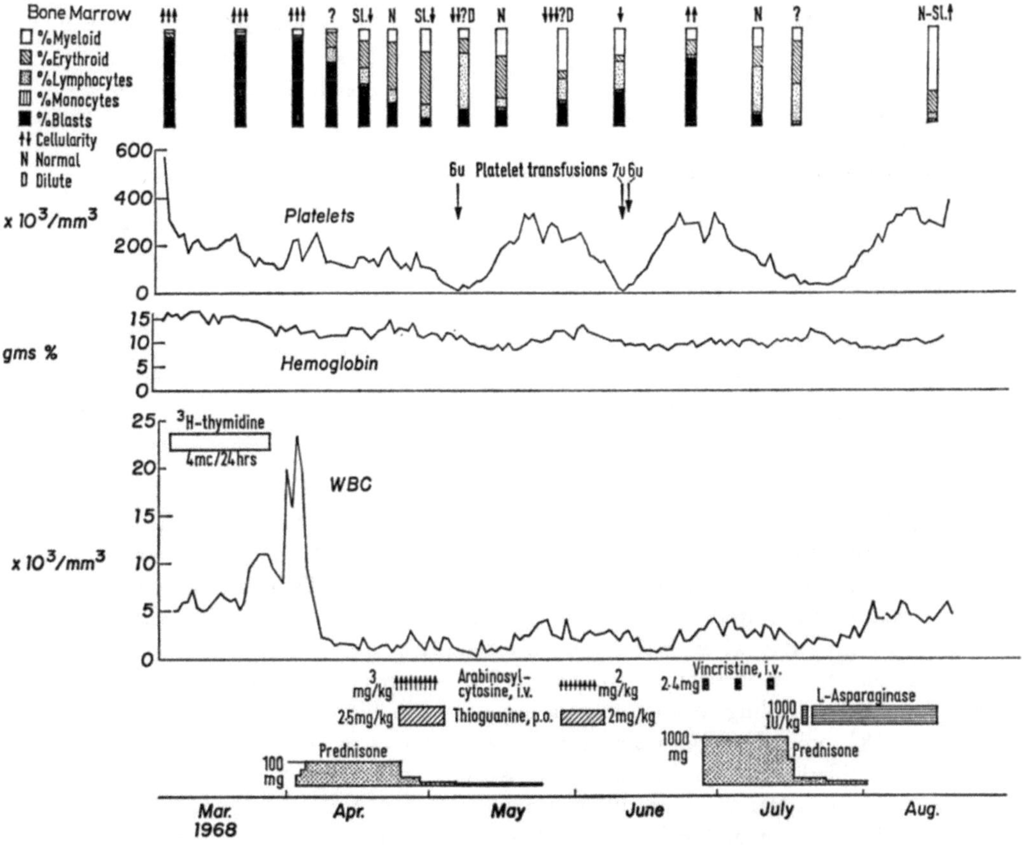

Fig. 1. Course of J. T. while at Memorial Hospital

Cytokinetic Studies

Leukemic Cells

The flash ^{3}H-TdR *(in vitro)* LIs of the marrow and blood blasts were 8% and 1%, respectively (Table 1); their labeling patterns during the ^{3}H-TdR infusion are shown in Fig. 2. After 20 days' infusion, 89% were labeled in the marrow and 94% in the blood; 2 days later 92% of marrow blasts were labeled.

Table 1. *J. T. ^{3}H-TdR labeling indices (LI) in vitro and in vivo, and grain count halving times of cells after stopping ^{3}H-TdR infusion*

Cell type	Marrow or blood	Flash ^{3}H-TdR LI *(in vitro)* [a] %	LI at end of ^{3}H-TdR infusion *(in vivo)* %	Therapy	Grain count halving time (hours) Median	Geometric mean
Leukemic cells						
Mitoses	M	0	100	None	147	133
	M	0	—	Prednisone	775	484
Interphase	M	8	92	None	297	389
	M	—	—	Prednisone	686	604
	B	1	94	None	230	214
	B	—	—	Prednisone	240	219
Erythrocyte precursors						
Pronormoblasts	M	84	100	None	18	18.5
Basophilic normoblasts	M	71	99	None	16	17
Polychromatic normoblasts	M	48	98	None	21	22
Orthochromatic normoblasts	M	0	87	None	35	30

[a] Determined just prior to ^{3}H-TdR infusion.

Fig. 3 shows the median grain counts of the mitotic and interphase leukemic cells after stopping the ^{3}H-TdR infusion (before and after prednisone) to illustrate the method used in determining T_G. The T_G of the interphase cells before treatment was twice that of the mitotic cells (Table 1), and indicates that many daughter cells entered a resting state after their parents divided [10].

The nuclear size distribution of the marrow blasts and their labeling frequency and intensity according to nuclear area are shown in Fig. 4. As in previous studies [10, 17, 18], only the large cells plus a few medium sized ones were labeled after 24 hours ^{3}H-TdR infusion, but their MGCs were similar, indicating similar rates of DNA synthesis. After 20 days' infusion most cells were labeled and the largest ones had significantly higher labeling intensities. This suggests that either the large cells went through more division cycles during the infusion than the others, or (more

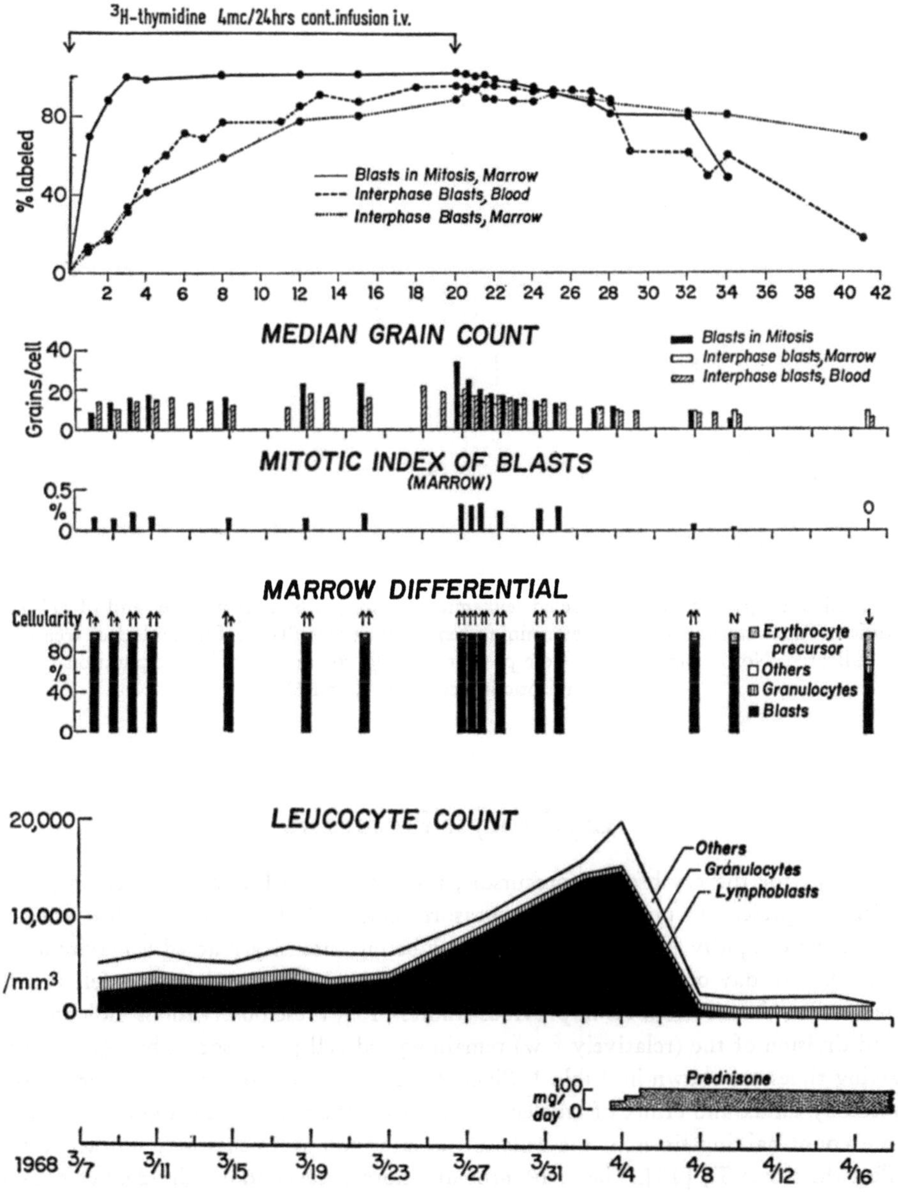

Fig. 2. Labeling pattern of interphase leukemic cells in marrow and blood, and of mitotic leukemic cells in marrow (no mitoses were found in the blood) of J. T. during and after continuous ^{3}H-TdR infusion. Autoradiographs exposed 12 weeks

probably) that a higher proportion of the former were in late S or G_2 and hence had a greater DNA content at the moment of sampling. A week after ending the infusion (before prednisone) the MGCs of all cells had dropped to an almost uniform level, indicating continual interchange between cells of different sizes due to growth and division.

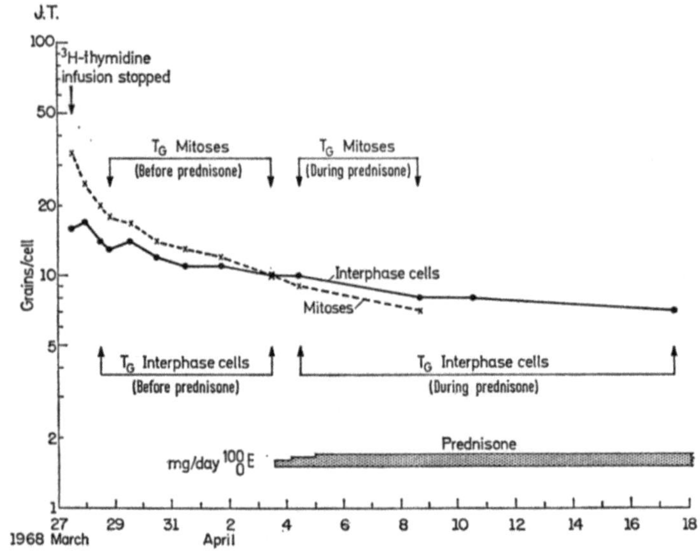

Fig. 3. Median grain counts of labeled leukemic cells in J. T.'s marrow after end of ^{3}H-TdR infusion. Time intervals used in determining generation times (T_G) before and after treatment are indicated. Not enough mitoses were present after $^{4}/_{9}$ to carry out the computation further (see mitotic indices, Figs. 2 and 6)

Erythrocyte Precursors

Except for the erythrocyte precursors, there were too few normal hematopoietic precursors present to obtain reliable measurements. All the earliest erythrocyte precursors were rapidly labeled (Fig. 5), their labeling intensity reached a maximum by about the 3rd day of the ^{3}H-TdR infusion, and their LI and grain counts fell rapidly after ending the infusion. As in previous studies [13], these observations indicate very rapid division of the (relatively few) remaining red cell precursors. Their grain count halving times are shown in Table 1. Since it is not possible to correct for pertubation caused by influx and efflux of labeled cells between the maturation compartments, the grain count halving times of the cells in the later compartments may not accurately reflect their true T_G [13]. The orthochromatic normoblasts do not divide, but because of their relatively short transit time in that compartment the fall in their grain count roughly reflects the T_G of their precursors.

The secondary rise in the LIs of the red cell precursors on day 32 (Fig. 5) is unexplained, but this was confirmed by counting a duplicate set of autoradiographs. Conceivably, it could be due to recruitment of prelabeled but unrecognized temporarily resting stem cells committed to red cell differentiation. As the concentration of leukemic cells was reduced in the marrow by prednisone, the resting stem cells could have been released from the inhibitory influence exerted by the leukemic cells (see discussion).

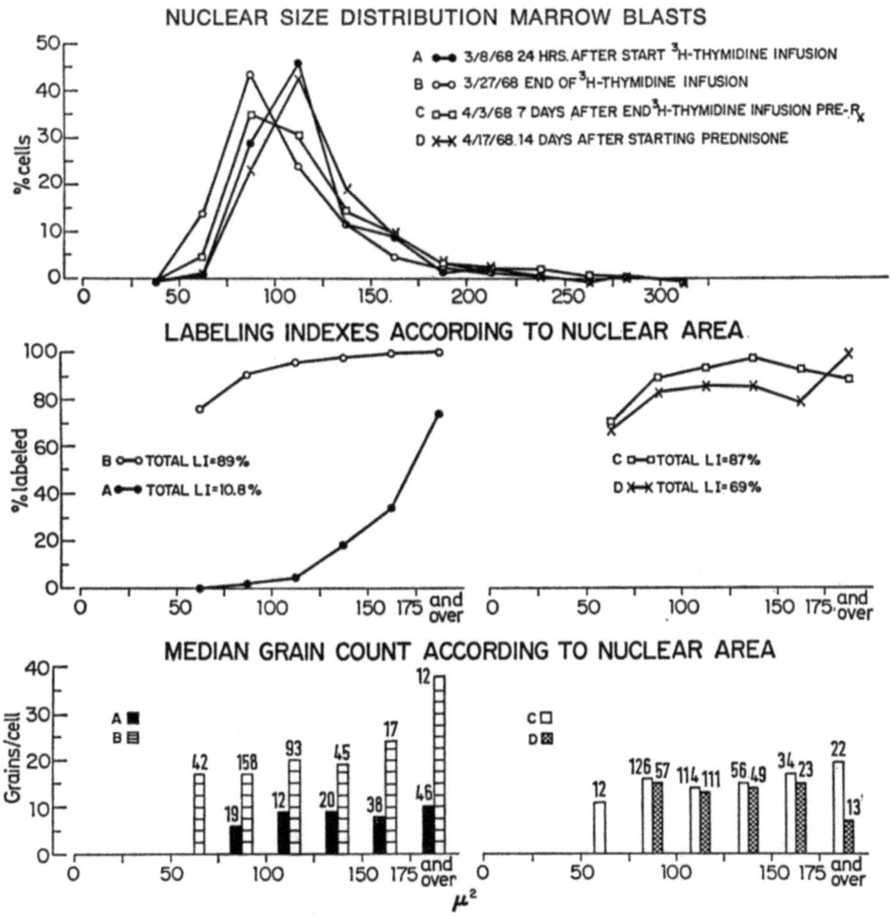

Fig. 4. Nuclear size distribution of marrow leukemic cells in J. T. and relation of nuclear size to ³H-TdR labeling frequency and intensity during the ³H-TdR infusion, and after ending it before and during prednisone. The areas of 400 or more nuclei were measured in each sample for the size distributions and labeling indices, and the number of labeled cells counted in each size category for labeling intensity are indicated above each column of grains per cell. Autoradiographs exposed 12 weeks

Effect of Chemotherapy

Although it failed to induce a complete remission, prednisone obviously killed many leukemic cells (Fig. 2), and temporarily almost completely arrested further division of the remaining ones. Their mitotic index fell to zero, the flash ³H-TdR LI fell significantly (Fig. 6), and the grain count halving times of both the mitotic and interphase blasts in the marrow were greatly prolonged (Table 1). However, the effect was incomplete and transient as about 35% leukemic cells persisted in the marrow and their LI and MI began to recover despite continuing the drug (Fig. 6).

During prednisone, the residual leukemic cells were more fragile on smearing, but the size distribution of the intact ones was almost unchanged, and, except for the very

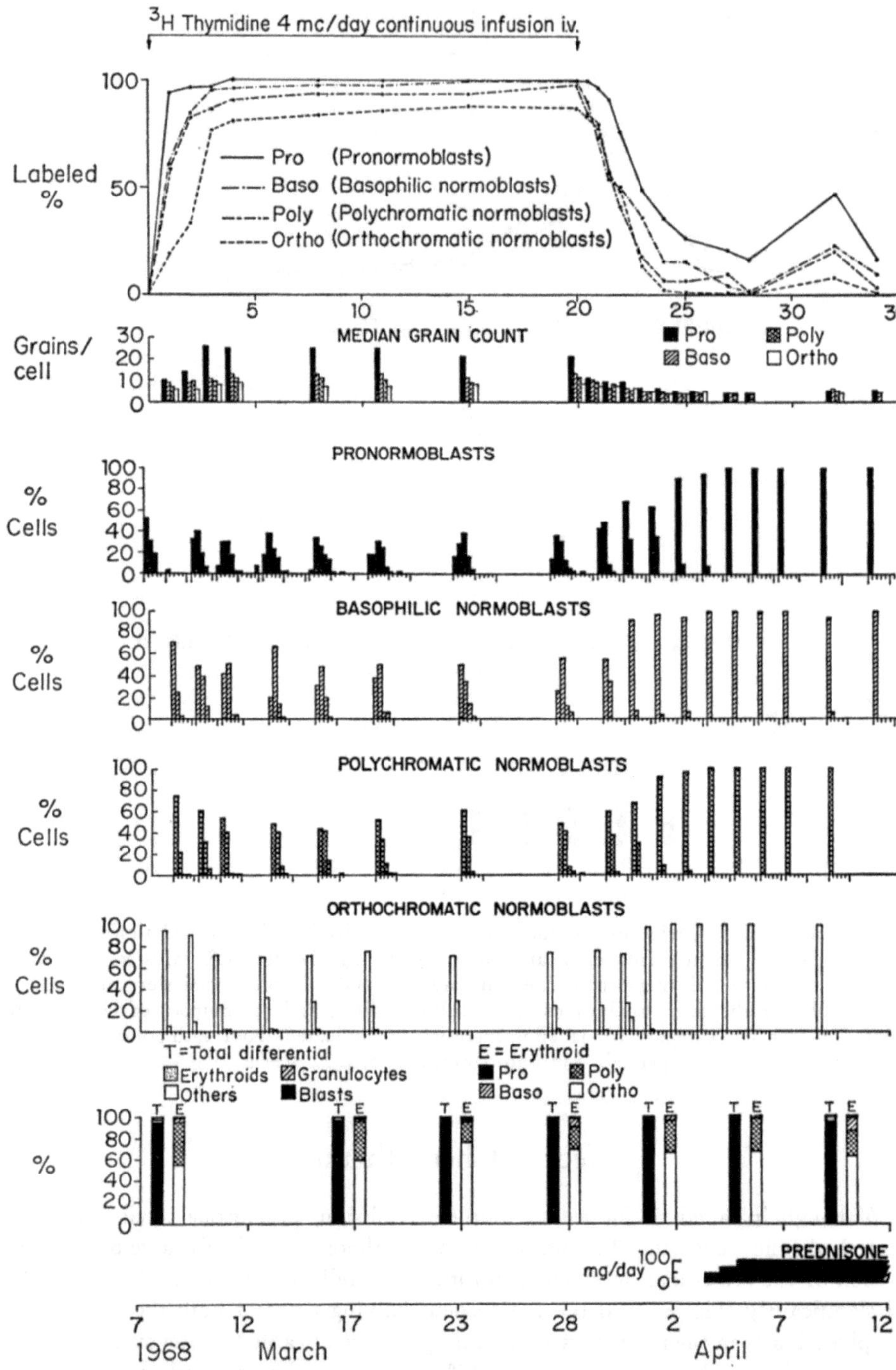

Fig. 5. Labeling pattern of erythrocyte precursors in J. T. during and after infusion of ^{3}H-TdR. The grain count distributions for each cell type are plotted from left to right in 5 groups: 4—10, 11—20, and so on up to 41—50, or (if necessary) in 10 groups up to 91 to 100 grains per nucleus. Very few cells contained over 80 grains

largest cells, there was little further reduction in grain count (i. e., between 4/3 and 4/17, Fig. 4). This suggests that killing was random with respect to cell size and that almost none of the surviving cells (except possibly the very largest ones) divided during the first 2 weeks on prednisone.

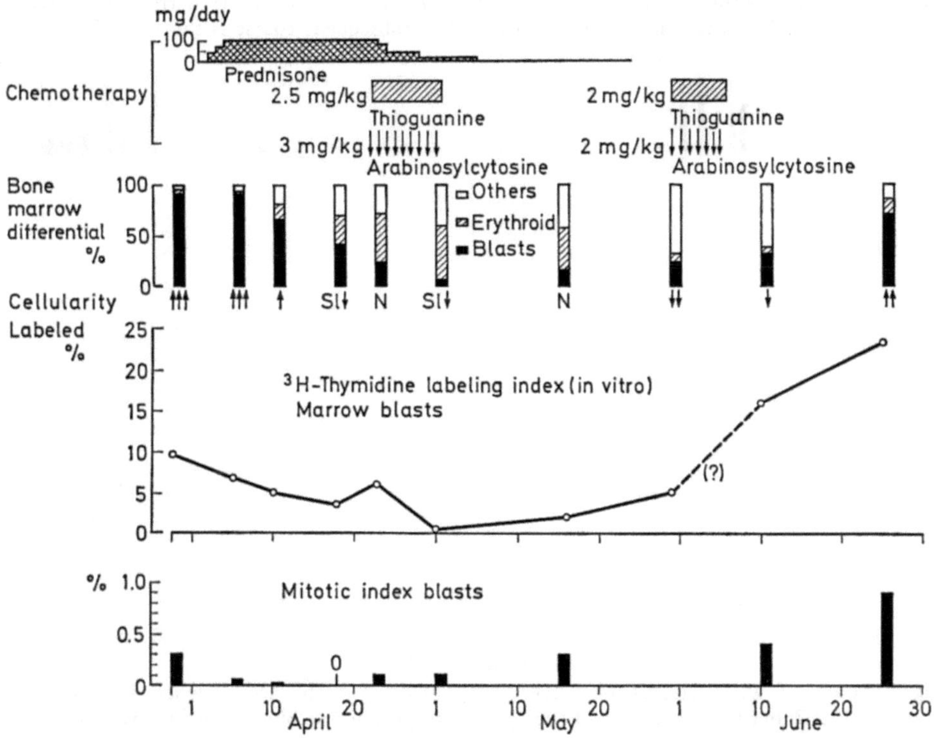

Fig. 6. Effect of chemotherapy on marrow cellularity and differential, on flash *(in vitro)* ^{3}H-TdR LI, and on mitotic index of marrow blasts of J. T.

Nine consecutive daily doses of arabinosylcytosine and thioguanine [19] were then given which further reduced the number of leukemic cells. The LI and MI of the surviving cells remained low (Fig. 6), but they recovered rapidly. A second 7-day course of therapy with the same drugs had little effect (these were given at lower dosage because of severe thrombocytopenia and leukopenia following the first course). After stopping therapy, both the LI and MI rose to more than double their pretreatment values as the marrow refilled with blasts.

A remission was subsequently induced with prednisone (in high dosage) and vincristine, and this was followed by a month of "consolidation" therapy with L-asparaginase [20] (Fig. 1). Following this, no treatment was given and relapse occurred about 2 months later. Further therapy with other drugs failed to reinduce a remission and he died in May 1969.

Second Case — Acute Myelomonoblastic Leukemia

W. J. was a 73-year old man who was well until February 1967 when he developed progressive anemia and a diagnosis of acute leukemia was established elsewhere. He was given no therapy except for about 20 blood transfusions during the next 8 months. At the time of his admission to Memorial Hospital in October 1967, review of his blood counts and periodic marrow slides from February through October revealed little change in his disease status except for a gradual increase in the fraction of leukemic cells in the marrow and blood; the platelet and WBC remained almost normal. His subsequent course is shown in Fig. 7.

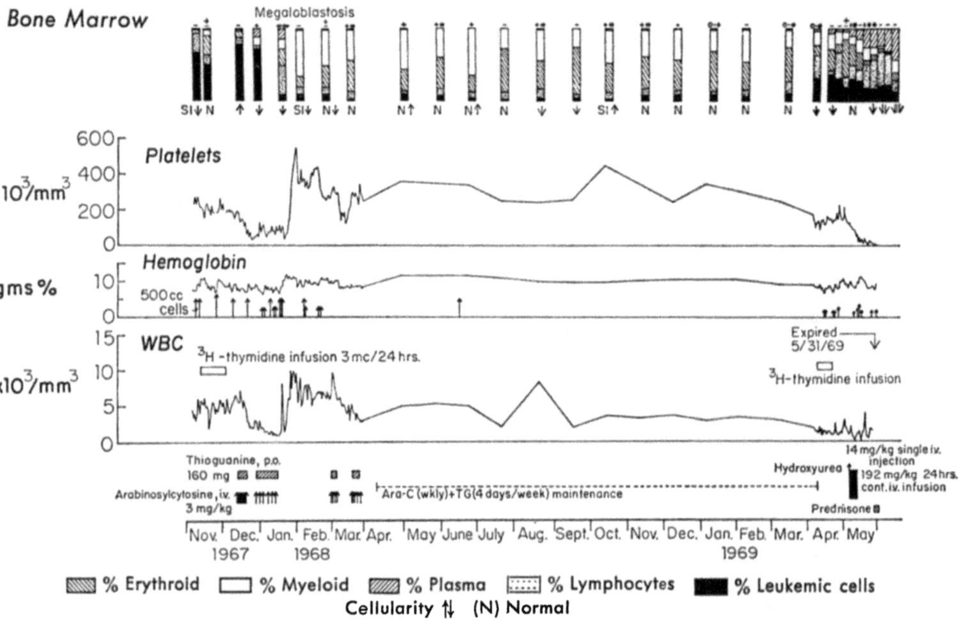

Fig. 7. Course of W. J. after October 1967. Diagnosis was established elsewhere in February 1967, but no treatment had been given except multiple blood transfusions

Cytokinetic Studies

Leukemic Cells. W. J.'s leukemic cells could be separated into 3 types based on their level of maturity (Fig. 8): I = most primitive blasts (small = I a; and large = I b); II = intermediate forms; and III = most mature forms recognizable. The Type I cells could of course not be distinguished from normal blasts. The division between large and small Type I cells was arbitrarily set at a nuclear diameter of 12 μ (nuclear area = 115 μ²). The flash ³H-TdR *(in vitro)* LIs of the leukemic cells are shown in Table 2. As in similar cases previously described (10,17), we have inferred that the Type III cells were no longer capable of dividing, owing to their mature appearance and zero flash LI.

The first ³H-TdR infusion was administered prior to any therapy in November '67 and continued without interruption for 21 days; the second infusion was given about 16 months after the first, shortly after his disease relapsed from a remission which had lasted about a year (Fig. 7).

During both continuous infusions, all mitoses (Types I and II cells combined) were labeled by the third day, and by the end of the first infusion 98% and 99% of

Table 2. *W. J.* *^{3}H-TdR labeling indices (LI) of marrow cells in vitro and in vivo, and median grain count (MGC) halving times after stopping ^{3}H-TdR infusion*

Cell type	Average differential during ^{3}H-TdR infusions Study I %	Study II %	Flash ^{3}H-TdR LI *(in vitro)* [a] Study I %	Study II %	LI at end of ^{3}H-TdR infusion *(in vivo)* Study I (21 days)	Study II (12 days)	MGC [b] halving time (hours) Study I	Study II
Leukemic cells								
Mitoses (Types I and II combined)			0	0	100	100	56	35
Interphase								
Total (marrow)	65	30	16.0	14.0	98	92	82	91
(blood) [c]	69	15	0	0	99	89	76	91
Type I a (marrow)	2	3	0	0	92	68	121	251
I b	8	6	35	21	99	95	53	54
II	52	19	14	18	99	97	76	97
III	3	1	0	0	98	90	79	149
Erythrocyte precursors	13	30						
Pronormoblasts	0.2	0.2	92	88	100	100	17	16
Basophilic	1.4	3.2	83	85	100	100	20	22
Polychromatic	4	13	46	51	100	97	28	26
Orthochromatic	7	14	0	0	98	92	45	28
Granulocytes	5	9						
Neutrophilic myelocytes	0.6	3.6	—	51	100	100	—	40
metas	2	2	0	0	} 100	} 97	—	} 69
bands	0.8	3	0	0			—	
polys	1.2	0.3	0	0			—	
Eosinophilic myelocytes	—	} 0.6	—	36	—	100	—	97
bands and polys			—	0	—	100	—	101

Table 2 (continued)

Cell type	Average differential during ^{3}H-TdR infusions Study I %	Study II %	Flash ^{3}H-Tdr LI (*in vitro*) [a] Study I %	Study II %	LI at end of ^{3}H-TdR infusion (*in vivo*) Study I (21 days)	Study II (12 days)	MGC [b] halving time (hours) Study I	Study II
Megakaryocytes								
Promegakaryocytes [d]	0.2 (all megakaryocytes)	1.0 (all megakaryocytes)	48 (promegakaryocytes and transitional mkc)	70	100	100	47 (all megakaryocytes)	57 (all megakaryocytes)
Transitional mkc with vacuolated cytoplasm				36	100	100		
Mkc with granular cytoplasm without platelets			0	0	100	100		
Mkc with platelets			0	0	100	100		
Lymphocytes	12	19	0	0	13	15	161	—
Plasma cells	5	8	2.0	4.0	39	47	111	130
Histiocytes	0.4	0.6	0	0	4	8	—	—

[a] Determined just prior to ^{3}H-TdR infusion.
[b] Use of the geometric mean grain count yielded similar results.
[c] Very few (large) type I b cells were found in the blood on either occasion.
[d] No megakaryoblasts were seen. See Fig. 11.

all interphase leukemic cells were labeled in marrow and blood respectively (Fig. 9 and Table 2). In Fig. 10, the different leukemic cell types are plotted individually. During the first infusion, the LI of the (large) Type I b cells rose fastest, while that of the (small) Type I a cells increased least rapidly. The MGC halving times of the mitotic and (large) Type I b cells were almost the same, while that of the (small) Type I a cells was significantly longer (Table 2). Although the Type III cells did not divide, their life span was sufficiently short so that their grain count decrease reflects the T_G of their precursors.

A lower percentage of leukemic cells was present during the second infusion and there were relatively more Type I and fewer Type II cells (Figs. 9 and 10, Table 2). The rate of labeling of the interphase leukemic cells was slightly slower than in the first study, and since the duration of the second infusion was only 12 days, the final LIs (especially of Type I a cells) were lower than at the end of the first infusion (Table 2). The MGC halving time of the mitoses was shorter, and those of the Type I a and Type III cells longer than those found in the first study, but because the method is not very precise, it is uncertain whether these differences are significant.

Because of the slow clinical progression of his disease, we had anticipated that W. J.'s leukemic cells would either have a very long T_G or that a relatively large fraction would be in a prolonged resting state. Since neither supposition proved correct, the most logical alternative explanation is that they must have had a high spontaneous death rate.

Normal Hematopoietic Cells

The differential counts and ^{3}H-TdR LIs of the normal precursors in the marrow and their MGC halving times are shown in Table 2, and their labeling pattern during the ^{3}H-TdR infusions in Fig. 11. As in J. T., the red cell precursors were dividing very rapidly. Not enough myelocytes were present at the time of the first study to obtain reliable data, but their labeling parameters during the second study indicate a fairly rapid turnover rate (Table 2). Only typical large normal myelocytes were counted to avoid confusion with the leukemic cells. The data on non-dividing granulocytes (metamyelocytes and later forms) were pooled because there were so few cells of each type; they have been plotted separately in prior studies [13]. The slower rate of labeling of eosinophilic myelocytes, their longer MGC halving times, and their slower rate of disappearance after the end of the infusion suggest that they divide more slowly than neutrophilic ones and also probably that mature eosinophils live longer than neutrophilic granulocytes; similar results have previously been found for basophils in chronic granulocytic leukemia [21].

Megakaryocyte precursors also showed a rapid rate of proliferation and maturation (Fig. 11). Since only the immature forms were labeled on flash exposure to ^{3}H-TdR (Table 2), the more mature cells apparently do not continue DNA synthesis, and the increasing lobulation of their nuclei is thus analogous to nuclear segmentation in polymorphonuclear leukocytes. Similar results have been reported for rat megakaryocytes [22—24].

Lymphocytes, plasma cells, and histiocytes (or their precursors) were clearly proliferating much less rapidly and had longer life spans as indicated by their rela-

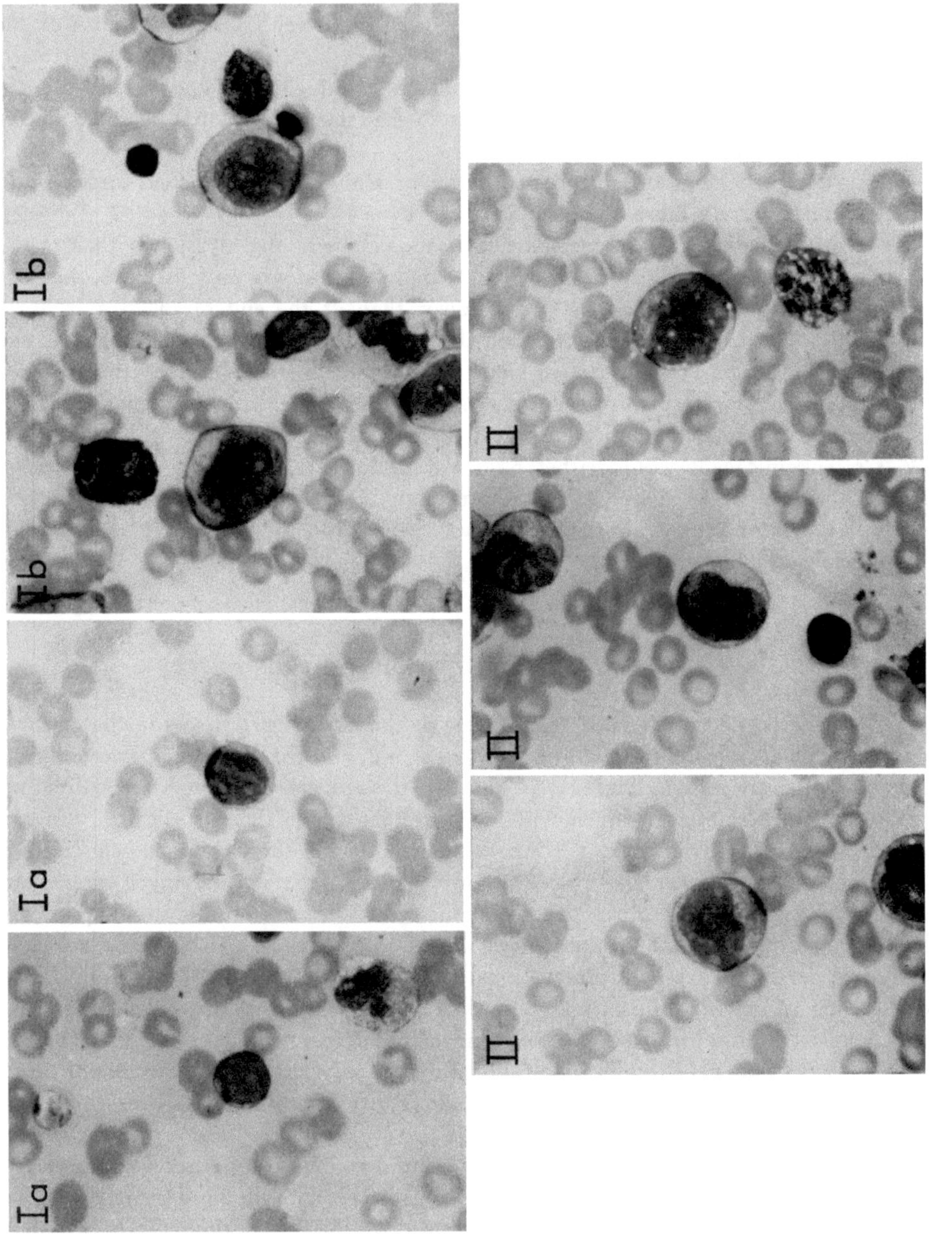
Ib
Ib
Ia
Ia
II
II
II

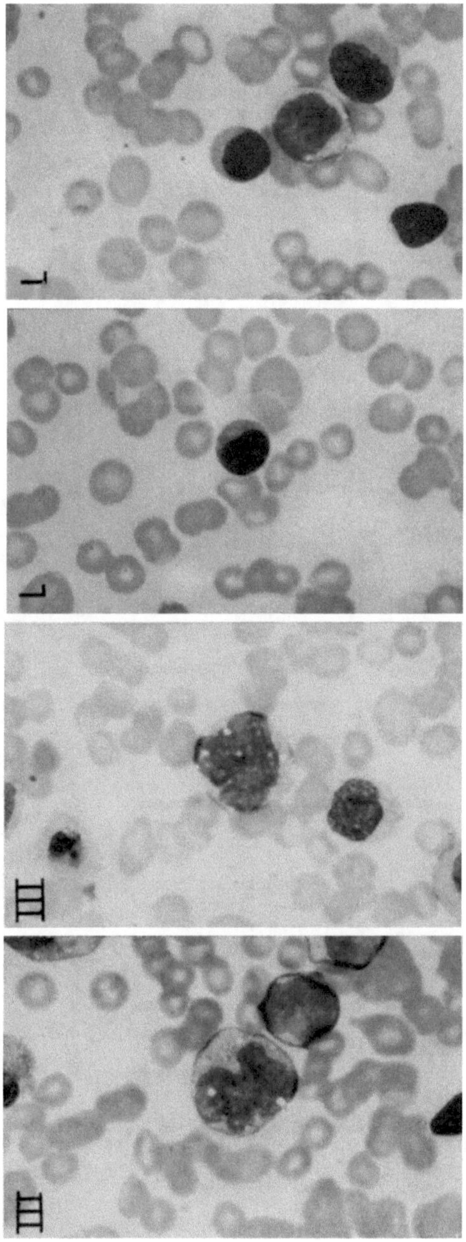

Fig. 8. Typical examples of 3 types of leukemic cells in W. J.: Two small (I a) and two large (I b) cells; three Type II cells; two Type III cells; two normal lymphocytes (L) (in center of photographs) for comparison. (For CLARKSON, B. D., et al.: Consideration of the cell cycle in chemotherapy of acute leukemia)

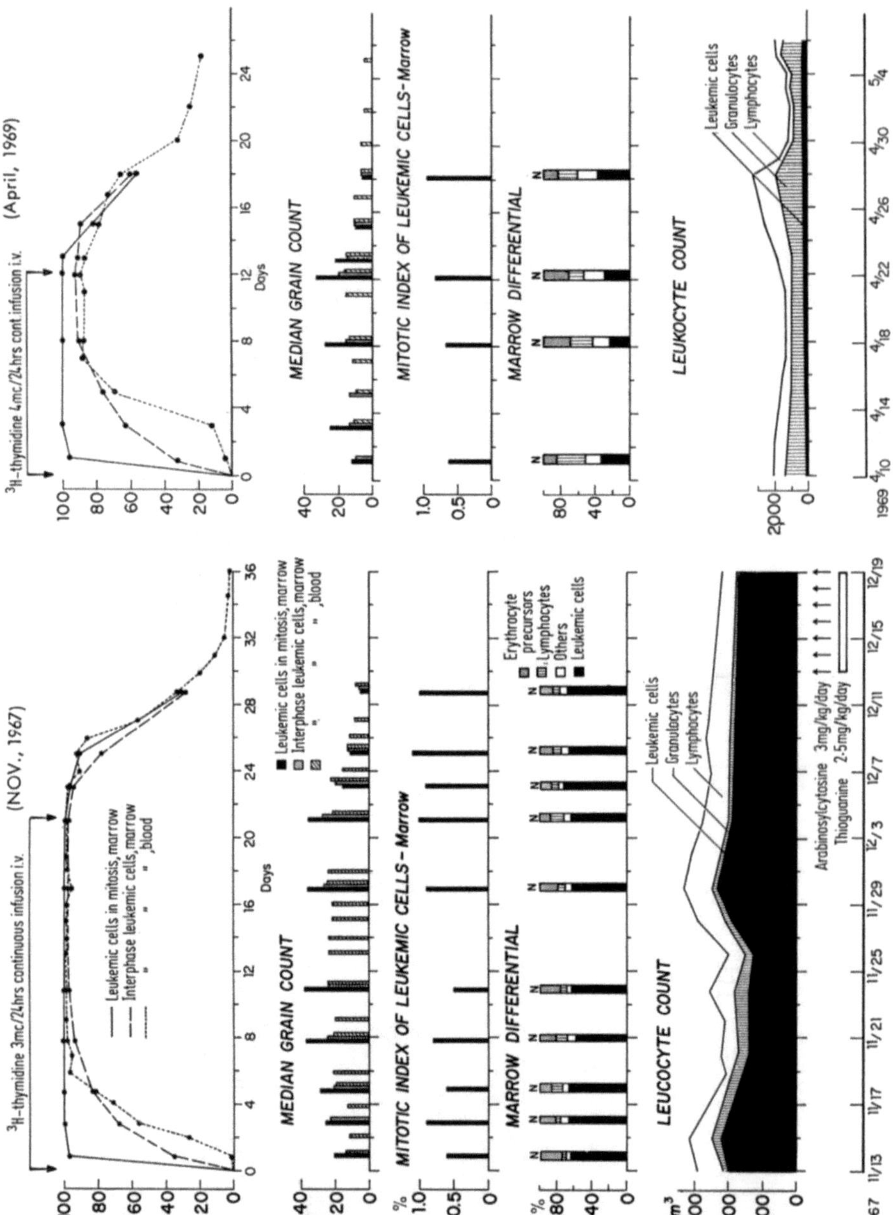

Fig. 9. Overall labeling pattern of total leukemic cells in W. J. in marrow and blood during and after continuous ³H-TdR infusion. The mitotic cells include both Types I and II cells as they could not be distinguished in the autoradiographs when in mitosis. The autoradiographs were exposed 20 weeks for the entire first study. For the second study, the labeling indexes were determined on autoradiographs exposed 20 weeks, but the grain counts were performed on autoradiographs exposed only 12 weeks because the latter were of superior quality

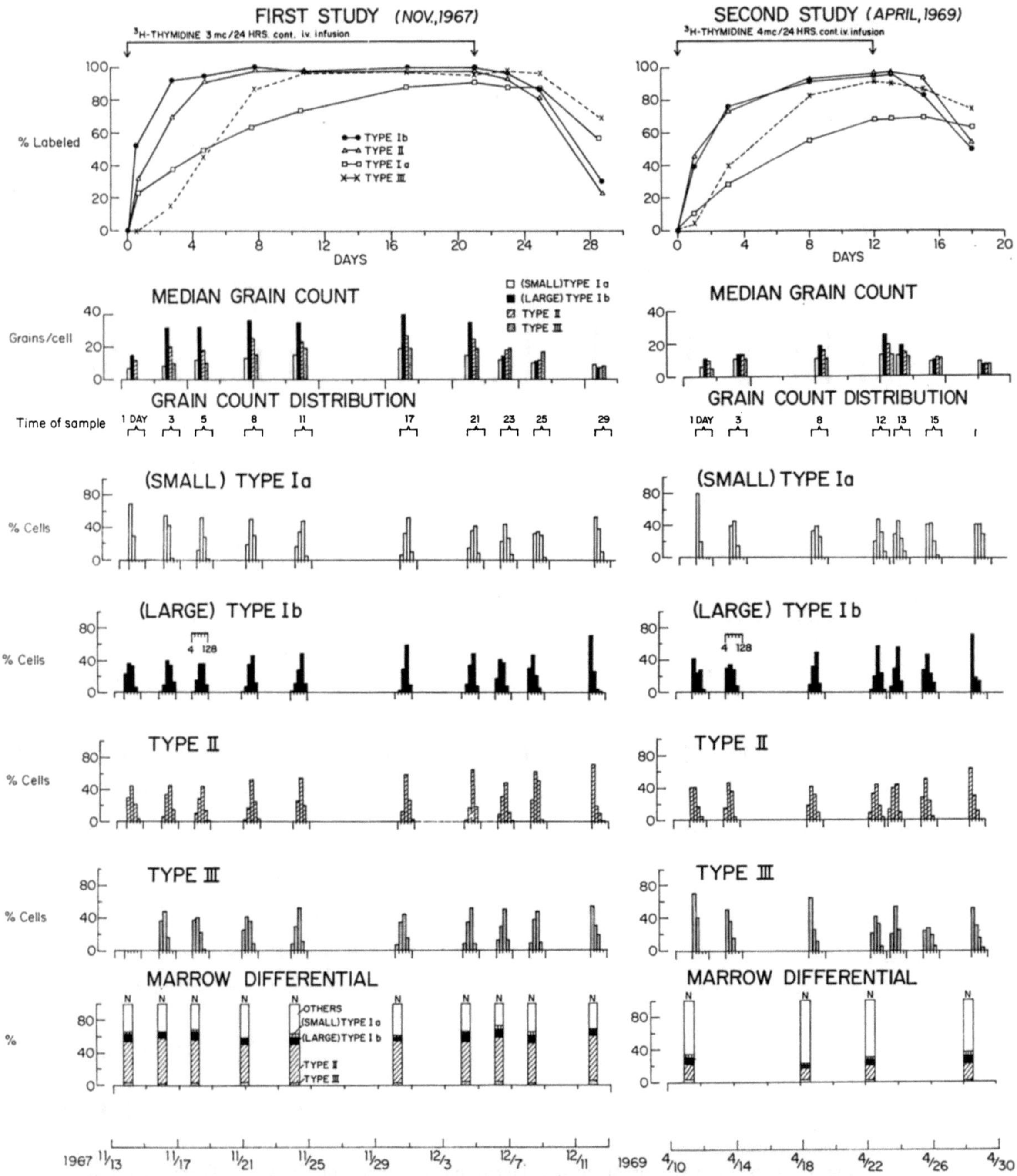

Fig. 10. Labeling patterns of 3 types of interphase leukemic cells in marrow of W. J. plotted individually. The grain count distributions are plotted from left to right in 5 groups: 4—8, 9—16, 17—32, 33—64, and 65—128 grains per nucleus. The average distribution of the different types of leukemic cells during the first and second ³H-TdR infusions were respectively: I a = 3.4 and 11%; I b = 11.6 and 23%; II = 80.5 and 61%; III = 4.5 and 5%. For autoradiographic exposure times, see legend of Fig. 9

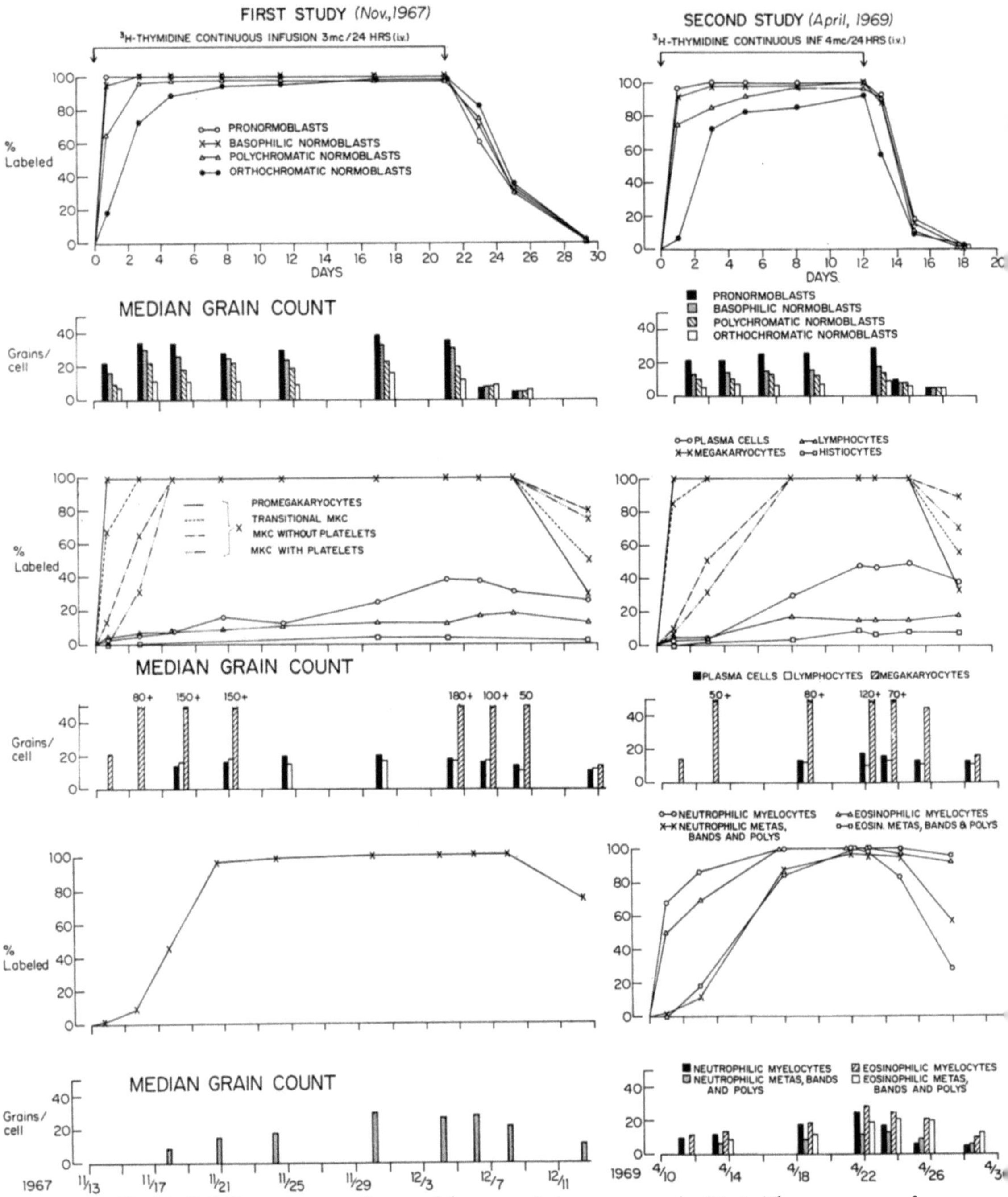

Fig. 11. Labeling patterns of normal hematopoietic precursors in W. J. There were too few normal myelocytes to obtain reliable data in the first study and earlier granulocyte precursors could not be distinguished from the leukemic cells. The megakaryocytes (mkc) are classified according to Diggs, L. W., Sturm, D., Bell, A.: The Morphology of Human Blood Cells. W. B. Saunders Co., 1956. Their distribution was: megakaryoblasts = 0; promkc = 7%; transitional mkc with vacuolated cytoplasm = 18%; mkc with granular cytoplasm without platelets = 42%; mkc with platelets = 21%; naked mkc nuclei = 12%

tively long grain count halving times and low LIs at the end of the infusions (Fig. 11, Table 2).

An increased percentage of plasma cells was present during both ^{3}H-TdR infusions (Table 2), but the reason is not known. There was no evidence of infection and the patient remained completely afebrile during both studies (until after chemotherapy). The serum gamma globulin was slightly and diffusely elevated and the liver function tests were normal. Serum and urine examined by Dr. LEONHARD KORNGOLD were negative for myeloma and Bence Jones proteins.

Less than 1% histiocytes was present on both occasions, but they exhibited prominent phagocytosis of cellular remnants; possibly this was related to the high spontaneous death rate of the leukemic cells.

Effect of Chemotherapy

Arabinosylcytosine and Thioguanine

Treatment was started 8 days after ending the first ^{3}H-TdR infusion, but the grain counts of the leukemic cells fell so rapidly below threshold that the effect of the drugs on the cells' T_G could not be measured (Fig. 9). Eight consecutive daily doses of both drugs were given [19] (Fig. 7), but 8 days after stopping therapy there was still about the same proportion (73%) of leukemic cells in the marrow as before treatment, although the marrow was much less cellular. He was then given 6 more doses of both drugs spaced at 3-day intervals; a marrow sample 2 days after the last dose (1/16/68) was still less cellular and contained only 9% leukemic cells and 23% erythrocyte precursors.

He developed severe thrombocytopenia and leukopenia and almost died as a result of a severe cellulitis of the left foot which progressed to gangrenous necrosis of the 3rd, 4th, and 5th toes and eventually necessitated open amputation of these toes (on 2/9/68). No antileukemic therapy was given during this period. After he recovered from the infection, the marrow (2/21/68) showed 9% leukemic cells and 34% erythrocyte precursors. Two short (4 and 5 day) "consolidation" courses of Ara-C and thioguanine were given in March (Fig. 7), following which he had a complete remission. During the next year he was given the same two drugs as maintenance therapy as often as tolerated [19], and the percentage of blasts in the marrow remained below 6% (blasts + monocytes = <10%) until 4/7/69 when 31% leukemic cells reappeared.

Hydroxyurea

Following the second ^{3}H-TdR study, he was given a continuous intravenous infusion of hydroxyurea (HU) for 119 hours at a dosage of 8 mg/kg/hour, immediately following an initial single "loading dose" of 14 mg/kg (Fig. 7). Blood levels obtained serially during this infusion showed a fairly constant drug level around 8—9×10^{-4} M. The patient developed severe ulcerative inflammation of the palate, pharynx and uvula, laryngitis, bronchopneumonia, a generalized petechial maculo-papular rash, proctitis and peri-anal ulcerations, and high spiking fever. Although no specific causative organism was identified, he was treated with multiple antibiotics. However he remained febrile and became progressively weaker and died in shock on 5/31/69. In addition to the lesions mentioned above, autopsy showed splenomegaly (450 gm) with increased connective tissue and infiltration of mononuclear cells, congestion and early periportal fibrosis of the liver, bilateral serous pleural effusions, and myocardial hypertrophy. The marrow was hypocellular.

The effects of HU on the leukemic and normal hematopoietic cells are shown in Figs. 7 and 12. The marrow became very hypocellular, but the percentage of leukemic cells fell only slightly; relatively more small (Type I a) blasts were present after HU

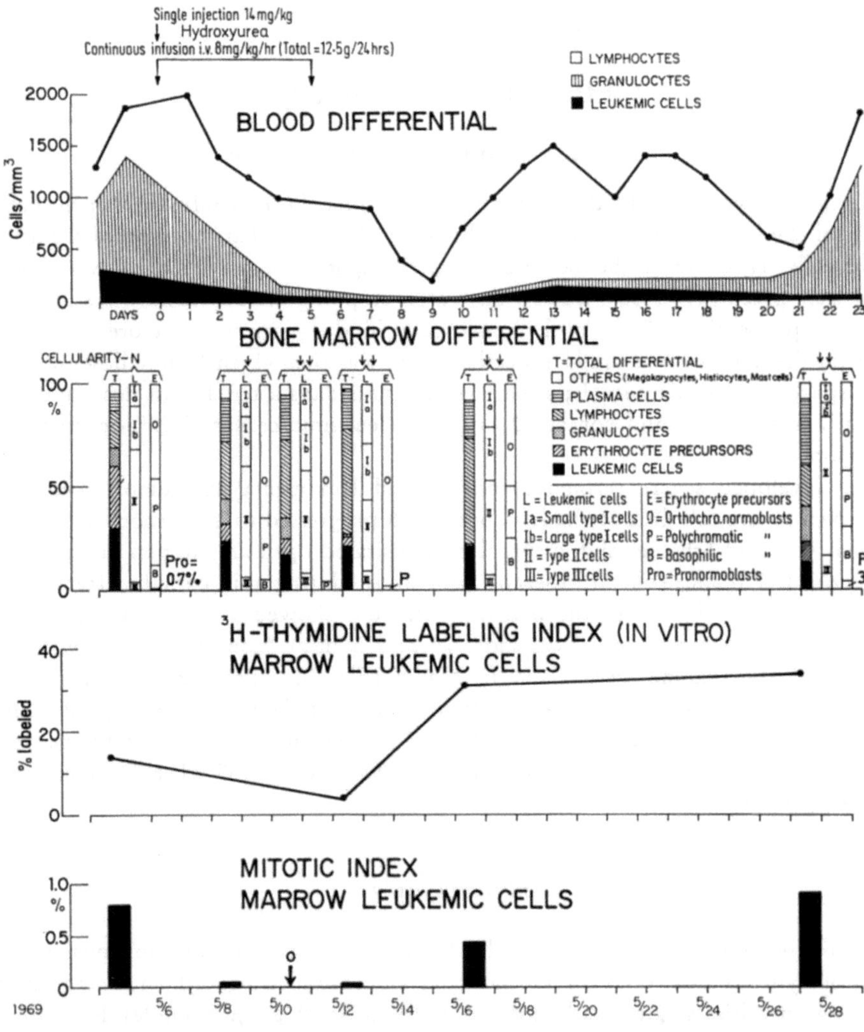

Fig. 12. Effect of 5 day infusion of hydroxyurea in W. J. on marrow cellularity and differential, and on flash *(in vitro)* ^{3}H-TdR LI and mitotic indices of marrow leukemic cells; too few remained after therapy to obtain reliable data for the different types of leukemic cells individually

(Fig. 12). The MI of the leukemic cells fell transiently to zero and their LI also decreased significantly, but both indices recovered rapidly. Five days after stopping the drug, the LI of the surviving leukemic cells was twice the pretreatment value, and both the LI and MI were still relatively high 2 weeks later; by this time the distribution of leukemic cells had again changed with fewer Type I and relatively more Types II and III cells.

The rapidly dividing normal precursors in the marrow also decreased rapidly following HU. The erythrocyte precursors fell from 30% to 1%, and the basophilic normoblasts and pronormoblasts disappeared entirely (Fig. 12). Myelocytes and later granulocytes also almost disappeared and the megakaryocytes fell from about 1% to zero (not shown in differentials). Five days after stopping HU, practically the only cells remaining aside from surviving leukemic cells were (slowly dividing) plasma cells, lymphocytes, and histiocytes.

Two weeks after stopping HU, the last marrow (4 days prior to death) showed that erythrocyte precursors (including 3.6% pronormoblasts) had begun to reappear as had normal granulocytes in both the marrow and blood. The proportion of leukemic cells had fallen to 13%, providing further evidence that the normal precursors were proliferating faster. The very high (30%) proportion of plasma cells at this time was presumably associated with his terminal infection; the serum gamma globulin rose to 5 gm% and immunoelectrophoresis showed normal Gamma-A and Gamma-M immunoglobulin levels but the Gamma-G was 3600 mg% (normal up to 1800 mg%).

Discussion

Before discussing the cytokinetics of human leukemia in relation to treatment, for comparative purposes some of the relevant basic principles that have been learned from the simpler L 1210 model system will be reviewed briefly.

Growth Characteristics and Chemotherapy of L1210 Leukemia of Mice

Skipper and his co-workers [1, 2, 4, 8] have demonstrated that a logarithmic relationship exists between the number of leukemic cells inoculated (from a single cell up to 10^6) and the time required to reach about 10^9 cells, which is a lethal number for the mouse. The inoculation of a single cell is known to cause death in about 15 days [8]; this corresponds to 30 generations required to reach 10^9 cells, for a population doubling time of about 12 hours. This is consistent with the results obtained by labeling methods, namely a generation time of about 12 hours (with relatively little variability) [7, 8]. Thus the growth fraction [25] is nearly 1.0, at least until the number of cells exceeds about 10^8. During early disease, the median duration of DNA synthesis is about 9 hours and therefore occupies about 75% of the cell cycle time [7]. Later in the course of the disease, the S-phase becomes slightly longer (10.7 hours), but the cell cycle time becomes proportionately even longer (21 hours), so that the S-phase then occupies only about 50% of the cell cycle [7].

If the disease is not too advanced (i. e., 10^6 or less cells), injection of effective lethal doses of arabinosylcytosine (Ara-C) every 3 hours for 24 hours (or about twice the median cell cycle time) will kill 99.99% or more of the cells (4 "log kill" or greater), and repeated courses of such treatment every 4 days will regularly provide cures [3, 4, 8, 9]. Repeated injections of Ara-C every 6 hours for 24 hours are still highly effective, but if the doses are spaced 9 hours or longer apart, no cures are effected [26]. Presumably this is because the duration of the S-phase is somewhat variable, and some cells are able to complete DNA synthesis in the interval between periods of effective blood drug concentration and hence escape being killed.

Hydroxyurea and several other S-phase specific drugs (e. g., guanazole, 5-hydroxy picolinaldehyde thiosemicarbazone) are also effective in curing early L 1210 leukemia when given in a similar treatment schedule, but a number of other antimetabolites (e. g., methotrexate, 6-mercaptopurine, and 5-fluorouracil), which cause a lethal inhibition of DNA synthesis but which also inhibit other metabolic pathways (i. e., protein or RNA synthesis), produce no cures. Skipper has postulated that this is because the latter effects are non-lethal, but may retard the rate of movement of cells from G_1 into S so that they are not killed [26].

It has not been possible to cure advanced L 1210 leukemia or spontaneous AK leukemia (which is advanced when diagnosed) with any treatment schedule using S-phase specific drugs. The growth fraction in such advanced leukemic populations is significantly less than 1.0. Some cells may die while others enter a resting state but retain the capacity to resume proliferation later; such resting cells are insensitive to drugs whose lethal action is restricted to S-phase events [2]. However, if the leukemic population is first substantially reduced by pretreatment with an agent which is not cell-cycle dependent (e. g., cyclophosphomide or 1,3-bis (2-chloroethyl), 1-nitrosourea), the residual disease is then quite sensitive to Ara-C [2, 5, 8, 9]. Presumably this is because the surviving cells, under lessened population pressure, are able to resume logarithmic growth; few cells persist in the (drug-insensitive) resting state and the growth fraction again approaches 1.0. Probably for the same reason, human hematopoietic cells in long-term established culture exhibit a similar increase in sensitivity to S-phase active drugs as they convert from stationary to log phase growth after their population density is lowered [27].

Cell Cycle in Human Leukemia

Killmann [28] has recently reviewed the proliferative kinetics of human leukemic cells in detail, and only the parameters of immediate relevance to therapy will be considered here. Most investigators [11, 29—34], on the basis of percent labeled mitoses curves, have obtained an estimate of DNA synthesis time of about 20 (16—22) hours for human leukemic cells *in situ* in the marrow (lymphoblastic and myeloblastic) [3]. These measurements were all made in patients whose marrows were fairly densely populated with leukemic cells. As in L1210 leukemia it is possible that the leukemic cells may have a shorter synthetic period during earlier disease when they

[2] There are undoubtedly other reasons for the failure to cure advanced disease, such as sequestration of leukemic cells in the brain and other sanctuaries where the drug may not penetrate in a lethal concentration.

[3] There have been several other reports [28, 35, 36] which indicate that the duration of the S-phase in acute leukemic cells may be much shorter (4.7 to 7 hours), but convincing evidence has not been published to substantiate these estimates.

are less crowded, perhaps closer to that reported for normal human erythrocyte and granulocyte precursors (13—16 hours) [31, 32]. However, because of the scarcity of blasts, their low mitotic index, and the inability to distinguish residual leukemic from normal blasts, it is almost impossible to obtain accurate measurements of S during early relapse.

In untreated patients, or in those not receiving chemotherapy during the study (which may temporarily cause prolongation as in J. T., Table 1, and in previous studies [11, 17, 18]), the *mean* generation time (T_G) has almost always been found to be between 2 and 10 days [10, 11, 17, 18, 28—31, 37—39]. Since in most patients in whom percent labeled mitoses curves were determined, no second wave of labeled mitoses was discernible, most of these T_G estimates are based on grain count halving methods similar to that used in the present studies. Only labeled cells are of course included in these measurements, but after continuous ^{3}H-TdR infusions of sufficient duration, the labeled cells constitute the majority of the population. The main objection that has been raised concerning the validity of the grain count-halving method is that the measured T_G includes cells which may have entered a resting phase following division of their parents. However, since there is substantial evidence that the resting state is only temporary and that the resting cells may later resume dividing [10, 39], it seems only reasonable that they should be included. The difference between the grain count halving times of the mitotic and interphase cells (before therapy), gives a rough indication of the magnitude of movement of actively proliferating cells into a (temporary) resting state. This apparently varies considerably in different patients and probably also in accordance with the stage of disease. In J. T., who had advanced disease and in whom the cells were proliferating very slowly, the grain count halving time of the interphase cells was twice that of the mitotic cells (Table 1), whereas in W. J., whose marrow was less impacted with leukemia and in whom the cells were dividing more rapidly, the MGC halving time of the mitoses and large primitive (Type I b) interphase blasts were similar (Table 2). Variable results in other patients have been reported previously [10, 39].

All of our studies [10, 11, 17, 18, 39, 40] have indicated that there is considerable variability in the generation time within any one population of leukemic cells. Since the durations of the S, G_2 and M phases appear to be reasonably constant (around 20, 2—3, and 1 hour(s) respectively), most of the variability occurs in G_1. That is, the cells remain in G_1 as "resting" cells for variable lengths of time [4].

Because of the variability in G_1 (and hence T_G), because of an unknown spontaneous death rate, and because of the lack of an accurate method to measure the doubling time of a human leukemic population *in vivo*, it is not possible to obtain a precise estimate of the growth fraction as in L 1210 leukemia. KILLMANN [28], on the basis of published data on human leukemia and using a variety of methods, has estimated that the growth fraction may be in the order of 13—35%. However these estimates were admittedly very crude and it was acknowledged that the growth

[4] The designation "G_0" will be avoided in this discussion because there is no accepted biochemical definition of the distinction between cells in a prolonged G_1 phase and those in G_0, nor any acceptable criterion of how long a cell must remain in a dormant state before being classified in G_0. Thus, until disproven by contrary information, we will assume that all long-term resting leukemic cells are in G_1, and that they either die or retain the potential to eventually resume dividing.

fraction probably changes during the course of disease. The traditional concept of growth fraction at any given moment in fact becomes much less meaningful if one's primary consideration is elimination of the entire leukemic population. In the latter instance it is essential to consider cells which are in a prolonged G_1 but which may later resume division. In the classical methods used to calculate the growth fraction, such cells are all assumed to be non-proliferating and thus the true (i. e., potential) growth fraction may be greatly underestimated.

The methods used to calculate T_G do not allow precise estimates of the extremes. However, it is unlikely that the minimum T_G is much less than about 18 hours, since this is the shortest T_G observed for human hematopoietic cells in culture during log phase growth [41]. It is almost certain that there is no distinct subpopulation of (large) cells which continue to divide at their most rapid potential rate for more than a few generations. If this were true, such cells would quickly outgrow the rest of the population and there is convincing evidence that this does not occur [10, 11, 39].

Regarding the upper limit of T_G, this is also unknown beyond the fact that it is almost certainly longer than 20 days, since a significant fraction of (apparently viable) cells were still unlabeled and therefore had remained in a prolonged G_1 phase for longer than the duration of the ^{3}H-TdR infusions. As in previous studies [10, 17, 18], almost all of these (unlabeled) long-term resting cells are small primitive cells. As none of the smallest cells are labeled on short-term exposure to ^{3}H-TdR (Fig. 4 and Table 2), it is probable that they must first attain a certain critical mass before they can begin DNA synthesis [10] [5]. The LI and median grain count of the small blasts rose gradually in both patients during the continuous ^{3}H-TdR infusions as unlabeled small cells grew and entered S and as new (labeled) small cells were formed after division of intermediate-sized cells (Figs. 4 and 10).

In W. J., the fraction of small resting (Type I a) cells was increased during the second ^{3}H-TdR study (Fig. 10) and they had a longer MGC halving time than at the time of the first study (Table 2). We have noted similar findings in one other patient (J. D.) who had received vigorous chemotherapy for over a year [17]. It is possible that protracted treatment leads to an increased proportion of small resting cells which remain in a resting state for extremely long periods, possibly functioning as a mechanism to enhance survival of the leukemic population. Further confirmation is obviously necessary, but if this postulate is true, it might account in part for the generally poorer therapeutic results during relapse from drug-induced remissions than upon first treatment. There may of course be other reasons, such as development of resistance to drugs which were initially effective.

Effect of Stage of Disease on Proliferative Activity

There are several reports [10, 30, 39, 42—44] which indicate that the proliferative activity of human leukemic cells may be greater during early than late disease. Higher flash ^{3}H-TdR LIs frequently occur during early relapse than at the time of diagnosis

[5] It is of course not possible to distinguish small leukemic blasts on morphological grounds from normal blasts, but because of their number and close association with the other leukemic cells, we have assumed they are all leukemic. It is probable that a significant number of leukemic stem cells (and perhaps also normal stem cells) are included within the "small blast" category, but there is as yet no proof of this.

when the disease is usually already advanced. The higher LIs during early relapse have been found to correlate with an increased percentage of large blasts [30, 43, 44] and, since the LI of the latter were found to remain fairly constant during different stages of disease, the decreased proliferative activity during advanced disease appears to be due to a larger fraction of small resting cells. Thus during late disease, although there are no accurate measurements, the growth fraction almost surely lessens significantly; KILLMANN [28] has come to the same conclusion.

As already indicated, it is as yet unknown whether the durations of the different phases of the cell cycle change with the stage of disease. However, if the resting or "extended G_1" phase is considered to be part of the mitotic cycle, this implies that the average duration of G_1 does increase significantly in late disease. If the resulting T_G distribution were bimodal [40], it would be meaningful to also consider whether the peak at shorter T_G's (corresponding to cells which spend only a relatively short time in G_1) changes with the stage of disease. However, in many cases there is no evidence for a second peak, and the experimental results may be consistent with a unimodal T_G distribution having a long tail towards higher T_Gs.

The spontaneous cell death rate also probably increases in late disease, as is true in most advanced experimental tumors, but again no direct measurements of this function have yet been made in human leukemia.

Application of Cytokinetic Principles to Chemotherapy of Acute Leukemia

It is apparent from the foregoing that the kinetic behavior of human leukemic cells is different in several crucial respects from that of long-transplanted L 1210 cells, and that these differences should be considered in formulating treatment schedules.

In most adults with acute leukemia, there are generally a trillion (10^{12}) or more leukemic cells at the time of diagnosis [45]. To bring about a complete remission [46], it is usually necessary to kill at least 99% (2 logs), and probably 99.9% when there is very extensive infiltration of the marrow and possibly other organs as in J. T. If a 2 log reduction occurs, the cells will return to their original number after only seven doublings; following a 3 log reduction, 10 doublings will be required. Since it is probable that there is a substantial spontaneous death rate and that only a relatively small fraction of the population (magnitude unknown) possesses unlimited proliferative potential (i. e., function as leukemic stem cells), it is probably not essential to actually achieve a 13 log reduction in order to eliminate the last cell. However, since we suspect that leukemic stem cells have a unique propensity for survival and that one or more of them is likely to persist among the last few survivors, we would guess that it is probably necessary to come close to this goal to achieve a cure [6].

[6] In this context, we have deliberately discounted hypothetical "host defense" mechanisms, since we consider it probable that human leukemia commonly originates from transformation of a single (stem) cell, and that this transformation bestows on it and its progeny the properties of unlimited proliferative potential coupled with relative unresponsiveness to normal homeostatic regulatory mechanisms. Whatever surveillance mechanisms might

(continued p. 112)

Since the duration of the S phase in human leukemic cells is about 20 hours (at least late in the disease), one *lethal* dose of an S-phase active agent per day should kill most of the cells transversing S and two doses spaced 12 hours apart should kill all of them. Providing isotopic conditions are adequate to label all cells in S, the configuration of the ascending LI curve of interphase cells during a continuous ^{3}H-TdR infusion gives some indication of the rate of movement of cells from G_1 into S. Division of labeled cells of course also contributes to the increase in LI, and in addition the curve is influenced by several other factors such as cell migration, maturation and death, and by cells which enter a prolonged resting (G_1) phase after division of their parents. The steepness of the curve varies in different patients [10, 17, 39] and possibly also during different stages of disease, although the latter is uncertain since serial infusions have not yet been done in individual patients. In any case, it is clear from inspection of the curve in J. T. (Fig. 2) that only about 60% of the interphase leukemic cells in the marrow are labeled after 9 days, and that one cannot logically expect to kill many more than this with 9 consecutive days of treatment with drugs whose lethal action is restricted to cells engaged in DNA synthesis. If there is a substantial spontaneous death rate it may of course not be necessary to continue treatment for as long as the corresponding time it takes for 99% of the cells to become labeled. Moreover, therapy probably alters the kinetics, i. e., as the rapidly dividing cells are selectively destroyed and the population density lowered, resting cells may be stimulated to enter the division cycle at an increased rate.

In J. T., the impact of therapy on the proliferative kinetics (Fig. 6) is difficult to interpret since prednisone probably killed cells in all phases of the cell cycle; it also probably slowed the rate of transition of resting cells (in G_1) into S, and therefore made them less susceptible to the 9 day course of Ara-C and thioguanine. The increasing labeling and mitotic indices (Fig. 6) indicate that the surviving leukemic cells were recovering rapidly when the second course of Ara-C and thioguanine was given, and the cells should have been quite sensitive. However, the duration of treatment was too short and the drug doses were probably sublethal so that little therapeutic effect occurred. In a previously reported case (G. S.), only about 80% of the leukemic cells were labeled after 9 days' continuous ^{3}H-TdR infusion (99% were labeled after 15 days), but 9 consecutive daily injections of Ara-C alone (at doses which were apparently lethal for her leukemic cells) caused a complete remission which lasted 2 months without maintenance therapy [39].

Ara-C and thioguanine in combination have been shown to be more effective than either drug alone [19], and it has been our experience that in order to induce complete remissions in most patients with these 2 drugs (given separately 6—8 hours apart), it has generally been necessary to continue treatment for 10 to 20 consecutive

---

(continued from p. 111)

normally be operative to dispose of such aberrant cells, they are presumably defective in patients who develop leukemia.

This may in truth be what leukemia is: To maintain a steady state, a given stem cell must normally (on the average) generate one daughter committed to differentiation after going through a limited number of divisions, and one daughter which remains as a stem cell in order to carry on the line. Instead, the transformed (leukemic) cell generates 2 daughters which both behave as stem cells, and the progeny of subsequent generations continues to have a greater than 1 : 1 ratio of stem : committed cells.

days (or nearly consecutive with no more than a few days' interruption). Since several billion leukemic cells may remain once "complete" remission is induced, repeated "consolidation" courses of therapy (with the same and/or other drugs) are recommended after the normal marrow elements have recovered in order to kill as many leukemic cells as possible.

W. J.'s leukemic cells were proliferating much faster than those in J. T., and it is probable that a substantial number were spontaneously leaving the active proliferative compartment as a result of maturation and death. On the eighth day of the first ^{3}H-TdR infusion, almost all the large blasts (Type I b) but only about 65% of the small ones (Type I a) were labeled (Fig. 10). Eight consecutive daily doses of Ara-C and thioguanine killed many cells but failed to cause a remission, but 6 more doses of both drugs spaced at 3 day intervals did induce a partial remission, probably as a result of killing Type I cells as they converted from resting (I a) to proliferative (I b) status. When W. J.'s disease relapsed, a 5 day infusion of hydroxyurea in high dosage almost certainly killed all proliferating leukemic cells, but those surviving shortly resumed proliferating before the patient had recovered from toxicity (Fig. 12).

We have treated over a dozen patients with acute leukemia with continuous infusions of (high dose) hydroxyurea or Ara-C for 4 or 5 days with similar results. All have developed moderate to severe toxicity and no remissions have occurred. On the other hand repeated 5 day infusions of Ara-C interrupted by treatment-free intervals have produced a fairly good remission rate [47], possibly because the growth fraction of the surviving cells increases and they are then more susceptible to subsequent courses of treatment. Our own results have been disappointing when we have deliberately tried to increase the growth fraction by reducing the population density [7] prior to beginning intensive chemotherapy. The best we have seen has been a doubling or at most a tripling of the mitotic and labeling indices. It is likely that the growth fraction is somewhat increased either by repeated short courses of therapy interspersed by treatment-free intervals or by non-interrupted daily consecutive treatment [8], but apparently neither regimen is fully effective in recruiting all resting cells into the (drug-sensitive) S phase. Certainly not all surviving (resting) cells begin immediately to proliferate synchronously once treatment is interrupted. They apparently retain their characteristic cell cycle (G_1) variability and continue to dribble slowly into S, but with a significant fraction remaining in G_1 for very extended periods; exactly how long is unknown and probably varies in different populations.

In acute myeloblastic leukemia, the available chemotherapeutic agents [48] have relatively little selectivity of action, and it is often impossible to continue treatment

[7] Attempts have been made to reduce the population density either by killing cells by pretreatment with 3—4 day infusion of hydroxyurea or Ara-C, or by repeated leukapheresis using an IBM cell separator. In patients with many circulating blasts, up to 3×10^{12} leukemic cells have been removed using the cell separator, but although the number of circulating blasts is greatly reduced, the population density in the marrow is apparently much less affected.

[8] It is technically almost impossible to obtain a reliable flash ^{3}H-TdR LI (of surviving cells) *during* effective chemotherapy. This is because many dead and dying cells are present and one cannot positively identify which cells are destined to survive. The MI characteristically drops to zero during antimetabolite therapy with S-phase active drugs since the proliferating cells are unable to complete S and therefore none reach mitosis. Other drugs (e. g., vincristine) of course may arrest cells in mitosis and the MI will increase transiently.

long enough to induce remission without prohibitive toxicity to rapidly dividing normal cells. The non-cell-cycle dependent agents are not very effective, and one is left with drugs which act primarily on proliferating cells. As is evident from the prior discussion, the rate of movement of leukemic cells from the non-vulnerable G_1 state into S is so slow, that it usually requires 10—20 days of therapy to kill the 2 logs necessary to achieve remission. This still usually leaves many billions of leukemic cells which can rather quickly repopulate the marrow before the normal hematopoietic precursors have recovered sufficiently to make it possible to resume treatment. In the meantime, the patient has a high risk of dying from infection or hemorrhage due to depletion of granulocytes and platelets.

In confirmation of previous work [13], the present studies have demonstrated that although they are reduced in number in acute leukemia, the remaining erythrocyte, granulocyte and megakaryocyte precursors are proliferating rapidly, probably at near maximum rates. Because of their faster proliferative rate, they are not only killed more rapidly than the leukemic cells by S-phase active drugs (Fig. 12), but after treatment is interrupted, they also may in some instances repopulate the marrow more quickly. There is indirect evidence [11, 13, 39] that normal hematopoietic stem cells are somehow inhibited by leukemic cells, although the mechanism of inhibition is unknown. During advanced leukemia a relatively large fraction of normal stem cells are probably in an inactive state (? G_1 or G_0) and hence are less vulnerable to drugs which act on proliferating cells. The inactive normal stem cells are quite comparable in this respect to the long-term dormant leukemic cells, and in fact the latter undoubtedly inherit this behavioral characteristic from their normal ancestor(s). Thus the problem of how to destroy the dormant leukemic cells while at the same time sparing sufficient normal stem cells and giving them enough time to repopulate the marrow remains a formidable one.

In lymphoblastic leukemia it is now relatively easy to induce remissions because the cells are more sensitive to the available agents [48]. Once a good remission has been accomplished in either type of leukemia, apparently the major remaining obstacle to achieving a cure is the problem of how to eliminate all the long-term resting leukemic cells. No way has yet been found to force them to reenter the division cycle, and even if some means were devised to do so, there is a strong probability that resting normal stem cells would also be stimulated. Some non-cell-cycle dependent agents are cytotoxic to resting as well as to proliferating cells [2, 5, 8, 9], and these agents are currently being used after remission has been induced. However, it is doubtful that doses large enough to destroy all leukemic cells can generally be tolerated. Until some better means is discovered, probably the best strategy at the present time is to continue aggressive treatment for many months after complete remission is induced, using intensive short courses of treatment interrupted by treatment-free intervals (as short as possible) to allow recovery of normal marrow elements. A number of drugs with proven anti-leukemic efficacy are now available, and to circumvent the development of resistance to any one, it would seem most logical to use combinations of drugs concurrently or sequential courses of treatment with different drugs with different mechanisms of action in as high dosage as tolerated. The aim of such continuing therapy is of course to kill as many of the residual leukemic cells as possible as they gradually reenter the drug sensitive proliferative state. At present, it is not known exactly what magnitude of "log kill" may be achieved by these means. However, on the assumption that some long-term resting leukemic cells may still persist despite several months of intensive "consolidation" therapy, our own current treatment protocols call for continuing less intensive chemotherapy for at least several years. Again in an attempt to avoid development of drug resistance, the design of the protocols is to use repeated short (4 to 5 day) courses of therapy with different drugs in sequence in as high dosage as tolerable. In order to prevent significant regrowth of the (presumed) surviving leukemic cells, the treatment courses are spaced as closely together as is compatible with maintenance of reasonable levels of the normal blood elements. Whenever possible, no more than 10—14 days is allowed to elapse between courses of therapy.

Acknowledgements

We are most grateful to the patients for permitting us to perform these kinetic studies. They were fully informed both verbally and in writing that they would derive no therapeutic benefit, but they consented willingly and endured the frequent marrow aspirations and other hardships associated with the ^{3}H-TdR infusions without complaint. We are also grateful to Mrs. Annabel Strife for compiling the data in Fig. 4 and to Dr. Frederick Philips and Dr. Sol Rubinow for helpful discussions and suggestions.

Summary

The similarities and differences in the proliferative kinetics of leukemic cells in experimental murine leukemia (L1210) and acute leukemia in man are discussed in relation to the greater difficulties encountered in treating the human disease. To illustrate the investigative methods used clinically, two representative cytokinetic studies are described in which the patients were given continuous intravenous infusions of ^{3}H-thymidine for 20 days and serial autoradiographic studies performed on their marrow and blood cells.

In early L1210 leukemia (i. e., 10^6 cells or less), almost all the leukemic cells are dividing with an S phase of about 9 hours and a fairly constant generation time of around 12 hours; it is thus relatively easy to kill them with an S-phase active drug such as arabinosylcytosine (i. e., 99.99% or 4 $\log_{10}$ cell kill during 24 hours' drug exposure). In human leukemia the disease is usually advanced when diagnosed (i. e., 10^{12} or more cells), and the leukemic cells are proliferating much less rapidly. G_1 is very variable, and a significant fraction of the cells remain in G_1 for at least several weeks, in which state they are invulnerable to such drugs. At least a 2 $\log_{10}$ cell kill is necessary to achieve a remission, but the cells' rate of conversion from G_1 to S is so slow that it generally takes at least 10 days of treatment with an S-phase active drug to kill 1 $\log_{10}$ (90%) of the cells. In some patients the leukemic cells have an appreciable spontaneous death rate, and the apparent cell kill may be higher than can be accounted for on the basis of the drug's cytotoxic effects. Because they are proliferating more rapidly than are the leukemic cells, the normal erythrocyte, granulocyte and megakaryocyte precursors are readily killed by such therapy, and the patient consequently has a high risk of dying from infection or bleeding. If he survives this critical period and a sufficient number of leukemic cells have been destroyed, the normal cells may repopulate the marrow faster than can the leukemic cells and a remission ensues. A possible strategy is suggested as to how it might be possible to destroy the residual leukemic cells after remission has been induced.

References

1. Skipper, H. E., Schabel, F. M., Jr., Wilcox, W. S.: Experimental evaluation of potential anticancer agents. XIII. On the criteria and kinetics associated with "curability" of experimental leukemia. Cancer Chemother. Rep. **35**, 1 (1964).
2. Schabel, F. M., Jr., Skipper, H. E., Trader, M. W., Wilcox, W. S.: Experimental evaluation of potential anticancer agents. XIX. Sensitivity of non-dividing leukemic cell populations to certain classes of drugs *in vivo*. Cancer Chemother. Rep. **48**, 17 (1965).
3. Kline, I., Venditti, J. M., Tyrer, D. R., Goldin, A.: Chemotherapy of leukemia L 1210 in mice with 1-β-D-arabinofuranosylcytosine hydrochloride. I. Influence of treatment schedule. Cancer Res. **26**, 853 (1966).
4. Skipper, H. E., Schabel, F. M., Jr., Wilcox, W. S.: Experimental evaluation of potential anticancer agents. XXI. Scheduling of arabinosylcytosine to take advantage of its S-phase specificity against leukemia cells. Cancer Chemother. Rep. **51**, 125 (1967).
5. Tyrer, D. D., Kline, I., Venditti, J. M., Goldin, A.: Separate and sequential chemotherapy of mouse leukemia L 1210 with 1-β-D-arabinofuranosylcytosine hydrochloride and 1,3-bis (2-chloroethyl)-1-nitrosourea. Cancer Res. **27**, 873 (1967).
6. Wheeler, G. P., Bowdon, B. J., Wilkoff, L. J., Dulmadge, E. A.: The cell cycle of leukemia L 1210 cells *in vivo* and *in vitro*. Proc. Soc. exp. Biol. (N.Y.) **126**, 903 (1967).
7. Yankee, R. A., De Vita, V. T., Perry, S.: The cell cycle of leukemia L 1210 cells *in vivo*. Cancer Res. **27**, 2381 (1967).
8. Skipper, H. E.: Cellular kinetics associated with "curability" of experimental leukemias. In: Perspectives in Leukemia. Eds.: W. Dameshek and R. M. Dutcher. New York-London: Grune & Stratton, p. 187, 1968.
9. Schabel, F. M., Jr.: In vivo leukemic cell kill kinetics and "curability" in experimental systems. In: The Proliferation and Spread of Neoplastic Cells. Baltimore: Williams and Wilkins, p. 379 (1968).
10. Clarkson, B., Fried, J., Strife, A., Sakai, Y., Ota, K., Ohkita, T.: Studies of cellular proliferation in human leukemia. III. Behavior of leukemic cells in three adults with acute leukemia given continuous infusions of ^{3}H-thymidine for eight to ten days. Cancer **25**, 1237 (1970).
11. Clarkson, B. D., Ohkita, T., Ota, K., Fried, J.: Studies of cellular proliferation in human leukemia. I. Estimation of growth rates of leukemic and normal hematopoietic cells in two adults with acute leukemia given single injections of tritiated thymidine. J. clin. Invest. **46**, 506 (1967).
12. Fried, J.: Estimating the median generation time of proliferating cell systems in steady state. Biophys. J. **8**, 710 (1968).
13. Clarkson, B. D., Fried, J., Strife, A., Sakai, Y., Ota, K., Ohkita, T., Masuda, R.: Studies of cellular proliferation in human leukemia. IV. Behavior of normal hematopoietic cells in three adults with acute leukemia given continuous infusions of ^{3}H-thymidine. Cancer **26**, 1 (1970).
14. Fried, J.: Mean, geometric mean, or median grain count in cell cycle studies. Exp. Cell Res. **59**, 447 (1970).
15. Philips, F. S., Sternberg, S. S., Schwartz, H. S., Cronin, A. P., Sodergren, J. E., Vidal, P. M.: Hydroxyurea I. Acute cell death in proliferating tissues in rats. Cancer Res. **27**, 61 (1967).
16. Nery, R.: The colorimetric determination of hydroxamic acids. The Analyst, the Journal of the Society for Analytical Chemistry **91**, 388 (1966).
17. Clarkson, B. D., Sakai, Y., Kimura, T., Ohkita, T., Fried, J.: Studies of cellular proliferation in human leukemia. II. Variability in rates of growth and cellular differentiation in acute myelomonoblastic leukemia and effects of treatment. In: The Proliferation and Spread of Neoplastic Cells. Baltimore: Williams and Wilkins Co. 1968, p. 295.
18. — Fried, J., Ogawa, M.: Magnitude of proliferating fraction and rate of proliferation of populations of leukemic cells in man. Monograph: Symposium on normal and malignant cell growth. In: Recent Results in Cancer Research, Vol. 17. New York: Springer 1969, p. 175.

19. GEE, T. S., YU, K.-P., CLARKSON, B. D.: Treatment of adult acute leukemia with arabinosylcytosine and thioguanine. Cancer **23**, 1019 (1969).
20. CLARKSON, B., KRAKOFF, I., BURCHENAL, J., KARNOFSKY, D., GOLBEY, R., OETTGEN, H., DOWLING, M., LIPTON, A.: Clinical results of treatment with E. coli L-asparaginase in adults with leukemia, lymphoma, and solid tumors. Cancer **25**, 279 (1970).
21. OTA, K., CLARKSON, B. D.: Unpublished observations.
22. FEINENDEGEN, L. E., ODARTCHENKO, N., COTTIER, H., BOND, V. P.: Kinetics of megacaryocyte proliferation. Proc. Soc. exp. Biol. (N. Y.) **111**, 177 (1962).
23. EBBE, S., STOHLMAN, F., JR.: Megakaryocytopoiesis in the rat. Blood **26**, 20 (1965).
24. ODELL, T. T., JACKSON, C. W.: Polyploidy and maturation of rat megakaryocytes. Blood **32**, 102 (1968).
25. MENDELSOHN, M. L.: Autoradiographic analysis of cell proliferation in spontaneous breast cancer of C3H Mouse. III. The Growth Fraction. J. nat. Cancer Inst. **28**, 1015 (1962).
26. SKIPPER, H. E.: Personal communication.
27. GEE, T. S., TODO, A., STRIFE, A., CLARKSON, B. D.: Effect of Hydroxyurea (HU) and arabinosylcytosine (Ara-C) on logarithmic (log) and stationary (stat) phase human lymphoid (SK-L7) cells *in vitro*. Proc. Amer. Ass. Cancer Res. **11**, 114 (1970).
28. KILLMANN, S.: Acute leukemia: the kinetics of leukemic blast cells in man. An analytical review. Ser. Haemat. **1**, 38 (1968).
29. OTA, K.: Kinetics of cellular proliferation in leukemia and cancer. Acta Haemat. Jap. **27**, 693 (1964).
30. SAUNDERS, E. F., LAMPKIN, B. C., MAUER, A. M.: Variation of proliferative activity in leukemic cell populations of patients with acute leukemia. J. clin. Invest. **46**, 1356 (1967).
31. TODO, A.: Proliferation and differentiation of hematopoietic cells in hematologic disorders. III. In vivo radioautographic study of leukemia including erythro-leukemia. Acta Haemat. Jap. **31**, 947—966 (1968).
32. STRYCKMANS, P. A., CRONKITE, E. P., FACHE, J., FLIEDNER, T. M., RAMOS, J.: DNA synthesis time of erythropoietic and granulopoietic cells in human beings. Nature **211**, 717 (1966).
33. GAVOSTO, F., PILERI, A., GABUTTI, V., MASERA, P.: Cell population kinetics in human acute leukemia. Europ. J. Cancer **3**, 301 (1967).
34. KEISER, G., WAGNER, H. P., FREY-WETTSTEIN, M.: Cytokinetic studies in two acute lymphoblastic leukemias. Helv. med. Acta **34**, 155 (1968).
35. MAUER, A. M., FISCHER, V.: Characteristics of cell proliferation in four patients with untreated acute leukemia. Blood **28**, 428 (1966).
36. LALA, P. K., MALONEY, M. A., PATT, H. M.: Measurement of DNA-synthesis time in myeloid-erythroid precursors. Exp. Cell Res. **38**, 626 (1965).
37. CLARKSON, B., OHKITA, T., OTA, K., O'CONNOR, A.: Studies of cellular proliferation in acute leukemia. J. clin. Invest. (abstract) **44**, 1035 (1965).
38. OGAWA, M.: Studies of cellular proliferation in acute leukemia using H^3-thymidine. Nagoya Med. Assoc. J. **90**, 91 (1967).
39. Clarkson, B. D.: Review of recent studies of cellular proliferation in acute leukemia. In: Human Tumor Cell Kinetics. Ed.: S. PERRY. Bethesda (Md.): National Cancer Institute (Monograph No. 30), p. 81 (1969).
40. FRIED, J.: A proposal for the determination of generation time variability and dormancy of proliferating cell populations by a modification of the grain count halving method. (Submitted to J. theor. Biol.)
41. TODO, A., FRIED, J., CLARKSON, B.: Kinetics of proliferation of human hematopoietic cells in suspension culture. Proc. Amer. Ass. Cancer Res. **10**, 93 (1969).
42. SCHMID, J. R., OECHSLIN, R. J., FRICK, P. G., MOESCHLIN, S.: Cell proliferation in leukemia during relapse and remission. II. DNA synthesis of leukemic cells in the peripheral blood in vitro. Acta Haemat. (Basel) **37**, 16 (1967).
43. PILERI, A., GABUTTI, V., MASERA, P., GAVOSTO, F.: Proliferative activity of the cells of acute leukemia in relapse and in steady state. Acta Haemat. (Basel) **38**, 193 (1967).
44. FOADI, M. D., COOPER, E. H., HARDISTY, R. M.: Proliferative activity of leukemic cells at various stages of acute leukemia of childhood. Brit. J. Haemat. **15**, 269 (1968).

45. FREI, E., III, FREIREICH, E. J.: Progress and perspectives in the chemotherapy of acute leukemia. In: Advances in Chemotherapy. Eds.: A. GOLDIN, F. HAWKING, and R. J. SCHNITZER. New York: Academic Press 1965, p. 269.
46. CLARKSON, B. D.: Clinical techniques for evaluating antileukemic efficacy. In: Animal and Clinical Pharmacologic Techniques in Drug Evaluation, Vol. 2. Eds.: P. E. SIEGLER, and J. H. MOYER, III. Chicago: Year Book Med. Publ. Inc. 1967, p. 836.
47. BODEY, G. P., FREIREICH, E. J., MONTO, R. W., HEWLETT, J. S.: Cytosine arabinoside (NSC-63878) therapy for acute leukemia in adults. Cancer Chemother. Rep. **53**, 59 (1969).
48. HENDERSON, E. S.: Treatment of acute leukemia. Seminars in Hematology **6**, 271 (1969).

Current Status of Therapy for Acute Leukemia[1]

Emil J Freireich, Gerald P. Bodey, Jacqueline S. Hart, John P. Whitecar, Jr., and Kenneth B. McCredie

Therapy for acute leukemia has improved so rapidly in the last 22 years that many clinical investigators are evaluating therapy regimens designed to be curative rather than merely palliative [1, 2, 3]. For the childhood form of acute lymphoblastic leukemia (ALL) the frequency of induction of at least one complete hematological remission is in excess of 85 per cent. Virtually every child with ALL treated with vincristine and prednisone with or without addition of a drug such as 6-mercaptopurine will demonstrate complete regression of all evidence of disease. This is associated with complete recovery of bone marrow function resulting in normal levels of the formed elements of the blood within 3 to 5 weeks following diagnosis. Chemotherapy has such a high degree of selectivity for the tumor that remission induction can be accomplished with little morbidity and virtually no mortality. The requirements for supportive therapy are minimal in the majority of children. The exceptional failures are recorded only in children with established, irreversible complications such as hemorrhage and infection. Thus, the job of inducing remission of disease for ALL is virtually accomplished.

However, if therapy is discontinued when children achieve complete remission, the disease recurs rapidly with virtually all children having recurrent disease in less than 9 months. The rapid recurrence of disease coupled with studies of cytogenetics, histopathological studies, and kinetic data indicate that the child in remission has persistent leukemic cells. Thus, chemotherapy for the patient in complete remission is strongly indicated. Maintenance chemotherapy given during remission can greatly prolong the duration of remission.

These findings in childhood acute lymphoblastic leukemia encourage therapy regimens designed to eradicate residual disease. Continuation of intensive chemotherapy analogous to remission induction therapy over periods of 3 to 4 months followed by discontinuation of therapy resulted in substantial prolongation of remission and in prolongation of the time required for recurrence of disease following discontinuation of therapy [4]. These studies indicated that such remission induction

---

[1] The University of Texas M. D. Anderson Hospital and Tumor Institute at Houston, Department of Developmental Therapeutics, 6723 Bertner Avenue, Houston, Texas 77025. — Supported in part by Grants No. CA 10376 and CA 05831 and CA 03754 from the National Cancer Institute, National Institutes of Health, U. S. Public Health Service, Bethesda, Maryland 20014.

therapy given early in remission can significantly reduce residual disease. In subsequent studies, periods of intermittent reinduction type of chemotherapy were extended to periods of 12 to 13 months. These studies also indicated further prolongation of duration of remission and in addition the interval between discontinuation of therapy and the recurrence of disease was further prolonged by this period of continuous reinduction and maintenance therapy [4, 5]. Combining techniques of remission maintenance and continuous reinduction of remission for a variety of agents have continued to result in significantly longer periods of remission and the appearance of detectable 5-year survival rates from several centers [1, 2, 5, 6, 7, 8].

Thus, chemotherapy for the childhood form of acute lymphoblastic leukemia has resulted in substantial palliation with median survivals in excess of 3 years being reported from many series and the occurrence of a detectable 5-year survival rate.

Table 1. *Acute myelocytic leukemia in adults: Remission induction by treatment program*

Patient categories	Ara-C	Ara-C + cyclo-phosphamide	COAP [a]	Total
Time of study	1966—1967	1967—1968	1968—1970	1966—1970
Total entered	16	40	33	89
Adequate trial [b]	13	34	25	72
Adequate trial/total entered	82%	85%	76%	81%
Complete remission (CR)	5	16	14	35
CR/adequate trial	45%	47%	56%	49%
CR/total entered	31%	40%	42%	39%

[a] COAP = cyclophosphamide, vincristine, Ara-C, prednisone.
[b] Adequate trial — 6 or more weeks of treatment.

However, the results of similar chemotherapeutic agents for acute myeloblastic leukemia (AML) have been significantly less effective at all ages. The two agents with the highest specificity for the control of ALL, vincristine and prednisone, have minimal efficacy in AML. Fortunately, AML constitutes less than 15 per cent of the patients with acute leukemia under the age of 15. However, it is the predominant form of acute leukemia in adults, over 85 per cent of patients over 15 years of age having AML. Prior to 1965 less than 15 per cent of patients with AML achieved complete remission as a result of therapy with thiopurines. However, in 1966 studies with cytosine arabinoside (Ara-C or Cytosar) indicated a sharp increase in the frequency of remission induction in AML [9] (Table 1).

Cytosine arabinoside offers important advantages for the therapy of adults with AML. The side effect associated with the use of this drug is primarily myelosuppression and even at high doses only a low degree of toxicity to other major organs such as the gastrointestinal tract and liver can be observed. Secondly, the drug has an extremely short *in vivo* biological half-life and as a result is sensitive to variations of schedule. The drug lends itself to utilizing the kinetics of leukemic cell proliferation, for designing therapy with greater selectivity. In a recent study from the Southwest

Cancer Chemotherapy Study Group it was found that the remission rate was significantly higher (p less than 0.05) when the drug was administered by continuous infusion over a period of 120 hours than when the drug was given continuously over 48 hours [10] (Table 2).

Another important property of cytosine arabinoside is the demonstration in experimental systems of true therapeutic synergism between Ara-C and the thiopurines,

Table 2. *Effect of schedule on response of adult acute leukemia to Ara-C*

Schedule	Patients entered [a]		Adequate trials [c]	
	No.	% CR[b]	No.	% CR
48 hours	83	17	44	32
120 hours	79	32	46	54
Total	162	24	90	43

[a] Evaluable patients. [b] Complete remissions.
[c] 3 Evaluable courses or 6 weeks.

or alkylating agents, such as cyclophosphamide, or nitrosoureas. We initiated studies of the combination of Ara-C and cyclophosphamide; after study of 40 consecutive patients (Table 1) we found an overall complete remission rate of 40 per cent [11]. These results encouraged us to evaluate a 4-drug combination (COAP) where vincristine and prednisone were added in full therapeutic dosage to the combination of Ara-C and cyclophosphamide. These 2 drugs could be added in full therapeutic dose without significantly enhanced myelosuppressive toxicity. The regimen is outlined in Table 3. Four-day courses of therapy were repeated at approximately 2-week intervals or when recovery from myelosuppression permitted another course of therapy.

Table 3. *COAP schedule*

Cytoxan	120 mg/M²/d q 8h IV x 4 days
Oncovin	2 mg IV on day 1
Ara-C	120 mg/M²/d q 8h IV x 4 days
Prednisone	200 mg/d orally X 4 days

The results of this pilot study are shown in Table 1. The COAP therapy resulted in further improvement in the response rate. Considering the period 1966—1970 for 89 consecutive patients with AML in adults, we had an overall response rate of 40 per cent (Table 1). The significant improvement in remission induction frequency was also reflected in a high fraction of patients who received an adequate trial, i. e., 6 weeks or more of therapy (81 per cent). Thus, inadequate trials, frequently due to early deaths in the first 6 weeks, were infrequent. The frequency of an inadequate trial was reduced to less than half of the values reported prior to 1965.

The effect of morphologic diagnosis on response of adults with acute leukemia to COAP therapy is shown in Table 4. The response rate was slightly but not significantly higher in acute lymphoblastic leukemia. It has been found that age has a significant effect on response to therapy [12]. Similarly for COAP therapy, the response rate decreased with increasing age and a disappointingly low response rate was observed in patients over 65 (Table 5). This effect of age was observed for both AML and ALL (Table 6).

Table 4. *Results of COAP therapy in patients with acute leukemia*

	Patients entered	Adequate trial	Complete remission	Response
Acute myelogenous	32	23 (72%)	12 (37%)	16 (50%)
Acute lymphocytic	17	16 (94%)	10 (59%)	14 (82%)
Acute undifferentiated	2	1 (50%)	1 (50%)	1 (50%)
Total	51	40 (79%)	23 (45%)	31 (61%)

Table 5. *Effect of age on response to COAP therapy in adult acute leukemia*

	Patients entered	Adequate trial	Complete remission	Response
< 35 years	20	17 (85%)	14 (70%)	17 (85%)
35—65 years	25	20 (80%)	9 (36%)	13 (52%)
> 65 years	6	3 (50%)	0	1 (17%)
Total	51	40 (79%)	23 (45%)	31 (61%)

Table 6. *Relationship of age and morphologic classification on the response to COAP therapy*

Age range	Acute myelogenous		Acute lymphocytic	
	No. of patients	Complete remission	No. of patients	Complete remission
< 35 years	9	56%	11	73%
35—65 years	18	39%	5	40%
> 65 years	5	0%	1	0%

For the COAP study, 17 of the 23 patients who achieved complete remission are still in remission and are being followed at the present time. The maximum duration of remission is 16 months and the patient is still in remission. If all patients presently in remission were to relapse today the median duration of remission would be 6¾ months. The median duration of remission projected by a life table analysis is 12 months.

These data indicate a dramatic change in the outlook for patients with AML. The increasing frequency of complete response will now permit initiation of clinical studies designed for prolongation of remission and for continuous reinduction of remission and thus, the potential eradication of residual disease [13].

In addition to the results with the combination of Ara-C and cyclophosphamide, improved response rates have been reported with the combination of Ara-C and thioguanine [14, 15].

Between 30 and 40 per cent of patients with acute leukemia have chromosome abnormalities which indicate a clonal origin. Thus, the majority of mitoses identified in the marrow contain identical cytogenetic abnormalities. Among patients with acute leukemia, each patient has a unique or different type of abnormality, indicating that a cytogenetic abnormality is associated with the leukemic cells. Following chemotherapy which results in cytologic and hematologic evidence of complete remission, repeat cytogenetic study indicates disappearance of the leukemic clone with recovery of the normal diploid clone [16]. These findings were originally reported in childhood lymphoblastic leukemia but with improving frequency of complete remission in adults similar findings have also been reported. Of 8 patients with adult acute leukemia who had cytogenetically identifiable clones of leukemic cells prior to therapy, 7 had disappearance of leukemic clones following therapeutically induced complete hematological remission [17]. In patients who have recurrence of their leukemic disease the cytogenetically abnormal line present prior to therapy reappears. Three patients with acute granulocytic leukemia showing disappearance of an aneuploid line have now been followed through recurrent disease and have also shown recurrence of the original cell line. These studies indicate that remission is associated with a sharp reduction in leukemic cell population of greater than 99 per cent associated with recovery of normal diploid marrow. At recurrence of acute leukemia virtually all patients who have been carefully studied reveal recurrence of the original tumor. Thus recurrence results from persistence of a small quantity of leukemic cells.

The high degree of effectiveness and specificity of the chemotherapy, although still primarily palliative, encourages further study aimed at eradication of the cellular phase of acute leukemia. Not only identification of new chemotherapeutic agents, but improvement in the tactics used with agents already established to be effective, such as alterations of schedule and use of combination and sequential chemotherapy, are areas being actively pursued by the clinical investigator. In addition, improvements in supportive therapy of leukemia patients such as control of infections with antibiotics and chemotherapy, the control of hemorrhagic complications by platelet transfusion and the prevention of infection with controlled environments are areas of supportive therapy which can extend the therapeutic index of existing compounds and provide additional approaches to the eventual control of this disease [18]. The potential for replacement of leukocytes by transfusion for both granulocytes and lymphocytes, the potential for allogeneic bone marrow transplantation to support the patient's bone marrow function temporarily through periods of intense myelosuppression and the exciting possibilities for immunotherapy provide additional leads for extending the therapeutic index for existing agents. Thus, the current status of the therapy for acute leukemia reflects a rapidly evolving and rapidly improving prognosis. Effective palliation with low morbidity is available for virtually every patient with this diagnosis. Frequency of complete response and the prolongation of effective life is clearly established and is optimal in the younger age groups. There seems to be little basis for pessimism or skepticism when approaching the therapy of a disease which only 22 years ago was uniformly fatal and hopeless. The results to date justify an optimistic approach to the therapy of every patient with acute leukemia.

Summary

The improved effectiveness of chemotherapy for induction and maintenance of complete remissions in childhood acute leukemia have encouraged clinical studies having the objective of eradication of the cellular phase of leukemia. For adult acute leukemia, the effectiveness of arabinosyl cytosine for remission induction has renewed the potential for combination chemotherapy. Remission induction rates in excess of 40 per cent of patients treated are reported for several regimens and combinations with arabinosyl cytosine. Age has a profound effect on response rate, the younger the patient the higher the frequency of response. This has encouraged clinical studies in young adults having the objective of eradication of residual leukemia cells. Thus, chemotherapy results in significant palliation of patients with acute leukemia and the potential for long-term control of this disease has continued to improve.

References

1. Holland, J. F.: Who should treat acute leukemia? J. Amer. med. Ass. **209** (10), 1511 (1969).
2. Burchenal, J. H.: Success and failure in present chemotherapy and the implication of asparaginase. Cancer Res. **29**, 2262 (1969).
3. Freireich, E. J., Bodey, G. P., Hart, J. S., Trujillo, J., Hersh, E. M., Curtis, J. E., Whitecar, J. P., Jr., Frei, E., III: Potential for eradication of the cellular phase of acute leukemia. In: Progress in Antimicrobial and Anticancer Chemotherapy. Proceedings of the 6th International Chemotherapy Congress, University of Tokyo Press, Tokyo, 1970, pp. 645—649.
4. — Henderson, E. S., Karon, Myron, Frei, E., III: The treatment of acute leukemia considered with respect to cell population kinetics. In: Proliferation and Spread of Neoplastic Cells, The University of Texas M. D. Anderson Hospital and Tumor Institute at Houston, 21st Annual Symposium on Fundamental Cancer Research. Baltimore (MD): Williams and Wilkins Co. 1968, pp. 441—453.
5. Henderson, E. S.: Treatment of acute leukemia. Seminars in Hematology **6**, 271 (1969).
6. Burchenal, J. H.: Long term survivors in acute leukemia and Burkitt's tumor. Cancer (Philad.) **21**, 595 (1968).
7. Jacquillat, Cl., Weil, M., Tanzer, J., Najean, Y., Boiron, M., Bernard, J. L.: Long term survival in 65 cases of acute leukemia. Proceedings of the American Association for Cancer Research **11**, 40 (1970).
8. Zuelzer, W. W.: Therapy of acute leukemia in childhood. In: Proceedings of the International Congress on Leukemia-Lymphoma. Ed.: C. J. Zarafonetis. Philadelphia: Lea and Febiger 1968, pp. 451—461.
9. Bodey, G. P., Freireich, E. J., Monto, R. W., Hewlett, J. W.: Cytosine arabinoside therapy for acute leukemia in adults. Cancer Chemother. Rep. **53**, 59 (1969).
10. Bickers, J. N., Freireich, E. J., Wilson, H. E., Stuckey, W. J., Jr., Coltman, C. A., Jr., Hewlett, J. W., Van Slyck, E.: Arabinosyl cytosine (ARA-C) in acute leukemia in adults: Effect of schedule on therapeutic response. SWCCSG. (In preparation.)
11. Bodey, G. P., Rodriguez, V., Hart, J., Freireich, E. J.: Therapy of acute leukemia with the combination of arabinosyl cytosine and cyclophosphamide. Cancer Chemother. Rep. **54**, 255 (1970).

12. FREIREICH, E. J., BODEY, G. P., HARRIS, J. E., HART, J. S.: Therapy for acute granulocytic leukemia. Cancer Res. 27, 2573 (1967).
13. WHITECAR, J. P., JR., BODEY, G. P., FREIREICH, E. J.: Combination chemotherapy (COAP) of adult acute leukemia. Proc. Amer. Ass. Cancer Res. 11, 83 (1970).
14. GEE, T. S., YU, K. P., CLARKSON, B. D.: Treatment of adult acute leukemia with arabinosyl cytosine and thioguanine. Cancer (Philad.) 23, 1019 (1969).
15. HOLLAND, J.: Leukemia Group B Preliminary Report.
16. REISMAN, L. E., MITANI, M., ZUELZER, W. W.: Chromosome studies in leukemia. I. Evidence for the origin of leukemic stem lines from aneuploid mutants. New Engl. J. Med. 270, 591 (1964).
17. HART, J. S., SHIRAKAWA, S., TRUJILLO, J., FREI, E., III: The mechanism of induction of complete remission in acute myeloblastic leukemia in man. Cancer Res. 29, 2300 (1969).
18. FREIREICH, E. J., BODEY, G. P., DEJONGH, D. S., CURTIS, J. E., HERSH, E. M.: Supportive therapeutic measures for patients under treatment for leukemia-lymphoma. In: Leukemia-Lymphoma (A Collection of Papers Presented at the Fourteenth Annual Clinical Conference on Cancer, 1969, at The University of Texas M. D. Anderson Hospital and Tumor Institute at Houston, Houston, Texas; Chicago, Ill.: Year Book Med. Publ. Inc. 1970, 275—284.

Burkitt's Tumor: A Comparative Study in Africa and the United States

Paul P. Carbone [1], John L. Ziegler [2], Richard Morrow [2], Sebastian Kyalwazi [2], Clarence H. Brown [1], Vincent T. De Vita [1], and Costan Berard [3]

With 2 Figures

Burkitt's tumor is a malignant neoplasm of the lymphoreticular system originally reported from Africa but subsequently identified in other parts of the world [1, 2, 3, 4]. The high incidence of this tumor in Africa [5], its unusual climatologic limitations [6], evidence for a specific immune host response to the tumor [7, 8] and its extraordinary responsiveness to chemotherapy [9] have evoked considerably scientific interest. Burchenal has called this tumor "the stalking horse for acute leukemia" proposing that knowledge gained from studies of Burkitt's tumor will prove to be important in combating other cancers, particularly acute leukemia.

Since 1967, there has been a coordinated research effort between the Medicine Branch, National Cancer Institute, and Makerere University, Kampala, Uganda, designed to define quantitatively the clinical and immunologic features and response to therapy for Burkitt's tumor in Africa and the United States. In addition there was a simultaneous effort to relate Burkitt's tumor to the typical childhood lymphosarcoma and acute lymphocytic leukemia seen in both areas of the globe. Preliminary results have already been reported from each center [10, 11]. The present paper updates, synthesizes and compares results from these two centers and relates them to information available in patients with acute lymphocytic leukemia.

Materials and Methods

Patients in Africa were studied at the Lymphoma Treatment Center, an 18 bed ward with associated laboratories and facilities for out-patient care and follow-up. None of the patients had received prior therapy; all had histopathological and cytologic diagnosis of Burkitt's tumor (BT) or lymphosarcoma, lymphoblastic type [12]. The clinical features, staging and response to treatment have been previously reported

[1] Medicine Branch, National Cancer Institute, National Institutes of Health, Bethesda, Maryland 20014.

[2] Lymphoma Treatment Center, Makerere University Hospital, Kampala, Uganda, East Africa.

[3] Pathologic Anatomy Branch, National Cancer Institute, National Institutes of Health, Bethesda, Maryland 20014.

in 57 patients designated as Uganda Burkitt's tumor (UBT) [10] and in six with Uganda lymphosarcoma (ULS) [13].

In the United States the criteria for diagnosis and clinical evaluation studies have also been previously reported for the first 14 of the 17 patients included in this report [11]. All of these patients have been seen since August 1965 and have been treated primarily with cyclophosphamide. The 17 American Burkitt's tumor (ABT) and five American lymphosarcoma patients (ALS) will be compared to the African patients.

For clarity the staging and therapeutic protocols will be briefly described. The staging classification for the patients is presented in Table 1. In Africa the UBT

Table 1. *Clinical staging of Burkitt's tumor*

Stage	Extent of disease
I	Single facial tumor mass
II	Two or more separate facial tumor masses
III	Intra-thoracic, intra-abdominal, paraspinal, or osseous tumor (excluding facial bones)
IV	Central nervous system (malignant cells in the CSF) or bone marrow involvement

patients received cyclophosphamide, 40 mg/kg, and were re-evaluated after two weeks. Those patients in partial remission were continued on cyclophosphamide for five more doses at two to three week intervals, whereas the patients in complete remission were randomized by stage either to no further therapy or to five repeated doses. Treatment for central nervous system involvement and for those patients not responding to cyclophosphamide has been previously reported [10, 11].

For the American patients with ABT and ALS the staging classification was the same but treatment included radiotherapy (3000 rads) to the local tumor site for Stage I and II patients and cyclophosphamide, 40 mg/kg, every three to four weeks for six doses in all patients. In the last three patients the dose of cyclophosphamide was raised to 75 to 100 mg/kg in an attempt to improve the results. The toxicity for cyclophosphamide therapy in the African and American patients has been reported [14].

Results

In Table 2 are listed the numbers, ages and sex in each category of patients. The median ages are similar as is the preponderance of males in all groups.

The anatomical sites of tumor on presentation are shown in Table 3. In UBT 37 of 57 (65%) patients had involvement of jaw or orbit as did five of six patients with ULS. Involvement of jaw or orbit was less common in both groups of American patients. Intra-abdominal involvement was more frequent in the ABT than the UBT. However, because of the small number of patients these differences are not statistically significant. In contrast, adenopathy was described in nine of 17 ABT but only one of

57 UBT, a highly significant difference. The enlarged lymph nodes in ABT were usually localized to one anatomical area such as the neck or abdomen and in only one patient was adenopathy considered to be generalized. In contrast the majority of patients with ALS had large mediastinal nodes.

For the UBT patients central nervous system involvement on presentation represented the most common basis for classifying them as Stage IV. In ABT patients bone marrow infiltration with abnormal cells was more often seen. However, only one patient with ABT had complete replacement of the bone marrow biopsy specimen with abnormal cells on admission [11].

Table 2. *Burkitt's tumor*

	UBT	ABT	ULS	ALS
No. patients	57	17	6	5
Age years median (range)	8 (4–60)	10 (2–23)	10 (3–15)	9 (5–14)
Male/female	36/21	11/6	5/1	3/2

Table 3. *Burkitt's tumor. Tumor distribution on presentation*

	UBT [a]	ABT	ULS	ALS
Jaw-orbit	37	5	5	1
Abdominal	27	10	3	2
Adenopathy	1	9	2	4
Central nervous system	6	2	1	0
Bone marrow	1	7	1	0
Total number of patients	57	17	6	5

[a] Number of patients.

The clinical classification of disease extent by stage for all patients is shown in Table 4. Most patients presented with abdominal or thoracic involvement (Stage III). The numbers of patients with Stage IV disease in the UBT and ABT groups are similar although the anatomical sites involved were different (see above).

Response to therapy with cyclophosphamide is shown in Table 5 for UBT and ABT patients according to stage. The response rates are remarkably similar for both groups. For patients with ULS and ALS there were two of six and two of five complete responses, respectively.

The effects of single versus multiple dose chemotherapy were tested in Africa by randomizing patients, who had achieved complete remission after one dose, either to no further therapy or to continued intermitten cyclophosphamide. We previously [10] have reported that Stage I and II patients persisted in remission equally well after single as well as multiple doses of cyclophosphamide. However, in patients with

Stage III disease, the relapse rate was 64% with a single dose and 36% with continued treatment. The duration of remission was considerably longer for the multiple as compared to single dose treatment groups. The Stage IV patients failed to be maintained in remission with either scheme of management.

As of the present time, 19 of 57 patients with UBT, 10 of 17 with ABT and four of five ALS have relapsed (Table 6). Central nervous system disease makes up the bulk of failures for all three groups. All patients with ALS have had recurrence

Table 4. *Burkitt's tumor. Disease extent*

Stage	UBT	ABT	ULS	ALS
I—II	12	3	0	1
III	38	7	5	4
IV	7	7	1	0
Totals	57	17	6	5

Table 5. *Burkitt's tumor. Complete responses to cyclophosphamide*

Stage	UBT	ABT
I—II	12/12	2/3
III	28/38	5/7
IV	2/7	3/7
Total	74%	59%

Table 6. *Burkitt's tumor: Relapse rate*

	Relapse No: UBT[a]	ABT	ALS
Central nervous system	9	5	3
Bone marrow	1	4	4
Total relapses	19	10	4

[a] Number of patients.

within seven months in the bone marrow as acute lymphoblastic leukemia. In ABT, massive involvement of bone marrow occurred in four of ten patients with relapses. All four died soon after relapse. Two of the six patients with ULS are in remission following cyclophosphamide.

It is of primary importance to compare the survival of these patient groups. Ziegler has reported an analysis of UBT and ULS in a previous publication [13].

Fig. 1 is a life table analysis of the UBT and ABT groups showing a similar flattening of the survival curves at about 64% for UBT and 55% for ABT. Survival curves for ABT and ALS are shown in Fig. 2. None of the patients with ALS is alive after 18 months. In contrast five patients with ABT are alive in excess of 30 months, with four of these being in persistent unmaintained remission.

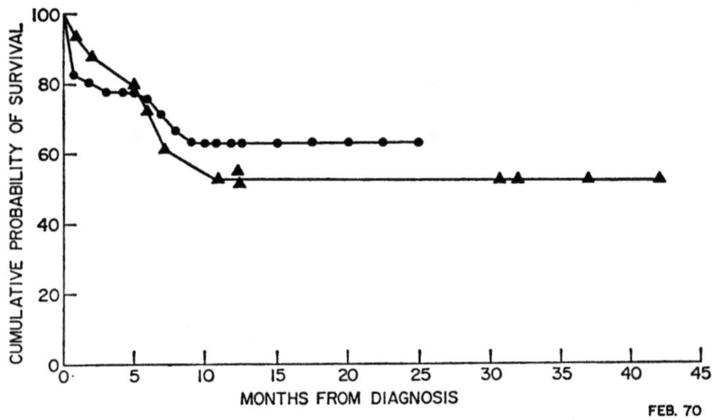

Fig. 1. Survival of patients with Burkitt's tumor in the United States and Africa. ▲—▲ American Burkitt tumor (17 patients); ●—● Uganda Burkitt tumor (57 patients)

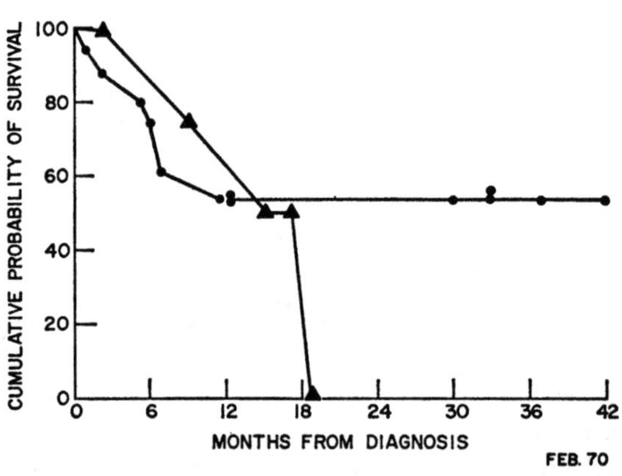

Fig. 2. Survival of patients with Burkitt's tumor and childhood lymphosarcoma in the United States. ●—● American Burkitt tumor (17 patients); ▲—▲ Lymphosarcoma (5 patients)

Immunologic Studies

Evaluation of host immunity in the UBT and ABT patients for antibody production, and delayed hypersensitivity reactions has been previously reported [11, 15]. Immunoglobulin levels were disturbed and antibody production was impaired whereas delayed hypersensitivity to primary or secondary stimulation was relatively intact for both groups of patients. In addition, Fass and coworkers have reported that a positive intradermal response could be elicited in approximately 50% of patients achieving clinical remission with preparations of tumor cell membranes [16]. There was a good correlation between these responses and the duration of remission.

Studies of serum EBV titers have been positive in all the patients with African Burkitt's tumor but in only about one-half of the American patients [17].

Discussion

The data presented in this paper represent a preliminary report of an ongoing collaborative effort to compare the clinical features and responses to cyclophosphamide of Burkitt's tumor and lymphoblastic lymphoma in Africa and in the United States. The results indicate that apparently identical histologic entities can be recognized in the United States and Africa. The clinical features, however, are less consistent, in that both similarities and differences exist between the disease characterized as Burkitt's tumor in the United States and Africa. In addition, ZIEGLER has reported that in Africa there is a group of patients whose biopsies are atypical for Burkitt's tumor, but who respond well to cyclophosphamide [10]. At present the ULS and ALS patients are too few to make meaningful clinical comparisons and more data must be collected.

Table 7

Etiology	UBT	ABT	ALL
Male preponderance	+	+	+
Clustering	+	–	+
Geographic limitations	++	–	–
Virus associated	?	–	–

In attempting to make comparisons between ABT, UBT and acute lymphoblastic leukemia of childhood (ALL), we collated reported data and derived approximate quantitative comparisons (Table 7). The information is grouped by topics and expressed as plus (+), minus (–) and question mark (?). The certainty and magnitude of the comparisons are recorded by the numbers of signs. UBT implies Uganda Burkitt's tumor, ABT, American Burkitt's tumor, and ALL, acute lymphocytic leukemia of childhood.

In the area of etiology all patient populations are associated with a male preponderance. Clustering phenomena have been described by PIKE and coworkers for Burkitt's tumor in the West Nile District [18]. A less positive but definite clustering for ALL has also been recorded [19, 20]. Geographic limitations of rain fall and temperature have been the rule for Burkitt's tumor in Africa and New Guinea but not for ABT or ALL. A virus candidate for etiology of UBT was originally attributed to the Epstein Barr Virus, a herpes type but subsequent studies have cast doubt on a direct relationship betwen this virus and the cause of Burkitt's tumor [21]. No likely candidate has been described for ABT or ALL.

The clinical features are summarized in Table 8. All three tumors occur predominately in children and have meningeal involvement. Extranodal presentation and rapid cell doubling times are characteristic of the Burkitt's tumor in Africa [22]. The hematologic features of leukemia are relatively absent in Burkitt's tumor compared to ALL.

Therapeutic responsiveness to various drugs is shown in Table 9. Burkitt's tumor in Africa and the United States is very responsive to alkylating agents, particularly

Table 8

Clinical features	UBT	ABT	ALL
Pediatric age group	++	++	++
Meningeal involvement	++	++	++
Extranodal presentation	++	++	−
Rapid growth	++	++	+
Bone marrow involvement	−	+	++
Thrombocytopenia	−	−	+
Leukocytosis	−	−	+

Table 9

Therapeutic responsiveness	UBT	ABT	ALL
Prednisone	−	?	+
Vincristine	+	+	+
Methotrexate	+	+	+
Cyclophosphamide	++	++	+
Phenylalanine mustard	++	?	+
L-asparaginase	−	−	+
Daunomycin	−	?	+
BCNU [a]	−	−	−
Cytosine arabinoside	+	+	+

[a] 1,3-bis(2-chloroethyl)-1-nitrosourea

cyclophosphamide [9, 10, 23], and phenylalanine mustard [24], but relatively resistant to asparaginase [25] and daunorubicin [10]. The antimetabolites have a limited effect against both UBT and ALL [26, 27].

Studies of host immune function and tumor specific antigens are summarized in Table 10. Studies of KLEIN [7] and HENLE [21] have indicated a common membrane and cytoplasmic antigen for UBT that is also detectable but with lower titer and frequency for ABT. These tests are not apparent in ALL. Studies by FASS [16] and HERBERMAN [28] have indicated a positive skin test to autochthonous tumor extracts in UBT and ALL. In Africa there is a positive correlation between skin test results and duration of unmaintained remission [16]. Antibody production has been found to be relatively normal in ALL and slightly depressed in UBT and ABT [11, 15]. In UBT immunoglobulin M levels have been found to be low and IGG levels high [15]. The levels of immunoglobulins have no consistent features in ABT [11]. Studies in patients with ALL have indicated normal levels early in the disease.

Of most importance is the proportion of patients achieving complete and durable remissions (Table 11). All three tumors are sensitive to initial therapy, with ALL being the most responsive to induction treatment. The proportion of patients alive at two years is again comparable. While figures can only be projected for five year

Table 10

Immunology	UBT	ABT	ALL
Common membrane antigen	++	+	–
Common cytoplasmic antigen	++	+	–
Autochthonus tumor reaction	+	?	+
Delayed hypersensitivity	+	+	+
Antibody production	+	+	+
IgG levels	++	+	+
IgM levels	–	+	+

Table 11

Prognosis	UBT	ABT	ALL
Percent complete remission	75%	60%	90%
Percent two year survivors	70%	55%	70%
Projected five year survival	50%	?	25%

survival, the experience for ABT and ALL may also be very similar, with UBT possibly being most likely to achieve durable long term remissions.

In attempting to assess the relationship of these diseases to each other and their relative importance to cancer research, several points are noteworthy. Burkitt's tumor is a world wide disease and must be considered when diagnosing lymphosarcoma of childhood not only in Africa but also in the United States.

Secondly, the geographic limitations and high incidence of Burkitt's tumor in Africa remain unexplained and offer investigators an excellent opportunity to explore for an etiologic virus agent. As yet few leads are available in the study of the etiology of ALL.

Thirdly, the durable responses to relatively low dose chemotherapy have also engendered a search for tumor specific immunity. Fass and coworkers have already obtained evidence for autochthonous host reactivity to tumor cell membranes. Similar studies are necessary in ALL and other diseases.

In addition the remarkable responsiveness to chemotherapy of Burkitt's tumor has been responsible for equally important studies. Unlike ALL where multiple, intensive, long term treatment appears to be necessary to achieve durable remissions, Burkitt's tumor is exquisitely sensitive to even single doses of cyclophosphamide [10] or phenylalanine mustard [24]. The reasons for this sensitivity are unknown. Studies by DE VITA and ADAMSON found no difference in the metabolism of cyclophosphamide in patients with Burkitt's tumor as compared to those less responsive tumor patients [29]. A very intensive study of tumor cell kinetics is presently underway in patients with ABT, UBT, and ALL that may elucidate at least some of the reasons for these therapeutic differences.

Finally, at present the successful treatment of cancer appears to be unique for each disease entity such as choriocarcinoma [30], Hodgkin's disease [31], adrenal carcinoma [32], testicular tumor [33], and now Burkitt's tumor [10]. Thus we must approach the more "resistant" tumors with more specific protocols and research programs. Unique measures may be essential for the successful treatment of tumors of each type.

Summary

Burkitt's tumor is a malignant neoplasm of the lymphoreticular system reported originally from Africa but subsequently shown to occur in other parts of the world. Since 1967 a coordinated research effort between the Medicine Branch, National Cancer Institute and Makerere University, Kampala, Uganda, has been underway to define the clinical and immunologic features and response to therapy for Burkitt's tumor in the United States and Africa. Using a relatively common protocol, 57 patients with Burkitt's tumor in Africa and 17 patients with Burkitt's tumor in the United States were evaluated and treated, primarily with cyclophosphamide, 40 mg/kg every three to four weeks. Involvement of the jaw occurred more frequently in the African patients whereas intra-abdominal disease was more frequent in the American patients with Burkitt's tumor. Central nervous system involvement was the primary reason for failure in Africa. More American patients had bone marrow involvement. Response to therapy with cyclophosphamide was similar for both the African and American patients. The portion of patients alive at two years for the American patients with Burkitt's tumor was 55%, and 64% for the African patients. Evaluation of immune response in the American and African patients indicated an impaired humoral response with relatively intact delayed hypersensitivity reactions. EBV antibody studies have been positive in all the African patients but only in one-half of the American patients. Thus, these studies indicate that Burkitt's tumor can be diagnosed in other parts of the world, and the response to cyclophosphamide appears to be as dramatic in the United States as in the African patients.

References

1. BURKITT, D.: Sarcoma involving jaws in African children. Brit. J. Surgery **46**, 218 (1959).
2. EDINGTON, G. M., MACLEAN, C. M. V., OKUBADEJO, O. A.: 101 necropsies on tumours of of the reticulo-endothelial system in Ibadan, Nigeria with special reference to childhood lymphosarcoma. In: Symp. Lymph. Tumours in Africa, Paris. Basel-New York: S. Karger 1964, p. 236.

3. TEN SELDAN, R. E. J., COOKE, R., ATKINSON, L.: Childhood lymphoma in the territories of Papua and New Guinea. Cancer **19,** 437 (1966).
4. CARBONE, P. P., BELL, W. R., GODWIN, H., O'CONOR, G. T.: New approaches to the treatment of Burkitt type tumor. In: Treatment of Burkitt's Tumor. Eds. J. H. BURCHENAL and D. P. BURKITT. Berlin-Heidelberg-New York: Springer 1967, p. 184.
5. BURKITT, D., O'CONOR, G. T.: Malignant lymphoma in African children: A clinical syndrome. Cancer **14,** 259 (1961).
6. — WRIGHT, D.: Geographical and tribal distribution of the African lymphoma in Uganda. Brit. med. J. **1966 I,** 569.
7. KLEIN, G., CLIFFORD, P., KLEIN, E., STJERNSWARD, J.: Search for tumor specific immune reactions in Burkitt lymphoma patients by the membrane immunofluorescence reaction. Proc. nat. Acad. Sci. (Wash.) **55,** 1628 (1966).
8. BURKITT, D.: Clinical evidence suggesting the development of an immunologic response against African lymphoma. In: Treatment of Burkitt's Tumour. Eds.: J. H. BURCHENAL and D. P. BURKITT. Berlin- Heidelberg-New York: Springer 1967, p. 197.
9. BURKITT, D. P., HUTT, M. S. R., WRIGHT, D. H.: The African lymphoma: Preliminary observations on response to therapy. Cancer **18,** 399 (1965).
10. ZIEGLER, J. L., MORROW, R. H., JR., Fass, L., KYALWAZI, S. W., CARBONE, P. P.: Treatment of Burkitt's tumor with cyclophosphamide. Cancer **26,** 474—484 (1970).
11. COHEN, M. H., BENNETT, J. M., BERARD, C. W., ZIEGLER, J. L., VOGEL, C. L., SHEAGREN, J. N., CARBONE, P. P.: Burkitt's tumor in the United States. Cancer **23,** 1259 (1969).
12. BERARD, C., O'CONOR, G. T., THOMAS, L. B., TORLONI, H.: Histopathological definition of Burkitt's tumor. Wld Hlth Org. Bull. **40,** 601 (1969).
13. ZIEGLER, J. L., MORROW, R. H., JR., TEMPLETON, A. C., BLUMING, A. Z., FASS, L., KYALWAZI, S. L.: Clinical features and treatment of childhood malignant lymphoma in Uganda. Int. J. Cancer (in Press).
14. BROWN, C. H., ZIEGLER, J. L., TEMPLETON, C., CARBONE, P. P.: Cyclophosphamide toxicity in American and Ugandan children with lymphomas. Cancer **26,** 462—467 (1970).
15. ZIEGLER, J. L., COHEN, M. H., MORROW, R. H., JR., KYALWAZI, S. K., CARBONE, P. P.: Immunologic studies in Burkitt's lymphoma. Cancer **25,** 734—739 (1970).
16. FASS, L., HERBERMAN, R., ZIEGLER, J. L.: Cutaneous hypersensitivity to Burkitt lymphoma cell extracts. New Engl. J. Med. **282,** 776—780 (1970).
17. CARBONE, P. P., BERARD, C. W., BENNETT, J. M., ZIEGLER, J. L., COHEN M. H., GERBER, P.: Burkitt's tumor. Ann. intern. Med. **70,** 817 (1969).
18. PIKE, M., WILLIAMS, E. H., WRIGHT, B.: Burkitt's tumor in the West Nile District of Uganda. **2,** 395 (1967).
19. KNOW, G.: Epidemiology of childhood leukemia in Northumberland and Durham. Brit. J. prev. soc. Med. **18,** 17 (1964).
20. HEATH, C. W., JR., HASTERLIK. R. J.: Leukemia among children in a suburban community. Amer. J. Med. **34,** 796 (1963).
21. HENLE, G., HENLE, W., DIEHL, V.: Relations of Burkitt's tumor associated Herpes-type virus to infectious mononucleosis. Proc. nat. Acad. Sci. (Wash.) **59,** 94 (1968).
22. COOPER, E. H., FRANK, G. L., WRIGHT, D. H.: Cell proliferation in Burkitt tumours. Europ. J. Cancer **2,** 377 (1966).
23. NGU, V. A.: Clinical experience in the therapy of Burkitt's tumour. In: Treatment of Burkitt's Tumour. Eds.: J. H. BURCHENAL and D. P. BURKITT. Berlin-Heidelberg-New York: Springer 1969, p. 71.
24. CLIFFORD, P. M.: Observations in the treatment of Burkitt's lymphoma. In: Treatment of Burkitt's Tumour. Eds.: J. H. BURCHENAL and D. P. BURKITT. Berlin-Heidelberg-New York: Springer 1969, p. 77.
25. CANELLOS, G. P., CARBONE, P. P., ZIEGLER, J. L.: L-asparaginase and Burkitt's lymphoma. Lancet **1969 II,** 380.
26. OETTGEN, H. F., BURKITT, D. P., BURCHENAL, J. H.: Malignant lymphoma involving the jaw in African children. Treatment with methotrexate. Cancer **16,** 161 (1963).
27. HENDERSON, E. S.: Treatment of acute leukemia. Seminars in Hematology **6,** 271 (1969).
28. HERBERMAN, R. B., OREN, M. E.: Delayed cutaneous hypersensitivity reactions to membrane extracts of human tumor cells. Clin. Res. **17,** 403 (1969).

29. DE VITA, V. T., ADAMSON, R. H.: The metabolism of ^{14}C cyclophosphamide Comparative drug metabolism studies on African and American patients with lymphosarcoma and Burkitt's tumor. Proc. Sixth Internat. Congress for Chemother. Tokyo, Japan (in Press).
30. HERTZ, R., LEWIS, R., JR., LIPSETT, M. B.: Five years experience with the chemotherapy of metastatic choriocarcinoma and related trophoblastic tumors in women. Amer. J. Obstet. Gynec. **82**, 631 (1961).
31. DE VITA, V. T., SERPICK, A. A.: Combination chemotherapy in the treatment of advanced Hodgkin's disease. Proc. Amer. Ass. Cancer Res. **8**, 13 (1967).
32. HUTTER, A. M., JR., KAYHOE, D. E.: Adrenal cortical carcinoma. Amer. J. Med. **41**, 572 (1966).
33. LI, M. C.: Management of choriocarcinoma and related tumors of uterus and testes. Med. Clin. N. Amer. **54**, 661 (1966).

Pharmacological Considerations of Alkylating Agents

GLYNN P. WHEELER

With 3 Figures

It has been experimentally demonstrated that implantation of one micromanipulator-isolated leukemia cell into a mouse can result in the leukemic death of the mouse [1, 2, 3]. Conversely, in order to cure a mouse of leukemia it will be necessary to eradicate every leukemia cell in the animal. Although the immunological mechanisms of the host might contribute toward eradication of the leukemia cell population, a major portion of the killing must be done by radiotherapy or chemotherapy. Since the magnitude of the immunological contribution is uncertain and since the immunological response might be altered by the administered therapeutic agents, one must aim at killing all of the leukemia cells by the agents. Among the factors involved in the achievement of this goal are the kinetics of cell killing, the chemical and biological persistence of the agent, the delivery of the agent to all loci in the body where leukemia cells might be, the sensitivity of the cells during the various phases of the cell cycle, the repair of sublethal damage, and the differential sensitivities of leukemia cells and host cells.

There is evidence that certain agents kill cells by first-order kinetics; that is, "A particular drug treatment eliminates about the same percentage of cells present at the start, not the same absolute number of cells [4]". A corollary to this statement is that equal percentages of the cell population are killed in equal increments of time if the concentration of the drug is constant [4]. WILKOFF et al. [5] obtained data (Fig. 1) illustrative of this when cultured leukemia L1210 cells were exposed to nitrogen mustard at designated concentrations for various periods of time and the surviving fraction was determined by bioassay in mice. Thus in order to kill all of the cells when low concentrations of nitrogen mustard are used, there must be an extended period of exposure to the agent. On the other hand, increased percentage of killing can be accomplished by increasing the concentration of the nitrogen mustard (Fig. 1 B). Similar results were obtained with 1,3-bis(2-chloroethyl)-1-nitrosourea (Fig. 2 A and B).

The time of exposure of leukemia cells in animals to the alkylating agent is dependent to a large extent upon the chemical reactivity of the agent and upon the period of time that it persists at significant levels in the circulating blood. Table 1 contains data for the chemical persistence for several commonly used alkylating agents. Although these data were obtained in several laboratories and by several

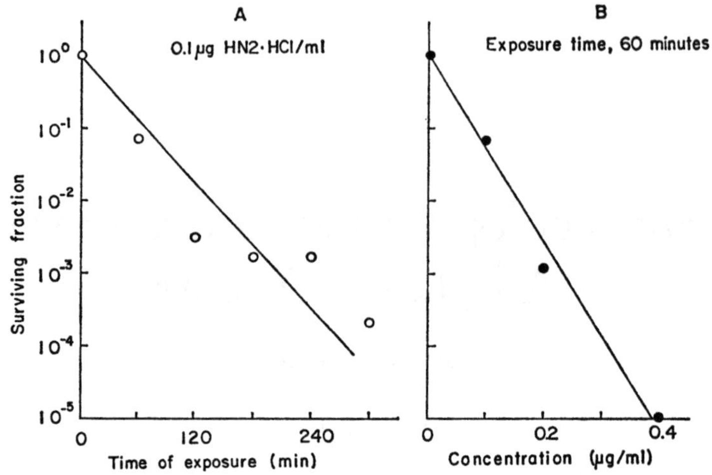

Fig. 1. Survival of cultured leukemia L1210 cells following treatment *in vitro* with nitrogen mustard hydrochloride (HN2·HCl). The viability of the treated cells was determined by *in vivo* bioassay in mice. (The data are those of WILKOFF et al. [5])

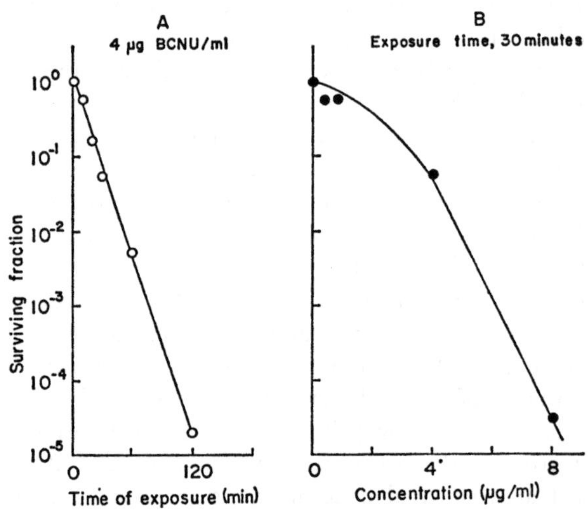

Fig. 2. Survival of cultured leukemia L1210 cells following treatment *in vitro* with 1,3-bis-(2-chloroethyl)-1-nitrosourea (BCNU). The viability of the treated cells was determined by *in vivo* bioassay in mice. (The data are those of WILKOFF et al. [5])

different methods, the data serve to show that these agents are chemically rather active and that even in isolated *in vitro* systems the concentrations decrease rather quickly. Nevertheless, as Figs. 1 and 2 show, if the initial concentration is high enough or the time of exposure is long enough essentially all of a population of cells can be killed *in vitro*. The data given in Table 2 show that the half-life of the agents in blood and plasma of animals following administration of the agents is often

Table 1. *Chemical persistence of some alkylating agents*

Agent	Medium	Observation	Reference
Nitrogen mustard	SRI-14 culture medium	$T_{0.5}=125$ min	6
	Fischer culture medium	$T_{0.5}=75$ min	7
	Dog blood	90% disappeared in 4 min	8
	Veronal buffer, pH 7.4	$T_{0.5}=30$ min	9
Phenylalanine mustard	Water, pH 7.0	$T_{0.5}=80$ min	10
	Blood	$T_{0.5}=105$—120 min	10
Myleran	Water, pH 7, 60° C	$T_{0.5}=117$ min	11
Triethylene thiophosphoramide	0.1 M phosphate buffer, pH 7.4	68% disappeared in 30 min	12
	Whole blood, pH 7.8	60% disappeared in 30 min	12
1,3-Bis(2-chloroethyl)-1-nitrosourea	Acetate buffer, pH 7.2	$T_{0.5}=103$ min	13
	Phosphate buffer, pH 7.2	$T_{0.5}=57$ min	13
	Phosphate buffer, pH 7.4	$T_{0.5}=52$ min	14
	Blood	$T_{0.5}=61.9$ min	13
	Serum	$T_{0.5}=45.4$ min	13
	Plasma	$T_{0.5}=20$ min	14

Table 2. *Biological persistence of some alkylating agents*

Agent	Animal	Observation	Reference
Nitrogen mustard	Dog	Blood level decreased 65—90% in 48 min	8
	Rabbit	Marrow-damaging concentration persisted in the blood for less than 15 min	15
	Rabbit	Marrow-damaging concentration persisted in the blood for less than 0.25 min	9
	Mice	Blood level decreased approximately 95% in 10 min	16
Phenylalanine mustard	Rabbit	Marrow-damaging concentration persisted in the blood for at least 60 min	15
Myleran	Human	Over 90% of the injected isotope disappeared from the blood within 2—3 min	16
Triethylene thiophosphoramide	Dog	Approximately 90% of the thio TEPA disappeared from plasma in 3 hours, but the generated TEPA persisted in the plasma for at least 6 hours	12
1,3-Bis(2-chloroethyl)-1-nitrosourea	Dog	$T_{0.5} < 15$ min in plasma *in vivo*	14
	Monkey	Disappeared from plasma within 5 min	17
	Man	Disappeared from plasma within 5 min	17
	Mouse	Retention of antileukemic activity indicated a biological half-life of about 1 hour	18
Cyclophosphamide	Mouse	$T_{0.5}=17$—25 min in plasma *in vivo*	19
	Hamster	$T_{0.5}=15$ min in plasma *in vivo*	19
	Dog	$T_{0.5}=32$—38 min in plasma *in vivo*	19
	Rat	$T_{0.5}=39$—43 min in plasma *in vivo*	19
	Monkey	$T_{0.5}=43$—48 min in plasma *in vivo*	19
	Human	$T_{0.5}=195$—210 min in plasma *in vivo*	19

significantly shorter than the chemical half-life. Probably a number of factors contribute to this fact, but the net result is that the period of exposure of leukemia cells in the animal, particularly those cells that have infiltrated into the various organs, to the agents will be very brief. Therefore, large doses at appropriate intervals might be more effective in killing leukemia cells than small doses at more frequent intervals.

Many efforts have been made to design potential alkylating agents that would require enzymatic alteration to generate the active alkylating agents. Hopefully, the necessary enzymes would be limited to, or more abundent in, cancer cells; and this would focus the toxic effects of the agents upon the cancer cells. To date these efforts have been unsuccessful. Cyclophosphamide is probably the best known compound that was designed for this purpose. It is inactive as an alkylating agent, but a series of modifications of the molecule occur in intact animals to yield one or more compounds having alkylating activity. The first modification is probably an enzymatic oxidation of the oxazaphosphorinane ring [20] by an enzyme that is most abundant in liver [21], and the subsequently derived compounds are transported by the blood to the other parts of the body. Although the goal of specific activation of the agent by the cancer cells was not attained, there are instances in which cyclophosphamide is more effective in therapy than other alkylating agents [22]. Perhaps this is at least partially due to the extended generation of the active compound by the liver with the resulting increase in biological persistence of the active compound and extended exposure time of the cancer cells. It has also been suggested that cancer cells might be more permeable to the activated metabolite than normal cells [21].

It is known that L1210 leukemia cells can extensively infiltrate into many organs of the mouse including the brain [23], and it has been demonstrated that the intracerebral implantation of a leukemia cell can lead to the leukemic death of the animal [2]. Therefore to kill all of the leukemia cells it is necessary that the agent arrive at the loci of the cells in sufficient quantity to give a lethal exposure. This requires that the agent pass the" blood-brain barrier". There is evidence that a number of commonly used anticancer agents including some alkylating agents (amethopterin, 6-mercaptopurine, 5-fluorouracil, azaserine, cyclophosphamide, and mitomycin C) are ineffective against intracerebrally implanted L1210 cells in mice [23], and that these agents do not eradicate L1210 cells that have infiltrated into the brain following intraperitoneal inoculation [24]. On the other hand, certain N-nitrosoureas, particularly 1,3-bis(2-chloroethyl)-1-nitrosourea (BCNU) and 1-chloroethyl-3-cyclohexyl-1-nitrosourea (CCNU), do effectively reduce the number of viable L1210 cells in the brains of mice [25]. Of the N-nitrosoureas tested, the more effective ones are essentially not ionized and have relatively high lipoid solubility [25], which probably facilitates passage of the "blood-brain barrier". If it is necessary for the clinician to assume that some leukemia cells have reached the brain of the patient, then it is important that he use a drug that can reach those cells or that he administer the agent intrathecally.

Even if the alkylating agent reaches the loci of the leukemia cells, all of the viable cells might not be equally sensitive to the agent, because they are in different phases of the cell cycle or perhaps not even proliferating during the time of exposure to the gaent. BRUCE and co-workers [26, 27] have presented evidence that nitrogen mustard will kill leukemia cells in all phases of the cell cycle and also noncycling leukemia cells, whereas cyclophosphamide and BCNU will kill leukemia cells in all phases of the cycle but will not kill non-cycling cells. DeWys and Kight [28] obtained data in *in vivo* experiments with L1210 leukemia which they interpreted to indicate that cells in different parts of the cell cycle had different sensitivities to cyclophosphamide. Experiments with cultured mammalian cells have shown that cells in the G_2 phase of the cycle are less sensitive to nitrogen mustard [29, 30], sulfur mustard [29, 31, 32], and BCNU [33] than cells in the other phases of the cycle. Then cells that are in the G_2 phase throughout the period of exposure to low concentrations of these agents will probably survive. At higher concentrations of nitrogen mustard [30] and BCNU [33] cells in G_2 can be lethally injured. Therefore the size of the fraction of the population of leukemia cells in G_2, the concentration of the agent, and the time of exposure can each be important factors in determining how large a portion of the population will be killed. If certain alkylating agents do not lethally affect non-cycling cells, the degree of cell kill will depend to some extent upon the growth fraction of the cell population. Very little information concerning the sensitivity of non-cycling cells to alkylating agents is presently available. The evidence of Bruce et al. [26, 27] has already been mentioned, but actually these data give only indirect evidence on the question. When suspensions of leukemia cells in ascitic fluid were treated *in vitro* with nitrogen mustard [33] or BCNU [35] and then inoculated into mice for bioassay, it was found that both agents were eftective in killing these "resting" cells. However, the state of these "resting" cells may not be the same as that of non-cycling or G_0 [36] cells *in vivo*. Thatcher and Walker [37] found that cultured hamster embryo cells that had multiplied to form confluent sheets on glass and then ceased multiplying were as sensitive to sulfur mustard and BCNU as cells of the same type that were multiplying exponentially. This result led them to conclude that the state of their non-replicating cells was different from the non-cycling (G_0) state of the cells used by Bruce et al., but it is not presently known how they differ. Since there is experimental evidence that the growth fraction of ascites L1210 leukemia cells decreases when the number of leukemia cells becomes large [38], it is possible that such a population of cells might be less sensitive to some alkylating agents than an exponentially growing population of cells. This fact might contribute to the difficulty in successfully treating advanced leukemia.

Plots of the surviving fraction of a population of cultured mammalian cells versus concentration of agent following treatment with nitrogen mustard [29, 30], sulfur mustard [29, 31, 32], and BCNU [33] are exponential after an initial shoulder. The presence of the shoulder is interpreted to be indicative of sublethal damage to the cells. There is evidence that the sublethal damage caused by sulfur mustard [32, 39, 40, 41] and dimethyl myleran [42] can be repaired by the cells, while there was less evidence of repair of sublethal damage caused by nitrogen mustard [42]. This repair is perhaps similar to, but not identical with, the repair of damage caused by X-irradiation [39, 40].

One of the essential steps in repair is elimination of alkylated bases from the damaged DNA. It has been shown that such elimination can occur in *Escherichia coli*, and strains resistant to growth inhibition by the alkylating agent eliminated the alkylated bases more extensively than the sensitive strains [43, 44, 45]. Alkylated bases can also be eliminated by treated cultured mammalian cells [46, 47] and non-semiconservative synthesis of DNA can occur [41].

The dose-response curve obtained in treating leukemia L1210 *in vivo* with cyclophosphamide has a shoulder, which is considered to be evidence for repair in this system also [28]. Then repair of damage to leukemia cells following low levels of damage might be a deterrent to success in using alkylating agents for chemotherapy. If repair is an important factor in the response of neoplasms, then prevention of such repair should increase the therapeutic response. GAUDIN and YIELDING [48] did increase somewhat the response of resistant hamster plasmacytomas to cyclophosphamide and to X-rays by pretreatment of the animals with caffeine or chloroquine, which have been shown to inhibit repair in damaged bacteria.

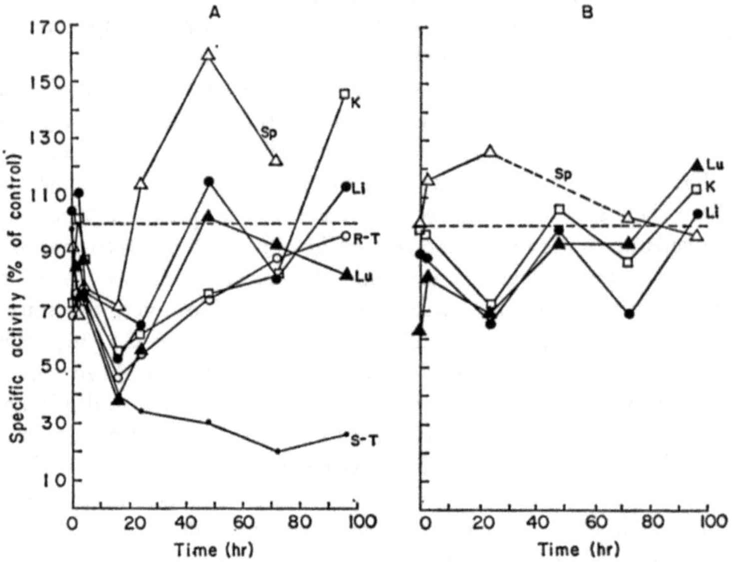

Fig. 3. Effects of a single intraperitoneal dose (20 mg/kg) of cyclophosphamide upon the *in vivo* fixation of ^{3}H of thymidine-C^3H_3 in the acid-insoluble fractions of tissues of hamsters (A) bearing bilaterally implanted cyclophosphamide-sensitive and cyclophosphamide-resistant plasmacytomas or (B) bearing no tumors. The thymidine-C^3H_3 was injected intraperitoneally at various times after the injection of the cyclophosphamide and 2 hours before killing the animals. Sp, spleen; K, kidneys; Li, liver; Lu, lungs; S-T, cyclophosphamide-sensitive plasmacytoma; R-T, cyclophosphamide-resistant plasmacytoma

In addition to repair of damaged DNA there are other factors, including sulfhydryl content and permeability, that might contribute to resistance to alkylating agents [49]. Recent reports have pointed to lower permeability of resistant cells to the agents [50, 51], but the observed differences in permeability of sensitive and resistant cells are not great enough to account for the observed degree of resistance.

At present there is little known concerning why alkylating agents preferentially kill cancer cells. It seems reasonable that the factors that contribute to resistance in resistant neoplasms might also contribute to resistance of host tissues, although the relative contributions of these individual factors might vary from tissue to tissue [49]. Fig. 3 A shows the effects of a single dose of cyclophosphamide upon the subsequent fixation of ^{3}H of thymidine-C^3H_3 into the acid-insoluble fraction of tumor and host tissues of hamsters bearing bilaterally implanted plasmacytomas. The data for the sensitive tumor are in agreement with previously obtained data [52] that show that maximum inhibition of nucleic acid synthesis does not occur until a number of hours after the administration of the cyclophosphamide. The curves in this figure show that at 16 hours after the administration of the cyclophosphamide there was decreased fixation of thymidine-C^3H_3 by the sensitive tumor, the resistant tumor, the liver, the lungs, the spleen, and the kidneys. By 48 hours there was significant recovery of the ability to fix this DNA precursors by all of the tissues except the sensitive tumor. This fact suggests that the differential toxicity of this agent for host tissues and plasmacytoma may be due to differences in ability of the tissues to recover from initial damage. Since it is known [53] that this tumor metastasizes extensively to the host tissues mentioned above, it seemed possible that the inhibitions for the host tissues shown in Fig. 3 A might be partially or totally accounted for by inhibition of the tumor cells present in the tissues. Therefore a similar experiment was performed with non-tumor-bearing hamsters. Fig. 3 B shows that at 24 hours there was inhibition of fixation of thymidine-C^3H_3 in liver, lungs, and kidneys, but there was less inhibition than in the tumor-bearing animals (Fig. 3 A); there was no inhibition in spleen. Thus it appears that cyclophosphamide caused some damage to the liver, lungs, and spleen and that these tissues soon recovered from this damage. The nature of this recovery is not known, but it might involve repair of damaged cells, loss of damaged or dead cells, and generation of new cells. More detailed information about these recovery phenomena might be useful for planning rational chemotherapy.

This discussion has pointed out a number of problems that must be recognized and overcome in order to accomplish cures of neoplastic diseases by means of alkylating agents. Perhaps recognition of the multiplicity of the problems leads to pessimism, but this pessimism can be counter-balanced by the knowledge that "cures" of certain experimental [3, 53, 54] and clinical [55, 56] neoplasms have been accomplished by the use of alkylating agents alone or in combination with other agents. One can be optimistic in expecting that rational approaches to overcoming the problems mentioned herein, which might involve utilizing optimum dosage levels, dosage schedules, and combinations of agents, will lead to extended clinical remissions and eventually to clinical cures of a number of kinds of human neoplasia.

Summary

Other investigators have shown that in order to effect cures of experimental leukemias it might be necessary to kill every leukemia cell in the host animal. Among the factors involved in the achievement of cures with chemotherapeutic agents, including alkylating agents, are the kinetics of cell killing, the chemical and biological persistence of the agents, the delivery of the agents to all loci in the body where leukemic cells might be, the sensitivity of the cells during the various phases of the cell cycle, the repair of sublethal damage, and the differential sensitivities of leukemia cells and host cells. These factors are discussed briefly in this paper with respect to alkylating agents, and some relevant data are presented.

References

1. FURTH, J., KAHN, M. C.: The transmission of leukemia in mice with a single cell. Amer. J. Cancer **31**, 276 (1937).
2. SKIPPER, H. E., SCHABEL, F. M., JR., WILCOX, W. S.: Experimental evaluation of potential anticancer agents. XIII. On the criteria and kinetics associated with "curability" of experimental leukemia. Cancer Chemother. Rep. **35**, 1 (1964).
3. SCHABEL, F. M., JR.: *In vivo* leukemic cell kill kinetics and "curability" in experimental systems. In: The Proliferation and Spread of Neoplastic Cells. Twenty-first annual symposium on fundamental cancer research. Houston: University of Texas M. D. Anderson Hospital and Tumor Institute 1967, p. 379.
4. WILCOX, W. S.: The last surviving cancer cell: the chances of killing it. Cancer Chemother. Rep. **50**, 541 (1966).
5. WILKOFF, L. J., DIXON, G. J., DULMADGE, E. A., SCHABEL, F. M., JR.: Effect of 1,3-bis-(2-chloroethyl)-1-nitrosourea (NSC-409962) and nitrogen mustard (NSC-762) on kinetic behavior of cultured L1210 leukemic cells. Cancer Chemother. Rep. **51**, 7 (1967).
6. WHEELER, G. P., SHADDIX, S. C.: Unpublished data.
7. GOLDENBERG, G. J., ALEXANDER, P.: The effects of nitrogen mustard and dimethyl myleran on murine leukemic cell lines of different radiosensitivity *in vitro*. Cancer Res. **25**, 1401 (1965).
8. MELLETT, L. B., WOODS, L. A.: The fluorometric estimation of mechlorethamine (Mustargen) and its biological disposition in the dog. Cancer Res. **20**, 518 (1960).
9. ULFOHN, A., KRAMER, S. P., DORFMAN, H., WITTEN, B., WILLIAMSON, C., SASS, S., MILLER, J. I., SELIGMAN, A. M.: The duration of the myelotoxic effects of alkylating agents. Cancer Res. **24**, 1659 (1964).
10. ROSS, W. C. J.: Biological Alkylating Agents. London: Butterworths 1962, p. 98.
11. — Biological Alkylating Agents. London: Butterworths 1962, p. 112.
12. MELLETT, L. B., WOODS, L. A.: The comparative physiological disposition of thioTEPA and TEPA in the dog. Cancer Res. **20**, 524 (1960).
13. MONTGOMERY, J. A., JAMES, R., MCCALEB, G. S., JOHNSTON, T. P.: The modes of decomposition of 1,3-bis(2-chloroethyl)-1-nitrosourea and related compounds. J. Med. Chem. **10**, 668 (1967).
14. LOO, T. L., DION, R. L., DIXON, R. L., RALL, D. P.: The anti-tumor agent, 1,3-bis(2-chloroethyl)-1-nitrosourea. J. pharm. Sci. **55**, 492 (1966).
15. ZHDANOV, G. L.: Duration of circulation of sarcolysin and several other chlorethylamines and ethylamines in the blood. Vopr. Khim. Zlobach. Opuk. **2**, 198 (1960).
16. SMITH, P. K., NADKARNI, M. V., TRAMS, E. G., DAVISON, C.: Distribution and fate of alkylating agents. In: Comparative Clinical and Biological Effects of Alkylating Agents. Ed.: D. S. Karnofsky. Ann. N. Y. Acad. Sci. **68**, 834 (1958).
17. DEVITA, V. T., DENHAM, C., DAVIDSON, J. D., OLIVERIO, V. T.: The physiological disposition of the carcinostatic 1,3-bis(2-chloroethyl)-1-nitrosourea (BCNU) in man and animals. Clin. Pharmacol. Ther. **8**, 566 (1967).
18. SCHABEL, F. M., JR.: Unpublished data.
19. MELLETT, L. B.: Comparative drug metabolism. In: Progress in Drug Research, Vol. 13. Ed.: E. JUCKER. Basel: Birkhäuser 1969, p. 136.
20. HILL, D. L., KIRK, M. C., STRUCK, R. F.: Isolation and Identification of 4-Ketocyclophosphamide, a Possible Active Form of the Antitumor Agent Cyclophosphamide. J. Am. Chem. Soc. **92**, 3207 (1970).
21. BROCK, N., HOHORST, H.-J.: Metabolism of cyclophosphamide. Cancer **20**, 900 (1967).
22. SCHMIDT, L. H., FRADKIN, R., SULLIVAN, R., FLOWERS, A.: Comparative pharmacology of alkylating agents. Part I. Cancer Chemother. Rep., Suppl. **2**, 1 (1965).
23. SKIPPER, H. E., SCHABEL, F. M., JR., WILCOX, W. S., LASTER, W. R., JR., TRADER, M. W., THOMPSON, S. A.: Experimental evaluation of potential anticancer agents. XVIII. Effects of therapy on viability and rate of proliferation of leukemic cells in various anatomic sites. Cancer Chemother. Rep. **47**, 41 (1965).

24. Skipper, H. E., Schabel, F. M., Jr., Trader, M. W., Thomson, J. R.: Experimental evaluation of potential anticancer agents. VI. Anatomical distribution of leukemic cells and failure of chemotherapy. Cancer Res. **21,** 1154 (1961).
25. Schabel, F. M., Jr., Johnston, T. P., McCaleb, G. S., Montgomery, J. A., Laster, W. R., Skipper, H. E.: Experimental evaluation of potential anticancer agents. VIII. Effects of certain nitrosoureas on intracerebral L1210 leukemia. Cancer Res. **23,** 725 (1963).
26. Bruce, W. R., Meeker, B. E., Valeriote, F. A.: Comparison of the sensitivity of normal hematopoietic and transplanted lymphoma colony-forming cells to chemotherapeutic agents administered *in vivo.* J. nat. Cancer Inst. **37,** 233 (1966).
27. — Valeriote, F. A.: Normal and malignant stem cells and chemotherapy. In: The Proliferation and Spread of Neoplastic Cells. Twenty-first annual symposium on fundamental cancer research. Houston: University of Texas M. D. Anderson Hospital and Tumor Institute 1967, p. 409.
28. DeWys, W. D., Kight, N.: Kinetics of cyclophosphamide damage — Sublethal damage repair and cell-cycle-related sensitivity. J. nat. Cancer Inst. **42,** 155 (1969).
29. Walker, I. G., Helleiner, C. W.: The sensitivity of cultured mammalian cells in different stages of the division cycle to nitrogen and sulfur mustards. Cancer Res. **23,** 734 (1963).
30. Wheeler, G. P., Bowdon, B. J., Adamson, D. J., Vail, M. H.: Effects of certain nitrogen mustards upon the progression of cultured H. Ep. No. 2 cells through the cell cycle. Cancer Res. **30,** 100 (1970).
31. Mauro, F., Elkind, M. M.: Differences in survival variations during the growth cycle of cultured Chinese hamster cells treated with sulfur mustard and X-rays. Cancer Res. **28,** 1150 (1968).
32. Roberts, J. J., Brent, T. P., Crathorn, A. R.: The mechanism of the cytotoxic action of alkylating agents on mammalian cells. In: The Interaction of Drugs and Subcellular Components in Animal Cells. Ed.: P. N. Campbell. Boston: Little, Brown and Co. 1968, p. 5.
33. Wheeler, G. P., Bowdon, B. J., Adamson, D. J., Vail, M. H.: Effects of 1,3-bis(2-chloroethyl)-1-nitrosourea and some chemically related compounds upon the progression of cultured H. Ep. No. 2 cells through the cell cycle. Cancer Res. **30,** 1817 (1970).
34. Burchenal, J. H., Cremer, M. A., Williams, B. S., Armstrong, R. A.: Sterilization of leukemic cells *in vivo* and *in vitro.* Cancer Res. **11,** 700 (1951).
35. Schabel, F. M., Jr., Skipper, H. E., Trader, M. W., Wilcox, W. S.: Experimental evaluation of potential anticancer agents. XIX. Sensitivity of nondividing leukemic cell populations to certain classes of drugs *in vivo.* Cancer Chemother. Rep. **48,** 17 (1965).
36. Lajtha, L. G., Gilbert, C. W., Proteous, D. D., Alexanian, R.: Kinetics of a bone-marrow stem cell population. Ann. N. Y. Acad. Sci. **113,** 742 (1964).
37. Thatcher, C. J., Walker, J. G.: Sensitivity of confluent and cycling embryonic hamster cells to sulfur mustard, 1,3-bis(2-chloroethyl)-1-nitrosourea, and actinomycin D. J. nat. Cancer Inst. **42,** 363 (1969).
38. Wheeler, G. P.: Unpublished data.
39. Mauro, F., Elkind, M. M.: Comparison of repair of sublethal damage in cultured Chinese hamster cells exposed to sulfur mustard and X-rays. Cancer Res. **28,** 1156 (1968).
40. Walker, I. G., Thatcher, C. J.: Studies on the lethal effects of sulfur mustard on dividing mammalian cells. Radiation Res. **34,** 110 (1968).
41. Roberts, J. J., Crathorn, A. R., Brent, T. P.: Repair of alkylated DNA in mammalian cells. Nature (Lond.) **218,** 970 (1968).
42. Goldenberg, G. J.: Repair of sub-lethal damage of L5178Y lymphoblasts *in vitro* treated with dimethyl myleran and nitrogen mustard. Biochem. Pharmacol. **17,** 820 (1968).
43. Lawley, P. D., Brooks, P.: Molecular mechanism of the cytotoxic action of difunctional alkylating agents and of resistance to this action. Nature (Lond.) **206,** 480 (1965).
44. Kohn, K. W., Steigbigel, N. H., Spears, C. L.: Cross-linking and repair of DNA in sensitive and resistant strains of *E. coli* treated with nitrogen mustard. Proc. nat. Acad. Sci. **53,** 1154 (1965).

45. Venitt, S.: Interstrand cross-links in the DNA of *Escherichia coli* B/r and B_8-1 and their removal by the resistant strain. Biochem. biophys. Res. Commun. **31**, 355 (1968).
46. Crathorn, A. R., Roberts, J. J.: Mechanism of the cytotoxic action of alkylating agents in mammalian cells and evidence for the removal of alkylated groups from deoxyribonucleic acid. Nature (Lond.) **211**, 150 (1966).
47. Reid, B. D., Walker, I. G.: The response of mammalian cells to alkylating agents. II. On the mechanism of the removal of sulfur-mustard-induced cross-links. Biochim. biophys. Acta (Amst.) **179**, 179 (1969).
48. Gaudin, D., Yielding, K. L.: Response of a "resistant" plasmacytoma to alkylating agents and X-ray in combination with the excision repair inhibitors caffeine and chloroquine. Proc. Soc. exp. Biol. (N. Y.) **131**, 1413 (1969).
49. Wheeler, G. P.: Studies related to mechanisms of resistance to biological alkylating agents. Cancer Res. **23**, 1334 (1963).
50. Rutman, R. J., Chun, E. H. L., Lewis, F. S.: Permeability difference as a source of resistance to alkylating agents in Ehrlich tumor cells. Biochem. biophys. Res. Commun. **32**, 650 (1968).
51. Wolpert, M. K., Ruddon, R. W.: A study on the mechanism of resistance to nitrogen mustard (HN2) in Ehrlich ascites tumor cells: Comparison of uptake of HN2-^{14}C into sensitive and resistant cells. Cancer Res. **29**, 873 (1969).
52. Wheeler, G. P., Alexander, J. A.: Effects of nitrogen mustard and cyclophosphamide upon the synthesis of DNA *in vivo* and in cell-free preparations. Cancer Res. **29**, 98 (1969).
53. Griswold, D. P., Jr., Schabel, F. M., Jr., Wilcox, W. S., Simpson-Herren, L., Skipper, H. E.: Success and failure in the treatment of solid tumors. I. Effects of cyclophosphamide (NSC-26271) on primary and metastatic plasmacytoma in the hamster. Cancer Chemother. Rep. **52**, 345 (1968).
54. Laster, W. R., Jr., Mayo, J. G., Simpson-Herren, L., Griswold, D. P., Jr., Lloyd, H. H., Schabel, F. M., Jr., Skipper, H. E.: Success and failure in the treatment of solid tumors II. Kinetic parameters and "cell cure" of moderately advanced carcinoma 755. Cancer Chemother. Rep. **53**, 169 (1969).
55. Luce, J. K., Bodey, G. P., Sr., Frei, E., III.: The systemic approach to cancer therapy. Hospital Practice **2**, 42 (1967).
56. Burchenal, J. H.: Formal discussion: Long-term survival in Burkitt's tumor and in acute leukemia. Cancer Res. **27**, Part I, 2616 (1967).

Management of the Chronic Leukaemias

David A. G. Galton

With 1 Figure

Chronic myelocytic and lymphocytic leukaemia have few features in common except their progressive and inevitably fatal course, the high leucocyte counts, and the fact that radiotherapy and some cytotoxic drugs are useful in controlling them but cannot cure them.

Chronic myelocytic leukaemia (CML) belongs to the group of primary myeloproliferative diseases that includes polycythaemia vera, essential thrombocythaemia, and myelosclerosis with myeloid metaplasia. It is convenient, though arbitrary, to limit our discussion to Ph^1-positive CML, which includes the majority of cases of presumptive CML. In the Ph^1-positive disease all or almost all the bone-marrow cells in metaphase in preparations for chromosome analysis contain one characteristic abnormal chromosome lacking a large part of the long arm in the pair of small acrocentric G-group autosomes; probably number 21. This abnormal chromosome is known as the Philadelphia chromosome. A minority of Ph^1-positive patients have atypical features such as myelosclerosis, or the combination of thrombocythaemia, only slightly elevated granulocyte counts, high alkaline phosphatase scores, absence of splenomegaly, poor response to treatment, and relatively short survival. Conversely, a few patients with apparently typical CML are Ph^1-negative. Most Ph^1-negative cases, however, have atypical features that permit their recognition before the chromosome analysis is made. Sometimes the only clues are minor cytomorphological abnormalities in the blood and bone-marrow films. It is also important to recognise hitherto symptomless CML presenting in blast-cell crisis because these patients respond badly to treatment. They usually present with a short history of febrile illness sometimes with loss of weight, and with symptoms resulting from anaemia and thrombocytopenia. Acute granulocytic leukaemia is often diagnosed because of the high blast-cell count, but the large spleen, the high absolute neutrophil and basophil counts point to a preceding CML. If we consider Ph^1-positive CML only, the disease, though variable, is sufficiently uniform to permit practical recommendations on management [1].

In contrast, chronic lymphocytic leukaemia (CLL) is a much more variable disease. It belongs to the group of primary lymphoproliferative diseases that includes all the malignant lymphocytic lymphomas the behaviour of which ranges from very slowly progressive, even benign disease, with a course spanning several decades, to the most highly malignant and rapidly fatal sarcomas. There is no single biological marker comparable to the Philadelphia chromosome that permits the separation of a group with relatively uniform features, and there is no single diagnostic feature that excludes other conditions. If we were to rely only on the height of the absolute blood lymphocyte count we should have to set an arbitrary lower limit, and we should have to include some cases of essential macroglobulinaemia, of nodular lymphocytic lymphoma, and of chronic lymphosarcoma-cell leukaemia, which would be missed if we did not study the serum proteins, the histological appearance of an excised lymph node, and the cytomorphology of the lymphocytes in the blood and bone marrow. If we were to rely only on demonstrating heavy lymphocytic infiltration of the bone marrow, we should have to include otherwise typical CLL patients whose blood lymphocyte counts may rise to high levels only after many years or may never rise, as well as many patients who would not ordinarily be diagnosed as suffering from CLL. These include the rare cases of pancytopenia unaccompanied by physical signs with reticulin-rich marrow in which marrow cannot be aspirated, and the lymphocytic infiltration can be demonstrated only by trephine biopsy [2]; some of these patients have a monoclonal IgM paraprotein in their serum. Even if we accept a diagnosis based on arbitrarily defined indispensible criteria such as an absolute lymphocyte count and a bone marrow lymphocyte count beyond agreed levels, and a histological picture of diffuse lymphocytic lymphoma in an excised lymph node, we are still in trouble, for many patients with otherwise typical CLL have no palpable lymph nodes; but if we dispense with the necessity of lymph-node biopsy we shall inevitably miss cases of nodular lymphocytic lymphoma, although a presumptive diagnosis might be possible if the characteristic notched-nucleus cells are seen in the blood and marrow films [3, 4]. If we accept the necessity of lymph-node biopsy we must decide whether to allow only cases of well-differentiated diffuse lymphocytic lymphoma. If we do, we shall miss a small number of patients with poorly-differentiated diffuse lymphocytic lymphoma whose disease in all other respects, including its response to treatment and long survival, is indistinguishable from typical CLL [5]. The same difficulty arises if we try to define limits for the cytological characteristics of the lymphocytes, for there is a surprising range of morphological variation in CLL, and it is difficult to relate the several patterns to the clinical picture except in one rare but well-defined type. This is prolymphocytic leukaemia [6] in which large prominent nucleoli are present in otherwise well differentiated though sometimes large lymphocytes. The patients are sometimes referred as cases of acute leukaemia, but they have large hard spleens, no palpable lymph nodes, and very high absolute lymphocyte counts. Unlike typical CLL in which enlarged lymph nodes bring the patient to the doctor at a relatively early stage, the patients with prolymphocytic leukaemia usually present at a late stage with symptoms resulting from bone-marrow failure. They are remarkably resistant to treatment often effective in typical CLL. Unlike Ph^1-positive CML in which almost all the patients present with symptoms, CLL is often discovered by chance from a routine blood count. The frequency depends on the quality of the medical services in the area, but is everywhere increasing. The difference between CML and CLL in this respect reflects the steadily progressive character of CML and the often static character of CLL in a subclinical stage. Different sets of survival figures for CML [7] are reasonably uniform and give a useful guide to the behaviour of the disease, but those for CLL vary so greatly as to be practically meaningless [8—13]. The differences are largely due to the lack of uniformity in diagnosis, in the stage of the disease from which survival is arbitrarily calculated, and in many sources of selection according to the provenance of the cases in each series. They are partly due to differences in treatment.

It is against this complex background that we must discuss the management of the chronic leukaemias.

Chronic Myelocytic Leukaemia (CML)

The 'Chronic' Phase

CML in its first 'chronic' phase is best regarded as a minimal-deviation tumour, a term first used to describe certain well-differentiated experimental liver-cell tumours apparently resembling normal liver tissue in all respects except one or a very few biochemical characteristics. In CML the normal bone marrow may be regarded as entirely replaced by a homogeneous, functional bone marrow, identifiable morphologically by its marker chromosome (Ph^1), and functionally by its partial loss of sensitivity to homeostatic control. The marrow produces apparently normal erythrocytes and platelets, and almost normal granulocytes, but it is persistently hyperplastic and differentiation is progressively directed towards granulopoiesis leading to a greatly expanded total granulocyte mass (TGM) which is responsible for the familiar clinical and haematological manifestations. It is not clear whether the proliferation of the Ph^1-bearing stem cells begins in the bone marrow, and the spleen has come under suspicion. With a few important exceptions to which I shall refer shortly, when the TGM has been reduced by appropriate treatment, and the spleen is no longer palpable, all the cells in marrow aspirates are still Ph^1-positive, and Ph^1-positive cells can still be identified in juice aspirated from the spleen [14].

Treatment of the 'Chronic' Phase

The aim of conventional treatment is first to reduce the TGM sufficiently to reverse the adverse features resulting from its overgrowth, and secondly to try to stabilize the advantageous position so gained by suitable maintenance therapy. No attempt is made to try to eradicate the Ph^1-bearing myeloid tissue in the hope that normal marrow will regenerate. We rely on the abnormal marrow to provide the required output of erythrocytes, granulocytes and platelets and the treatment is intended only to minimize the pathological sequelae of a greatly increased TGM. The total leucocyte count is roughly proportional to the TGM and the trend of the count reflects the change in size of the TGM. Treatment therefore is directed first to reducing the leucocyte count and then to prevent it from rising again. As the leucocyte count falls, the spleen shrinks, the symptoms of hypermetabolism recede, and the haemoglobin concentration rises. As long as the character of the disease remains unchanged, the favourable position brought about by reducing the leucocyte count may be maintained by stabilizing the count at approximately normal levels.

The precise means of reducing the TGM may well be of secondary importance. My own preference is still for busulphan, because of long familiarity with it, because there is a precise relationship between the dose and the effect on the leucocyte count and because the great majority of patients respond without experiencing side effects. Others prefer splenic X-irradiation, radiophosphorus, or the newer drugs dibromomannitol and hydroxyurea. In a comparative trial of busulphan and radiotherapy involving 102 patients carried out under the auspices of the Medical Research Council, both the length and the quality of survival were superior in the busulphan group [15].

As already mentioned, most patients with CML present with symptoms resulting from hypermetabolism, anaemia, or splenomegaly, and they should be treated as soon as the diagnosis is established. A few symptomless patients are diagnosed by chance, and if observed without treatment, most develop symptoms within 1 year, though occasional patients remain well for as long as 5 years [16]. Most symptom-free patients who are treated, however, claim to feel much better and say they did not realise how unwell they had been before treatment. In general, therefore, one should not defer treatment too long in symptomless cases, though an observation period of several months may sometimes be justified to discover the rate of progression of the disease.

The details of each treatment method vary in respect of the rate of fall of the leucocyte count to be aimed at, the rate of increase in the count to be expected when treatment is discontinued, and the type of maintenance therapy necessary to stabilize the count. In the case of busulphan, the first course, at a daily dose of 0.065 mg/kg of body weight usually requires from 12 to 24 weeks of treatment, administration being discontinued when the leucocyte count approaches 15,000/μl. Patients vary in the rate at which the leucocyte count subsequently increases, and when the doubling time of the count is longer than 70 days there is no urgency to begin maintenance therapy. One of my patients required no treatment after the end of the first course of busulphan in September 1966 until February 1970 when the leucocyte count had risen to 80,000/μl and the spleen had again become palpable; but this is exceptional. In general the patients with long leucocyte-count doubling times after the initial course of treatment have a better prognosis [7]. Some patients remain well controlled for many years but only 20% remain alive after 5 years, and 50% are dead within 3½ years [15]. The disease changes its character and is no longer amenable to control. To some extent the resistance to treatment is specific in that some measure of control may be regained by changing the treatment. For example a patient who has become resistant to busulphan administered at increasing daily dosage may respond again for a time to dibromomannitol, hydroxyurea or mercaptopurine, but the response is rarely as complete as when the patient was first treated and is usually shortlived. We must now examine the later phase of CML.

'Transformed' CML

The most dramatic and rapidly fatal change in the character of CML is the acute blast-cell crisis in which the patient is overwhelmed by an explosive proliferation of undifferentiated blast cells which replace the only slightly abnormal myeloid tissue which I have likened to a minimal-deviation tumour. However, this hyperacute termination is rare, and only the most extreme manifestation of the malignant transformation of the minimal-deviation disease of the chronic phase. In many cases the gradual evolution of the blast-cell phase over a period of as long as 2 years can only be appreciated by retrospective inspection of the haematological charts and an examination of successive blood films. In some cases no increase in the blast-cell counts occurs in the blood or marrow but the progressively downhill course of the patient and the features of the blood-count trends leave no doubt that the disease has changed its character and has become a malignant neoplasm. The nature of this progression towards autonomous neoplasia has been clarified by cytogenetic studies which reveal the Ph^1-bearing myeloid tissue as a genetically unstable population from its inception, with the inevitable consequence that competition for survival among varying cell lines leads to the dominance of stable clones having a selective advantage. The cells of these clones are usually but not necessarily recognisable as blast cells, and usually but not necessarily have demonstrably abnormal karyotypes in addition to the original Ph^1 abnormality. Serial karyotype examinations during the course of the disease often reveal the emergence of successful clones [17, 18, 19]. There is a certain regularity with which additional chromosomal abnormalities appear, and the Ph^1 chromosome itself may be the first recognisable and inevitable progression in a preceding but as yet unidentified abnormality. This is suggested by the existence of the Ph^1 chromosome in both cell lines of an XY/XXY mosaic [20] and by the frequency with which second Ph^1 chromosomes appear during the course of the disease. The progressive evolution towards malignancy is reflected in the survival curves of different series of patients, untreated, or treated by different methods, all of which show that the chance of dying in any given period is greater than in the preceding period. There is no doubt that treatment has prolonged life, and probably does so by slowing the rate of genetic mutation, but the practical gain is regrettably little.

Patients with transformed CML are difficult to treat. A few with an acute blast-cell transformation on a 'chronic' phase with a rapidly proliferating blast-cell clone have responded to prednisone and vincristine administered in combination. Several drugs administered in combination on the lines used in the treatment of lymphoblastic leukaemia have been tried but no regularly effective regime is available.

Possibility of Radical Therapy

The possibility of preventing the inevitable progression towards malignancy by selective elimination at an early stage of the original Ph^1-bearing clone is attractive, but evidence provided by the fate of patients unusually sensitive to or overdosed with busulphan is discouraging because it indicates that the Ph^1-bearing myeloid stem cell is more resistant to busulphan than is the normal myeloid stem cell [21]. The dose of busulphan required to control CML is higher than non-leukaemic patients tolerate, but this was not appreciated when the contrary statement was made because the non-leukaemic patients were treated for too short a time [22]. Most patients with CML who are overdosed with busulphan die but some who have been kept alive in a state of pancytopenia with hypoplastic fatty bone marrows have subsequently relapsed with chronic-phase disease or have died in blast-cell crisis with persistently fatty marrow. A few long surviving patients whose leucocyte counts fell unusually rapidly during busulphan therapy were found subsequently to have cells of normal karyotype in their bone marrow, but in every case known to me, Ph^1-positive cells were present also. Three patients in unmaintained remission with a mixed population of normal and Ph^1-positive cells and a normal blood picture were alive 5, 10, and 15 years after the initial treatment, but relapse of the leukaemia took place in the 4th year in a fourth case [21]. The increased resistance of the Ph^1-bearing myeloid stem cell is not specific for busulphan. When triethylenemelamine was used the doses necessary to control of CML were far higher than could be tolerated by non-leukaemic patients [23].

The prospects for improving the results of treatment of CML by more aggressive chemotherapy are thus not encouraging.

Chronic Lymphocytic Leukaemia (CLL)

Just as the clinical disability of CML results from the greatly increased TGM, much of the clinical disability of CLL results from a greatly increased body burden of lymphocytes. They infiltrate and gradually replace the bone marrow with consequent impairment of bone-marrow function. They infiltrate the lymph nodes throughout the body, the splenic white and red pulp, and the portal tracts of the liver. Patients with very large spleens, unlike those with CML, suffer the effects of hypersplenism. In varying degree all these infiltrative effects can be reversed by treatment. The enlarged lymph nodes and spleen decrease in size, though the enlarged liver rarely responds to a comparable extent, and bone-marrow function is restored, although focal aggregates of lymphocytes more numerous than are found in normal marrow persist. There is, however, a second feature of CLL, not explicable in terms of the total lymphocyte mass (TLM), that becomes progressively severe during the course of the disease, however well the infiltrative features are controlled. This is the impairment of immunological capacity which leads to increasing susceptibility to infections not only to common bacterial and viral pathogens, but also to organisms not normally pathogenic for healthy subjects. Live vaccines may be highly dangerous to CLL patients. Smallpox vaccination for example may cause vaccinia gangrenosa with rapidly fatal viraemia. All patients should be told that they must not be vaccinated against smallpox. Non-living vaccines and toxoids are not harmful, but neither are they beneficial because CLL patients cannot make antibodies when challenged. During the course of the disease the serum immunoglobulin levels fall. Unlike the infiltrative propensity of CLL, the immunological defect cannot be reversed by any form of treatment, though some passive protection against infection may sometimes be conferred by regular injections of human gammaglobulin.

Indications for Treatment

The fact that treatment can reverse only some of the adverse features of CLL is a major consideration in formulating the indications for treatment. Other crucial factors are the natural history of the disease itself, the necessity for striking a compromise between the possible benefits and the adverse effects of treatment, and the fact that patients often become resistant to treatment.

The Natural History of CLL

In clinical practice there is a striking difference between those patients whose disease seems to have no obvious adverse effect on their well-being and shows little evidence of progression for one or two decades whether or not the patients are treated, and those whose disease behaves aggressively from the time of diagnosis, responds poorly to treatment and runs a relatively short course. It is difficult to decide whether these differences represent two distinct forms of the disease [24, 25, 26], or only the extremes of a continuous spectrum of variation [13]. In practice it is important to recognise the slowly progressive disease because treatment should be withheld. The patients have no symptoms attributable to the disease, though they may have sought advice because they found enlarged lymph nodes, and they have well preserved bone-marrow function even though aspirated samples of bone marrow are often heavily infiltrated with lymphocytes. Their condition remains essentially unchanged during many years of observation, though they may begin to suffer from infections as their immunological capacity deteriorates. The lymphocyte counts of many of these patients fluctuate above and below a constant mean value for many years, without showing an upward trend. Rarely, (Fig. 1) a spontaneous lowering of the absolute lymphocyte count establishes an equilibrium at a lower level for some years after which the count rises to its previous level. The subject of Fig. 1 has received no treatment in 10 years of observation. He has had an attack of herpes zoster, and has subnormal levels of serum immunoglobulins.

The chief general indication for treatment is evidence of progressive disease, and in particular, of impairment of bone-marrow function. The trends in the haemoglobin

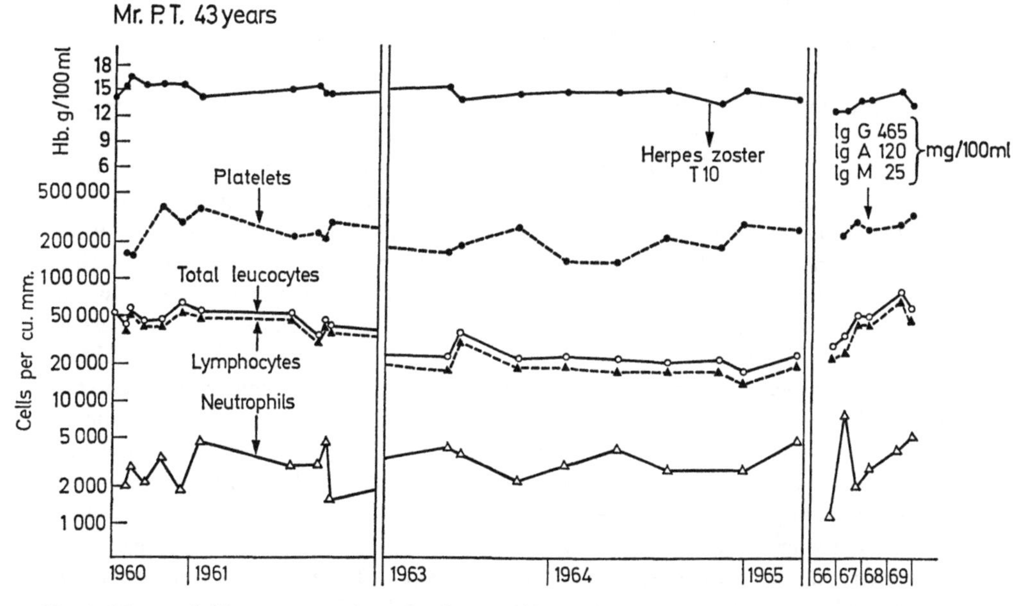

Fig. 1. Haemoglobin concentration, platelet, total leucocyte, lymphocyte and neutrophil counts of a 43-year old man suffering from chronic lymphocytic leukemia. The patient received no treatment during an observation period of almost 10 years

concentration, platelet and neutrophil counts provide better evidence of the state of marrow function than the appearance of films of aspirated bone marrow. Treatment should be started as soon as it is clear that marrow function is declining, because bone marrow failure is a threat to life. Some patients present in bone-marrow failure. A few present with an autoimmune haemolytic anaemia, and yet others present with thrombocytopenia not accounted for by marrow failure due to lymphocytic infiltration. Each of these situations requires active treatment.

The chief special indication for treatment in patients with well-preserved bone-marrow function is the presence of infiltrations in such organs as the skin, tonsils, conjunctivae, salivary glands, and stomach. These manifestations are best treated by local radiotherapy and will not be further considered, except to mention that patients with skin infiltrations are often particularly refractory to treatment by any of the available methods.

Methods of Treatment

The most useful methods of treatment are (1) external radiotherapy and radiophosphorus, (2) the alkylating agents chlorambucil and cyclophosphamide, (3) the steroid hormones, and (4) splenectomy. The place of extracorporeal irradiation of the blood has been discussed already in this Symposium by Dr. E. P. CRONKITE.

The aim of treatment is to reduce the TLM sufficiently to clear the bone marrow as far as possible of excess lymphocytes, and so to permit the recolonisation of the marrow by haemopoietic cells. In contrast to CML, where the trend of the total leucocyte count reflects that of the TGM, the trend of the lymphocyte count does not reflect that of the TLM. It is usually easy to reduce the lymphocyte count to normal levels by radiotherapy or by treatment with alkylating agents, but in some cases there is little or no reduction in the size of the lymph nodes or spleen or of improvement in bone-marrow function. However, in some of these apparently refractory cases, repeated courses of treatment, or in the case of the alkylating agents continuous treatment at appropriate dosage, eventually bring about regression of the spleen and of most of the lymph nodes, and return to normal levels of the haemoglobin concentration, neutrophil and platelet counts. OSGOOD [27] found that the median time required to achieve optimal conditions with treatment by radiophosphorus was 27 months, and this is true also for the alkylating agents. Thus it is important not do abandon treatment as useless at too early a stage. In practice it is worth continuing with the first planned treatment as long as the patient's condition is not deteriorating. Patients on long-term treatment thus respond in one of three main ways: first, there is continued, though sometimes slow and only partial improvement which is maintained until the disease becomes refractory to treatment, or the patient succumbs to uncontrollable infection; second, there is little change sometimes over a period of years, and it is difficult to assess the value of the treatment; lastly, there is steady deterioration.

There have been no long-term comparative therapeutic trials of radiotherapy and chemotherapy comparable with the Medical Research Council's Trial in CML, and there is no convincing evidence in favour of any one of the methods mentioned. The main point to emphasize is that patients who present in bone-marrow failure should not be treated in the first instance with radiotherapy or with alkylating agents. This is because the failing marrow cannot tolerate further assault from myelosuppressive agents. These patients should be treated first with steroids.

Use of Adrenal Corticosteroids

Steroid therapy has 4 major effects in hitherto untreated CLL patients who present in bone-marrow failure. An immediate effect on the capillary endothelium may reduce purpura in patients with thrombocytopenia. Within 2 weeks and sometimes within a few days the spleen and enlarged lymph nodes shrink, the lymphocyte count rises. The proportion of lymphocytes in the bone marrow falls, and lastly, bone-marrow regeneration begins with an ensuing rise in the reticulocyte counts, haemoglobin concentration, platelet and neutrophil counts.

Because of the hazards of long-term steroid therapy, particularly in immunologically incompetent patients, steroid therapy is best reserved for emergency treatment as already outlined, with the object of rescuing the patient from bone-marrow failure. When the marrow is regenerating, usually within 8 weeks, treatment with an alkylating agent may be started and the administration of the steroid tailed off.

A situation in which steroid therapy is effective but alkylating agents are very harmful is that of haemolytic anaemia that is compensated, or not quite compensated. The erythropoietic capacity has no reserve, but in the former case, the haemoglobin level is steady while in the latter it is falling. Treatment with an alkylating agent causes an immediate fall in red-cell production, and because the red-cell life span is reduced, a catastrophic fall in the haemoglobin concentration ensues. This situation accounts for some though not all [28] of the reports of the induction of a haemolytic crisis by alkylating agents. Autoimmune haemolytic anaemia is also an indication for steroid therapy, but here also an alkylating agent should be substituted for the steroid as soon as it is safe to do so.

A difficult problem is that of profound thrombocytopenia not accounted for by lymphocytic replacement of the bone marrow. There is usually only minimal enlargement of the lymph nodes and spleen, the lymphocyte count is only moderately raised, and there is only moderate lymphocytic infiltration of the bone marrow. It is not clear whether the thrombocytopenia is related to the CLL. It is probably best to treat these patients as if they had idiopathic thrombocytopenia, having regard to the special danger of long-term steroid therapy. Splenectomy should be considered at an early stage.

Splenectomy

Patients with very large spleens and hypersplenism are difficult to treat with radiotherapy or alkylating agents. Elective splenectomy is often successful and after the operation the CLL may be well controlled by alkylating agent therapy.

Treatment-Resistant CLL

A minority of patients fail to respond to any of the methods of treatment mentioned, and they do not respond when other types of chemotherapeutic agents are tried. But the great majority of treatment-resistant patients are those who have previously responded well, sometimes for many years, to treatment. Resistance usually develops gradually and may not be recognised until several years have elapsed. It occurs whether chemotherapy has been administered on an intermittent or a continuous schedule. One of my patients who had received a single course of chlorambucil and prednisone in combination 6 years previously was completely resistant to a second identical course of treatment. Patients resistant to chlorambucil are resistant to cyclophosphamide and to other alkylating agents. When the state of resistance is obvious it is not in the patient's interest to persist with chemotherapy in the hope that it might do some good or might at least retard the progress of the disease. At this stage the alkylating agents act only as myelosuppressant and immunosuppressant agents and have no therapeutic value, while the dangers of ineffective steroid therapy need no further emphasis. Even local irradiation to lymph nodes, often grossly enlarged at this stage, may cause thrombocytopenia and neutropenia. It is in this situation that extracorporeal irradiation of the blood has sometimes conferred some temporary benefit.

Richter's Syndrome

Unlike CML, in which a progressive change or metamorphosis [29] towards florid malignant behaviour is part of the natural history of the disease, CLL only rarely provides evidence of a comparable change. Even when a manifestation usually regarded as malignant appears such as widespread osteolytic skeletal deposits [30], the lymphocytes still appear well differentiated morphologically.

One rare termination of CLL is the appearance of a malignant pleomorphic histiocytic lymphoma, associated with intractable pyrexia, and sometimes with an 'M' protein, usually a monoclonal IgM or Bence Jones protein in the serum or urine. Bernard [31] attributed the first description of this condition to Richter [32], and because of the presence of multinucleated giant cells in the tumour, and of the pyrexia, considered the tumour to be Hodgkin's disease. This syndrome should be suspected whenever a CLL patient develops persistent pyrexia for which no cause can be found, and if an 'M' protein is found in the blood or urine. If no accessible tumour is available for biopsy, confirmation may be sought by lymphography, or even laparotomy. I have observed no benefit from local irradiation or from treatment with vinca alkaloids.

Summary

The treatment of CML is directed first to reducing the greatly enlarged total granulocyte mass (TGM), and secondly to preventing it from enlarging again by appropriate maintenance therapy. The abnormal symptoms, signs, and haematological findings are abolished by reducing the TGM but the karyotypically abnormal marrow stem cells persist. Treatment loses its effect as the disease changes its character and becomes more frankly malignant. Malignant transformation is occasionally a one-step acute event ('blast-cell crisis') but is more often a multi-step process; in either case treatment is relatively ineffective.

Treatment of CLL may be considered in terms of the greatly increased total lymphocyte mass (TLM) in the body. This causes topographical effects by infiltration of tissues and enlargement of organs, and functional effects, chiefly bone-marrow failure, autoimmune effects, and immunological incompetence. All but the last can be reversed in varying degree by treatment. Symptomless patients with well preserved bone-marrow function should be observed without treatment; alkylating agents are used when bone-marrow function begins to decline, and steroids are used to start treatment in cases of bone-marrow failure, to be replaced by an alkylating agent as marrow function improves. Long-term steroid therapy should be avoided. Resistance to alkylating agents develops between 4 and 15 years after starting treatment; therefore these agents should not be used without a clear indication. Splenectomy is often helpful in cases of gross splenomegaly with secondary hypersplenism. Radiotherapy is useful to reduce troublesome local manifestations.

References

1. GALTON, D. A. G.: The treatment of chronic myelocytic leukaemia. Seminars in Hematology **6**, 323 (1969).
2. DUHAMEL, G., GUERRA, L.: Un syndrome hématologique difficile à définir: La myelofibrose lymphoide. Presse méd. **74**, 585 (1966).
3. ANDAY, G. J., SCHMITZ, H. L.: Follicular lymphoma with transient leukemic phase. Arch. intern. Med. **89**, 621 (1952).
4. ROSENTHAL, N., DRESKIN, O. H., VURAL, I. C., ZAK, F. G.: The significance of haematogones in blood, bone marrow and lymph node aspiration in giant follicular lymphoblastoma. Acta haemat. (Basel) **8**, 368 (1952).
5. GALTON, D. A. G.: Chronic lymphocytic leukaemia: its pathogenesis and relationship to lymphosarcoma. In: Symposium on Lymphatic Tumours in Africa, Paris. Basel-New York: S. Karger, p. 163.
6. GOLDENBERG, G. J., GALTON, D. A. G.: In: British Empire Cancer Campaign. Annual Report 1964, p. 25.
7. BERGSAGEL, D. E.: The chronic leukemias: a review of disease manifestations and the aims of therapy. Canad. med. Ass. J. **96**, 1616 (1967).
8. MINOT, G. B., ISAACS, R.: Lymphatic leukemia; age incidence, duration, and benefit derived from irradiation. Boston med. Surg. J. **191**, 1 (1924).
9. TIVEY, H.: The prognosis for survival in chronic granulocytic and lymphocytic leukemia. Amer. J. Roentgenol. **72**, 68 (1954).
10. OSGOOD, E. E., SEAMAN, A. J., KOLER, R. D.: Results of the 15-year program of treatment of chronic leukaemias with titrated regularly spaced total body irradiation, with phosphorus 32 or X-ray. In: Proceedings of the Sixth International Congress for the International Society of Hematologists. Boston: Grune and Stratton 1958, p. 44.
11. GREEN, R. A., DIXON, H.: Expectancy for life in chronic lymphatic leukemia. Blood **25**, 23 (1965).
12. GALTON, D. A. G.: Trends in the therapy of leukaemia. In: Modern Trends in Radiotherapy. Eds.: T. J. DEELEY and C. A. P. WOOD. London: Butterworths 1967, p. 292.
13. BOGGS, D. R., SOFFERMAN, S. A., WINTROBE, M. M., CARTWRIGHT, G. E.: Factors influencing the duration of survival of patients with chronic lymphocytic leukemia. Amer. J. Med. **40**, 243 (1966).
14. SPIERS, A. S. D.: Personal communication.
15. Medical Research Council: chronic granulocytic leukaemia: comparison of radiotherapy and busulphan therapy. Brit. med. J. **1968 I**, 201.
16. WINTROBE, M. M., in: Clinical Hematology, 6th Ed. London: Kimpton 1967, p. 995.
17. DE GROUCHY, J., DE NAVA, C., CANTA, J.-M., BILSKI-PASQUIER, G., BOUSSER, J.: Models for clonal evolution: a study of chronic myelogenous leukemia. Amer. J. hum. Genet. **18**, 485 (1966).
18. PEDERSEN, B.: Cytogenetic evolution in chronic myelogenous leukaemia. Copenhagen: Munksgaard 1969.

19. BAIKIE, A. G.: Chronic granulocytic leukaemia: the metamorphosis of a conditioned neoplasm to an autonomous one (in press).
20. TOUGH, I. M., COURT BROWN, W. M., BAIKIE, A. G., BUCKTON, K. E., HARNDEN, D. G., JACOBS, P. A., KING, M. J., MCBRIDE, J. A.: Cytogenetic studies in chronic myeloid leukaemia and acute leukaemia associated with mongolism. Lancet **1961 I**, 411.
21. GALTON, D. A. G.: The possibility of radical chemotherapy in chronic myelocytic leukaemia. Haematologica Latina **12**, 703 (1969).
22. — The use of Myleran and similar agents in chronic leukemias: In: Advances in Cancer Research. Eds.: J. P. GREENSTEIN and A. HADDOW. New York: Academic Press 1956, p. 73.
23. BOND, W. H., ROHN, R. J., DYKE, R. W., FOUTS, P. J.: Clinical use of triethylenemelamine. Report of 75 cases. Arch. intern. Med. **91**, 602 (1953).
24. REINHARD, E. H., NEELY, C. L., SAMPLES, D. M.: Radioactive phosphorus in the treatment of chronic leukemias: long-term results over a period of 15 years. Ann. intern. Med. **50**, 942 (1959).
25. GUNZ, F. W., CAMPBELL, A. J., GOLDSTEIN, A. M.: The treatment of chronic leukaemia. N. Z. med. J. **60**, 441 (1961).
26. GALTON, D. A. G.: The pathogenesis of chronic lymphocytic leukemia. Canad. med. Ass. J. **94**, 1005 (1966).
27. OSGOOD, E. E.: Treatment of chronic leukemias. J. nucl. Med. **5**, 139 (1964).
28. YONET, H. M., VIGLIANO, E. M., HOROWITZ, H. I.: Acute hemolytic anemia associated with administration of alkylating agents: report of two cases due to cyclophosphamide and review of the literature. Amer. J. med. Sci. **254**, 71 (1967).
29. BAIKIE, A. G.: Chromosomes and leukaemia. Acta haemat. (Basel) **36**, 157 (1966).
30. Clinicopathological Conference. A case of chronic lymphocytic leukaemia presented at the Royal Postgraduate Medical School. Brit. med. J. **1970 I**, 546.
31. LORTHOLARY, P., BOIRON, M., RIPAULT, P., LEVY, J. P., MANUS, A., BERNARD, J.: Leucémie Lymphoïde Chronique Secondairement Associée à une Réticulopathie Maligne, Syndrome de Richter. Nouv. Rev. franç. Hémat. **4**, 621 (1964).
32. RICHTER, M. N.: Generalized reticular cell sarcoma of lymph nodes associated with lymphatic leukemia. Amer. J. Pathol. **4**, 285 (1928).

Chemotherapy of the Lymphomas

VINCENT T. DEVITA

With 1 Figure

Introduction

The lymphomas, as a group, are among the most responsive of neoplastic diseases man falls heir to. The modern period of the chemotherapy of the lymphomas began in the early 1940's with the appearance of the prototype alkylating agent, nitrogen mustard. While these agents have proven useful in the therapy of these diseases, there is no hard evidence that the life of patients with lymphomas has been significantly prolonged. In the twenty-five years that followed the introduction of nitrogen mustard, oncologists have been concerned primarily with the identification of new active drugs, at first new alkylating agents, but then other classes of antitumor drugs without cross resistance to the alkylating agents. In addition, a great deal of effort has been spent accumulating knowledge about the optimum way of employing each drug. Now that several classes of drugs with independent antilymphoma activity are available, recent studies have been more properly concerned with the best ways to employ them as a group, either used concomitantly, or in sequence in cyclical fashion, to prolong the life of patients, or if possible, to totally eradicate the disease.

This review will be concerned with recent results of chemotherapy of Hodgkin's disease, lymphosarcoma and reticulum cell sarcoma.

The Role of Histology in Evaluating Results of Therapy

It is quite apparent that the histologic appearance of the lymphoma in part plays a role in determining the prognosis of the patient [1, 2, 3]. In the past it seemed sufficient to delegate to the pathologist the responsibility of confirming the fact that the patient indeed had a malignant disease. While this task was often difficult enough, in the future it appears that clinicians may also be relying on the pathologists for histologic classification of the lymphoma in question to relegate the patient to appropriate treatment program. This point is best illustrated by the relatively favorable prognosis conferred on patients with Hodgkin's disease classified as lymphocyte predominant and/or nodular sclerosis [4]. In the case of lymphosarcoma, the giant follicular variety has generally been associated with a longer survival [5]. The validity of this diagnostic category as a separate entity is open to question. Patients with lymphosarcoma with all degrees of cellular differentiation may present with either a diffuse or a nodular pattern within the lymph node [2]. Cases classified as giant follicular lymphosarcoma, in the past, have probably represented all types of lymphosarcoma presenting with a nodular pattern. Although there is a suggestion that a nodular pattern and the degree of cell differentiation in patients with lymphosarcoma may indicate a more favorable overall prognosis, not enough information is available as to how the histologic picture influences the response of the tumor to X-irradiation or chemotherapy. Future studies should direct their attention increasingly to these points.

Staging and Therapy

The Rye classification is presently the most commonly used staging classification for Hodgkin's disease [6]. A similar staging classification can be used for the non-Hodgkin's lymphomas except that the distribution of cases into categories A (asymptomatic) or B (symptomatic with fever, night sweats or pruritus) seems less important.

At the present time, Stages I and II in all categories of lymphoma should be treated with radiotherapy. In lymphosarcoma and reticulum cell sarcoma, the pattern of clinically observed spread is much less predictable than in Hodgkin's disease [7, 8]. Recurrence in noncontiguous sites tends to be the rule rather than the exception. This is consistent with the failure of Peters to observe improved results with prophylactic X-irradiation of areas contiguous to the primary clinically involved area [9] and suggests that the disease is less often as locally involved as it appears. Many of the experimental therapeutic programs are concerned with the development of improved treatment for patients with advanced disease still confined to lymph nodes (Stage III). If stage and histology combine to influence both the response to therapy and overall survival many of these patients may have an inherent favorable prognosis for this relatively advanced stage. Since comparative radiotherapeutic and chemotherapeutic data are not available, conclusions regarding the appropriate therapy for this group of patients for all types of lymphomas should await the results of controlled clinical trials.

At the present time, all patients who have extended their disease into organ systems (Stage IV), are best treated with chemotherapy. Patients who have their primary lymphoma in the gut with involvement only of local draining nodes should, however, be regarded as having local disease and, following resection, should receive radiotherapy [10].

When to Treat

Most patients with lymphomas present to a physician because of enlarging lymph nodes, organ invasion, or symptoms of systemic disease. While some patients can pursue an indolent course without therapy, the continued presence of untreated, enlarged, or enlarging nodes, serves as a source of annoyance and despair, if they are aware of the significance of their diagnosis. If the risk of therapy can be kept to a minimum, all patients with advancing disease should be offered some available form of treatment. Waiting until the disease has advanced to the point of bulky tumors and/or debilitation decreases the chance of successful control and increases the risks of therapy.

The Approach to Treatment

Since the 1940's, many types of drugs have been tried in the treatment of the lymphomas. Four classes of drugs have been developed which are not cross-resistant and have clinical usefulness. These are, the alkylating agents, the corticosteroids, the vinca alkaloids, and the methylhydrazine derivatives. At least one member of each class is now available for clinical use. While the available agents are not ideal, and the search for new, more effective drugs continues, the availability of these drugs, and their effective use, involves a decision to embark on one of three major approaches to treatment as illustrated in Fig. 1. Program A involves the use of each drug singly, in an optimal fashion, until tumor resistance is apparent, before changing to the next available agent in sequence. The obvious questions posed by this type of treatment program are: 1. What is the optimal method of using each drug? 2. In what order should the drugs be used? 3. Should patients be continually maintained on therapy or intermittently retreated as needed? Program B involves the use of one agent at a time, each for a finite period of time, with recycling until resistance is demonstrated to all available agents. Again, the question of the sequence of drug usage assumes importance. Program C involves the use of the available effective drugs concomitantly. How to combine the drugs in an acceptable fashion poses the greatest problem with program C.

Available Effective Drugs

Table 1 summarizes pertinent details of some of the more commonly used drugs. The subject of the therapy of lymphomas has been recently reviewed in detail by Ultmann and Nixon [10 a]. For details on the pharmacology of the effective antitumor agents, the reader is referred to the review by Oliverio and Zubrod [10 b].

Nitrogen mustard is the prototype alkylating agent and is still a useful drug; it can only be given intravenously, is quite unstable and rapidly reactive with biologic materials [11]. As with all of the alkylating agents bone marrow suppression is dose limiting. Severe nausea and vomiting makes continuing repeated administration unpopular. Chlorambucil, on the other hand, can only be given orally but besides bone marrow suppression, has few side effects [11]. It is common practice to begin treatment initially with nitrogen mustard until a satisfactory response has been achieved and then attempt to maintain the response with chlorambucil.

Cyclophosphamide is inactive *in vitro* and has to be oxidatively metabolized to an unknown active moiety [11, 12]. Studies on metabolism of the compound in humans have not revealed as active degradation as is found in mice where the compound is more effective; excellent responses in patients with lymphoma have not been correlated with increased ability to metabolize the drug [13]. There are distinct advantages with the use of cyclophosphamide; first, it is completely absorbed orally and can also be given intravenously; second, it has a distinct platelet sparing effect even with large intravenous doses [14]. Since it is converted to its active form by microsomal enzymes, its metabolism can be increased or decreased nonspecifically by other drugs known to induce or inhibit microsomal metabolism and this can lead to inadvertent combination chemotherapy if this point is not kept in mind. To date, this

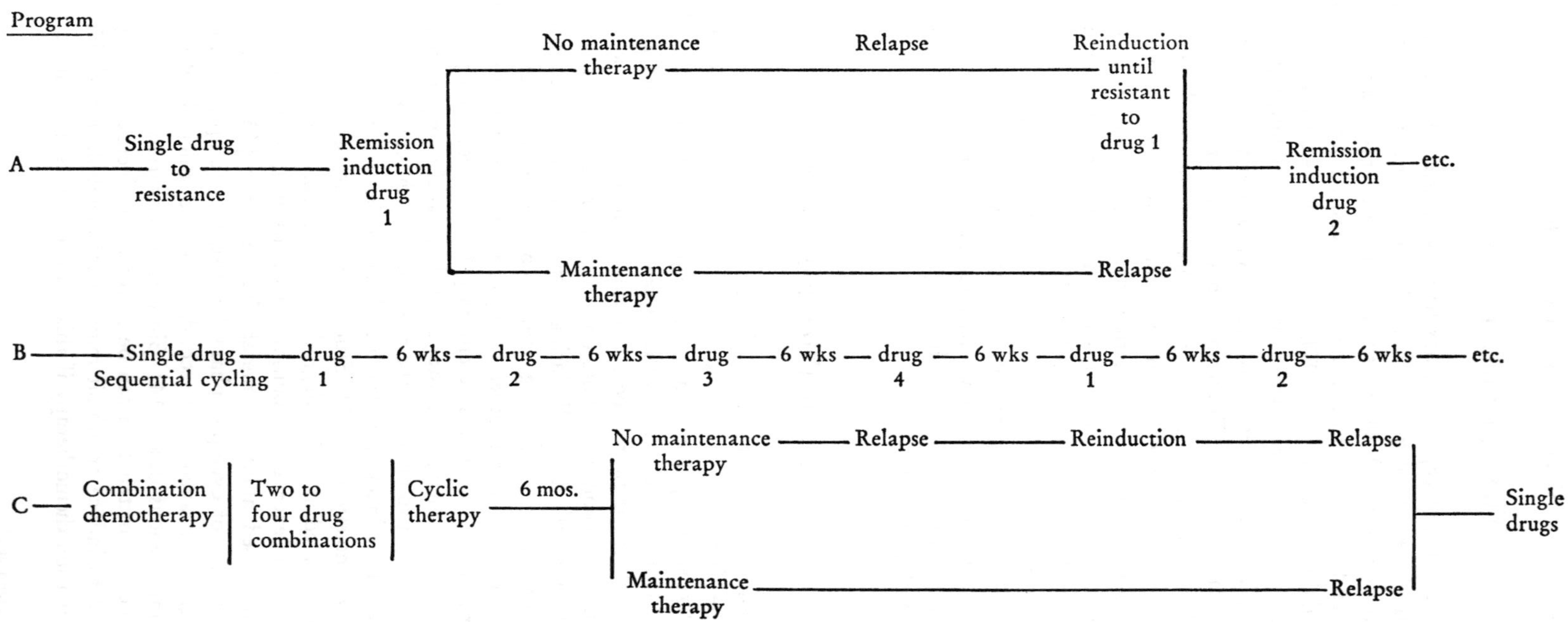

Fig. 1. Schematic representation of three possible approaches to using the available effective drugs in the treatment of lymphomas

Table 1. *Effective drugs generally available for the treatment of the lymphomas*

Drug	Routes of administration	Dose	Dose limiting toxicity	Other major side effects Acute	Chronic
Nitrogen mustard	IV	0.4 mg/kg single dose repeated q 3—4 weeks	Leukopenia Thrombocytopenia	Nausea and vomiting	Bone marrow depression
Chlorambucil	Oral	0.2—0.1 mg/kg/day	Leukopenia Thrombocytopenia		Bone marrow depression
Cyclophosphamide	Oral	4—1 mg/kg/day	Leukopenia		Hemorrhagic cystitis Epilation Marrow suppression
	IV	40 mg/kg single dose repeated q 3—4 weeks	Leukopenia	Nausea and vomiting Hemorrhagic cystitis Epilation	Epilation Marrow suppression
	IV	15 mg/kg/week	Leukopenia	Nausea and vomiting Epilation Hemorrhagic cystitis	Epilation Hemorrhagic cystitis Marrow suppression
Vinblastine	IV	0.1—0.3 mg/kg/week	Leukopenia Thrombocytopenia	Myalgias	Marrow suppression
Vincristine	IV	0.025—0.05 mg/kg/week	Peripheral Neuropathy Obstipation	Myalgias	Epilation Severe neuropathy
Procarbazine	Oral	5—3 mg/kg	Leukopenia Thrombocytopenia	Nausea and vomiting	Marrow suppression Drug eruptions Abnormal liver function
Prednisone	Oral	1 mg/kg/day	Osteoporosis Diabetes GI Bleeding	Euphoria Fluid retention	Osteoporosis Diabetes Cushing's syndrome Increased risk of infections

feature of cyclophosphamide has not been exploited clinically. On the negative side of the ledger, cyclophosphamide causes more epilation than other alkylating agents and can cause troublesome, and sometimes severe, hemorrhagic cystitis. Again, initial therapy is best begun with larger intravenous doses and either continued intermittently until resistance is apparent or the patient switched to treament by an oral maintenance program. There is cross resistance among the various alkylating agents but what occasionally appears to be drug resistance may be overcome by changing the dose and schedule (schedule resistance).

The vinca alkaloids are only generally available for parenteral administration [15—18]. Bone marrow suppression is the major dose limiting effect of vinblastine, but some patients develop a mild peripheral neuropathy with continued use. Generally, vinblastine is given weekly until a satisfactory response is obtained and then maintenance doses can be given either weekly or at intervals of two weeks or more. Vincristine is used in a similar fashion but peripheral and autonomic nervous system neuropathies are the dose limiting side effects, and after two to six doses in adults, treatment must either be stopped or doses given at wider intervals to allow for recovery from the neuropathy. Peripheral neuropathy, constipation or obstipation are more severe in older patients than in children. Unlike the alkylating agents, there appears to be little cross resistance between vinblastine and vincristine [19, 20].

The corticosteroids have generally been reserved for treatment in the late stages of illness or for treatment of complications such as hemolytic anemia or thrombocytopenia. They do, however, possess a significant degree of activity in patients with advanced disease and can be given orally or intravenously [21—23]. Their side effects are well-known. Large doses given every other day, rather than daily, have not been sufficiently evaluated in the treatment of the lymphomas, but this schedule has a certain appeal when one is faced with fairly long term usage of large doses.

Procarbazine, a substituted monomethylhydrazine, is the newest of the drugs with known effectiveness against Hodgkin's disease [24—28]. It is only available for oral use. Nausea and vomiting occur frequently with initial administration but these side effects clear with continued usage. Bone marrow suppression, sometimes lingering after cessation of therapy, is the dose limiting side effect. The drug is known to inhibit the enzyme monoamine oxidase [29, 30] and interfere with pyridoxine metabolism [31]. Aggravation of nausea and vomiting, rather than relief, with the usual antiemetics and sedatives has been reported from Europe and is consistent with our experience as well. There does not appear to be any cross resistance between procarbazine and other available agents. Procarbazine is less effective in the treatment of lymphosarcoma and reticulum cell sarcoma than in therapy of Hodgkin's disease.

New Drugs

Several new drugs have shown promise of future usefulness in the treatment of the lymphomas but are not yet available for general use. The nitrosourea derivative, 1,3-bis(2-chloroethyl)-1-nitrosourea (BCNU), has been shown to produce useful responses in about half of patients treated with advanced Hodgkin's disease resistant to available drugs including alkylating agents [32, 33]. The latter point is of interest since the nitrosoureas have been thought to have biologic alkylating activity. Some responses have been dramatic enough in patients with advanced, resistant disease, to suggest that the drug should be given a trial earlier in the course of Hodgkin's disease. Like procarbazine, BCNU is less effective in the treatment of lymphosarcoma and reticulum cell sarcoma than in treatment of Hodgkin's disease.

The enzyme asparaginase [34] and the antitumor antibiotic streptonigrin [35, 36] have had some usefulness in lymphosarcoma and represent new drugs not cross resistant to available agents. Many of the standard chemotherapeutic agents such as the folic acid, purine, and pyrimidine antagonists have had inadequate clinical trials in lymphomas to accurately state their true usefulness.

Patients resistant to the standard available agents listed in Table 1 are generally treated with new experimental antitumor agents.

Results of Therapy

Most of the available chemotherapy literature has been concerned with the type of treatment outlined in program A Fig. 1. In the last several years, the use of drugs in combination has provided interesting results. There are no data in the literature on the use of drugs as outlined in program B but such clinical trials are in progress. Since survival is the ultimate endpoint of all treatment programs, comparative trials of the three different approaches are necessary and to some extent in progress, but such comparative results are not available at present. Available chemotherapy data for lymphomas suggest that patients who respond live longer than nonresponders [37], and that the magnitude of the response is important. Patients achieving complete remissions have longer duration of remission whether maintained with drugs or left unmaintained [38]. Earlier reports of clinical trials have concentrated on the overall response rate usually indicating a response as shrinkage of tumor masses of greater than 50 percent with doses and schedules that produce comparable toxicity. Less emphasis has been placed on complete responses primarily because they occurred infrequently.

The two alkylating agents cyclophosphamide and nitrogen mustard have been compared in clinical trial with Hodgkin's disease, lymphosarcoma, or reticulum cell sarcoma by Jacobs et al [39], with no significant difference in response rate apparent. In another study by Stutzman et al. [40], vinblastine, while superior to cyclophosphamide in Hodgkin's disease, compared unfavorably with cyclophosphamide against reticulum cell sarcoma and lymphosarcoma. In Hodgkin's disease, a random trial of nitrogen mustard and vinblastine revealed equivalent response rates but a superiority of the sequence nitrogen mustard—vinblastine over the alternate sequence [41].

The overall response rate in these studies ranged from 40 to 60 percent but different criteria for grading response make these results difficult to interpret collectively. It seems that either nitrogen mustard or vinblastine can be used as the initial drug in the treatment of Hodgkin's disease with a slight advantage to the use of nitrogen mustard first. In lymphosarcoma and reticulum cell sarcoma, vinblastine or vincristine are less effective than alkylating agents and cyclophosphamide appears to be the single agent of choice. In the study by Carbone and Spurr [38] the vinca alkaloids were compared to cyclophosphamide in the treatment of the lymphomas. Vincristine was used in lymphosarcoma and reticulum cell sarcoma and vinblastine in Hodgkin's disease. Patients were divided according to whether they received prior therapy or not. Although both forms of therapy were effective there was a significant difference in their ability to induce responses, as illustrated in Table 2. Vinblastine induced a response in 75% of patients with Hodgkin's disease who had received no prior chemotherapy, while cyclophosphamide did so in 54%. Vinblastine also induced a greater proportion of complete responses. In previously treated cases no preference for vinblastine was shown. Again, in lymphosarcoma and reticulum cell sarcoma, although both therapies were effective, cyclophosphamide was superior. Notice as

Table 2. *Remission induction — no prior treatment*

	Number of patients	Response rate (percent)	Complete response rate (percent)
Hodgkin's disease			
Cyclophosphamide	54	54	18
Vinblastine	56	75	27
Lymphosarcoma			
Cyclophosphamide	41	71	14
Vincristine	35	46	9
Reticulum cell sarcoma			
Cyclophosphamide	31	52	13
Vincristine	27	37	15

indicated in Table 2, that the percentage of complete responses is small; this was particularly true in previously treated patients. There is a general impression that vinblastine is superior to vincristine in the treatment of Hodgkin's disease and the reverse is true of lymphosarcoma and reticulum cell sarcoma [38]; there are no comparative data available in previously untreated patients with Hodgkin's disease to support this clinical impression.

In patients previously treated with the vinca alkaloids and alkylating agents procarbazine produces response in as many as 70 percent of patients treated [24—28, 42, 43]. Use of this agent earlier in the course of the disease, as a remission inducer, seems indicated, since the duration of remissions obtained with procarbazine is short.

Hall has reviewed the literature on the use of steroids in Hodgkin's disease and other lymphomas [23]; about half of patients with lymphomas treated with large doses of corticosteroids show objective responses of short duration. Their lack of overlapping toxicity with the other drugs makes them ideal for use in combination. From the published data on the primary treatment of the lymphomas just reviewed it seems that when these drugs are used singly they should be used in the most optimal fashion (usually parenteral intermittently) to obtain as nearly a complete response as possible. Comparative trials on the effect of maintenance therapy on the duration of a response have not been conducted often. Scott [44] induced remissions with nitrogen mustard and randomized patients to either no maintenance therapy or treatment with chlorambucil. The results indicated a significant prolongation of remission in the chlorambucil treated group (37 weeks) when compared to the group on no further therapy (12 weeks).

A similar comparison was made in the study of CARBONE and SPURR [38] where patients were randomized to maintenance with oral cyclophosphamide or placebo after induction of a response with either a vinca alkaloid or cyclophosphamide. The results in this study are summarized in Table 3. Unmaintained remissions were short, averaging 5 weeks, while maintenance therapy prolonged remission significantly, particularly in Hodgkin's disease. Although maintenance therapy is more satisfactory from the patient's point of view, time to drug resistance was similar in both groups, and survival of both groups was not significantly different; there was, however, a trend in favor of intermittent reinduction therapy in patients with lymphosarcoma.

Median survivals of patients with generalized disease have been reported to be less than two years for Hodgkin's disease and shorter for lymphosarcoma and reticulum cell sarcoma, but the data are difficult to interpret [5, 37—40]. Most patients referred to large institutions have had previous therapy and calculating survival from time of entrance into a study may give falsely short results. In a study of Hodgkin's disease by RAPPAPORT et al [45] survival was measured from diagnosis to onset of chemotherapy (time I) and from onset of chemotherapy to death (time II). Median time II survival was 23 months which is similar to the survival of patients with Hodgkin's disease reported by CARBONE and SPURR [38]. Analysis of older data indicate that a small percentage of patients with Hodgkin's disease presenting with advanced disease will live for 5 years [46]. Similar figures are available in lymphosarcoma, but few people with advanced reticulum cell sarcoma have survived five years on chemotherapy alone. In Gellhorn's study, where life table analysis of survival data is presented, survival of all the lymphomas was clearly related to stage and histologic type [46].

Table 3. *Lymphoma — remission maintenance median duration — weeks*

	Cyclophosphamide	Placebo
Hodgkin's disease	33	5
Lymphosarcoma	15	6
Reticulum cell sarcoma	13	5

Combination Chemotherapy

In 1963, a pilot study using four drugs in combination for the treatment of Hodgkin's disease was performed at the National Cancer Institute; the results indicated a high complete response rate (80%) with reasonable cost in toxicity [47, 48]. LACHER and DURANT in 1964 [49] reported the use of vinblastine and chlorambucil in combination for Hodgkin's disease with a complete response rate of 40%. The NCI study was modified in 1964 to include the newly available procarbazine [50]. Therapy with this program consists of six two week cycles of treatment each separated by a two week rest interval for recovery from toxicity. Each cycle consists of vincristine 1.4 mg/m² (0.033 mg/kg) and nitrogen mustard 6 mg/m² (0.2 mg/kg) intravenously on days 1 and 8. Procarbazine is given at a dose of 100 mg/m²/day (3 mg/kg/day) for 14 days of each cycle and prednisone at 40 mg/m² (1 mg/kg) for 14 days of cycles 1 and 4 only. From June 1964 to July 1967, 43 previously untreated patients with advanced Hodgkin's disease were placed on study. Since 1967, the study has continued but patients entering a state of complete remission are randomized to maintenance or retreatment programs. Over 100 patients have now been treated and there are two drug related deaths, both due to rapid necrosis of tumor. The toxicity, although occasionally severe, is tolerable and therapy is given in the outpatient department. The results are encouraging in that of the first 43 patients, all patients responded and thirty-five of 43 (81%) had complete remissions. With no maintenance therapy and with duration of remission calculated from the end of all treatment, the median duration of unmaintained remission had exceeded previously preported survivals and will be between 29 and 42 months. Eighteen of 35 have relapsed with a median time to relapse of 11 months. The median survival of the group entering complete remission, as of February 1970, is 42+ months with twenty-seven of 35 living and seventeen of 35 still in their first unmaintained remission. The median survival of the group that responded but did not achieve a complete remission is 20 months with only one patient living. An additional 15 patients with generalized lymphosarcoma and 8 patients with generalized reticulum cell sarcoma were treated with the same combination of drugs [50]. Of the 15 patients with lymphosarcoma, there were 7 complete remissions and 5 partial responses. Among the 8 reticulum cell sarcoma patients 3 achieved a complete remission and 2 a partial response. For reticulum cell sarcoma patients, as of February 1970, survival is 42+, 54+ and 54+ months, for the three patients achieving a complete remission, and all three continue free of their disease. The 2 partial responders and 3 nonresponders died at 6, 4, 3, 3 and 1 month(s), respectively. For lymphosarcoma patients, the median duration of remission from the end of therapy is 9 months. One of the 7 patients achieving a complete remission remains in a complete remission at 37+ months and is surviving 43+ months. Two of the seven are still living. The median survival for those patients achieving less than a complete remission is 11 months. The median survival for those patients achieving a state of complete remission is 42 months. For the entire group of 15, the 1, 2 and 3 year survivals are 73, 46 and 40 percent, respectively. Five of 7 complete responders (71%) have survived three years.

Thus, the use of effective drugs in combination appears to yield a higher percentage of complete remissions, particularly in Hodgkin's disease. These remissions appear to last longer with no maintenance therapy than complete remissions obtained with single drugs, even when single drug induction is followed by continued maintenance therapy. It also appears that the longer complete remissions are translated into more prolonged disease free survivals.

Summary

The chemotherapy of the lymphomas has changed radically over the past 25 years with the development of several independent classes of drugs with antitumor activity. During this interval the importance of staging, particularly in reference to Hodgkin's disease, has become more apparent as have the potential benefits of radiation therapy of local tumor. The use of single drugs in the treatment of all the lymphomas has yielded the following data: (1) The overall response rate is from 50 to 70 percent for each drug. (2) Complete remissions are uncommon, occurring in 15 to 25 percent of cases. (3) Maintenance of remissions with drugs prolongs the duration free of disease but does not affect survival when compared to intermittent reinduction treatment. (4) Median survival has rarely exceeded two years even for Hodgkin's disease. Recently, the available drugs have been used in combination; studies have indicated that the complete response rate can be improved, the disease free period after all therapy is discontinued can be increased, and survival may be prolonged. Comparative studies between radiation and drug therapy in intermediate stages are in progress.

Acknowledgment

The author would like to express his appreciation to Miss Myra Stull for her assistance in the preparation of this manuscript.

References

1. Gall, E. A., Mallory, T. B.: Malignant lymphoma: A clinicopathologic survey of 618 cases. Amer. J. Path. **18**, 381 (1942).
2. Rappaport, H.: Tumors of the hematopoietic system. Armed Forces Institute of Pathology. 91 (1966).
3. Lukes, R. J.: Relationship of histologic features to clinical stages in Hodgkin's disease. Amer. J. Roentgenol. **90**, 944 (1963).
4. — Butler, J. J.: The pathology and nomenclature of Hodgkin's disease. Cancer Res. **26**, 1063 (1966).
5. Rosenberg, S. A., Diamond, H. D., Craver, L. F.: Lymphosarcoma: The effects of therapy and survival in 1269 patients in a review of 30 years experience. Ann. intern. Med. **53**, 877 (1960).
6. — Report of the committee on the staging of Hodgkin's disease. Cancer Res. **26**, 1310 (1966).
7. Banfi, A., Bonadona, G., Carnevali, G., Oldini, C., Salvini, E.: Preferential sites of involvement and spread in malignant lymphomas. Europ. J. Cancer **4**, 319 (1968).
8. Han, T., Stutzman, L.: Mode of spread with localized malignant lymphoma. Arch. intern. Med. **120**, 1 (1967).
9. Peters, M. V.: The contribution of radiation therapy in the control of early lymphomas. Amer. J. Roentgenol. **90**, 956 (1963).
10. — Hasselback, R., Brown, T. C.: The natural history of the lymphomas related to the clinical classification. In: Proceedings of the International Conference on Leukemia-Lymphoma. Ed.: C. J. D. Zarafonetis. Lea and Febiger 1968, p. 357.

10 a. Ultmann, J. E., Nixon, D. D.: The therapy of lymphoma. Seminars in Hematology **6**, 376 (1969).

10 b. Oliverio, V. T., Zubrod, C. G.: Clinical pharmacology of the effective antitumor drugs. Ann. Rev. Pharmacol. **5**, 335 (1965).

11. Goodman, L. S., Gilman, A.: The Pharmacologic Basis of Therapeutics, 3rd Ed. New York: Macmillan Co. 1965, p. 1345.
12. Brock, N., Hohorst, H. J.: Über die Aktivierung von Cyclophosphamide *in vivo* und *in vitro*. Arzneimittel-Forsch. **13**, 1021 (1963).
13. DeVita, V. T., Adamson, R. H.: The metabolism of ^{14}C cyclophosphamide: Comparative drug metabolism studies in African and American patients with lymphosarcoma and

Burkitt's tumor. In: Proceedings of the Sixth International Congress of Chemotherapy, 1969. (In press.)
14. Calabresi, P., Welch, A. D.: Chemotherapy of neoplastic diseases. Ann. Rev. Med. **13**, 147 (1962).
15. Frei, E. III, Carbone, P. P., Shnider, B. I., Gold, G. L., Colsky, J., Franzino, A., Krant, M. J., Brena, G. P., Owens, A. H., Holland, J. F., Costa, G., Hull, T. C., Hosley, H., Horton, J., Tan, N., Salvin, L. G.: A study of vinblastine in the treatment of patients with neoplastic disease. Arch. intern. Med. **117**, 846 (1965).
16. Frost, J. W., Goldwein, M. I., Bryan, J. A.: Clinical experience with vinca leukoblastine in far advanced Hodgkin's disease and various malignant states. Ann. intern. Med. **56**, 854 (1962).
17. Wright, T. L., Hurley, J., Korst, D. R., Monto, R. W., Rohn, R. J., Will, J. J., Louis, J.: (Midwest Cooperative Chemotherapy Group) Vinblastine in neoplastic diseases. Cancer Res. **23**, 169 (1963).
18. Bleehan, N. M., Jelliffe, A. M.: Vinblastine sulphate in the treatment of malignant disease. Brit. J. Cancer **19**, 268 (1963).
19. Bohanan, R., Miller, D., Diamond, H.: Vincristine in the treatment of the lymphomas and leukemias. Cancer Res. **23**, 613 (1963).
20. Carbone, P. P., Bono, V., Frei, E. III, Brindley, C. O.: Clinical studies with vincristine. Blood **21**, 640 (1963).
21. Freymann, J. G., Vander, J. B., Marler, E. A., Meyer, D. G.: Prolonged corticosteroid therapy of chronic lymphocytic leukemia and the closely allied malignant lymphomas. Brit. J. Haemat. **6**, 303 (1960).
22. Kofman, J., Perlia, C. P., Boesen, E., Eisenstein, R., Taylor, S. G. III: Role of corticosteroids in treatment of malignant lymphomas. Cancer **15**, 338 (1962).
23. Hall, T. C., Choi, O. S., Abadi, A., Krant, M. J.: High dose corticoid therapy in Hodgkin's disease and other lymphomas. Ann. intern. Med. **66**, 1144 (1967).
24. Bollag, W., Grunberg, E.: Tumour inhibitory effects of a new class of cytotoxic agents: methylhydrazine derivatives. Experientia **19**, 130 (1963).
25. Mathé, G., Schweisguth, O., Schneider, M., Amiel, J. L., Berumen, L., Brule, G., Cattan, A., Schwarzenberg, L.: Methylhydrazine in the treatment of Hodgkin's disease. Lancet **1963 II**, 1077.
26. Todd, I. D. H.: Natulan in management of late Hodgkin's disease, other lymphoreticular neoplasms and malignant melanomas. Brit. med. J. **1965 II**, 628.
27. Brunner, K. W., Young, C. W.: A methylhydrazine derivative in Hodgkin's disease and other malignant neoplasms. Ann. intern. Med. **63**, 69 (1965).
28. DeVita, V. T., Serpick, A., Carbone, P. P.: Preliminary clinical studies with Ibenzmethyzin. Clin. Pharmacol. Ther. **7**, 542 (1966).
29. — Hahn, M. A., Oliverio, V. T.: Monamine oxidase inhibition by a new carcinostatic agent N-isopropyl-a-(2 methylhydrazine)-p-toluamide (MIH). Proc. Soc. exp. Biol. (N.Y.) **120**, 561 (1965).
30. Bichel, J.: Procarbazine and cheese. Lancet **1968 II**, 877.
31. Chabner, B. A., DeVita, V. T., Considine, N., Oliverio, V. T.: Plasma pyridoxal depletion by the carcinostatic procarbazine. Proc. Soc. exp. Biol. (N. Y.) **132**, 1119 (1969).
32. Lessner, H. E.: BCNU [1,3-bis(B chloroethyl)-1-nitrosourea]: Effects on advanced Hodgkin's disease and other neoplasia. Cancer **22**, 451 (1968).
33. DeVita, V. T., Carbone, P. P., Owens, A. A., Gold, G. L., Krant, M. J., Edmonson, J.: Clinical trials with 1,3-bis(2-chloroethyl)-1-nitrosourea, NSC 409962. Cancer Res. **25**, 1876 (1965).
34. Haskell, C. M., Canellos, G. P., Leventhal, B. G., Carbone, P. P., Block, J. B., Serpick, A. A., Selawry, O. S.: L-asparaginase: Therapeutic and toxic effects in patients with neoplastic disease. New Engl. J. Med. **281**, 1028 (1969).
35. Hackenthol, C. A., Golbey, R. R., Tani, H. C., Karnofsky, D. A., Burchenal, J. H.: Clinical observations on the effects of streptonigrin in patients with neoplastic disease. Antibiot. and Chemother. **11**, 178 (1961).
36. Harris, N. A., Medrek, T. J., Golumb, F. M., Gumport, S. C., Postel, A. A., Wright, J. C.: Chemotherapy with streptonigrin in advanced cancer. Cancer **18**, 49 (1965).

37. Ultmann, J. E., Cunningham, J. K., Gellhorn, A.: The clinical picture of Hodgkin's disease. Cancer Res. **26,** 1047 (1966).
38. Carbone, P. P., Spurr, C.: Management of patients with malignant lymphoma. A comparative study with cyclophosphamide and vinca alkaloids. Cancer Res. **28,** 811 (1968).
39. Jacobs, E. M., Peters, F. C., Luce, T. K., Zippen, C., Wood, D. A.: Mechlorethamine HCl and cyclophosphamide in the treatment of Hodgkin's disease and the lymphomas. J. Amer. med. Ass. **203,** 104 (1968).
40. Stutzman, L., Ezdinli, E. Z., Stutzman, M. A.: Vinblastine sulfate vs. cyclophosphamide in the therapy for lymphoma. J. Amer. med. Ass. **195,** 111 (1966).
41. Ezdinli, E. Z., Stutzman, L.: Vinblastine vs. nitrogen mustard therapy of Hodgkin's disease. Cancer **22,** 473 (1968).
42. Bonadonna, G., Monfardini, S., Oldini, C.: Comparative effects of vinblastine and procarbazine in advanced Hodgkin's disease. Europ. J. Cancer **5,** 393 (1969).
43. Fairley, G. H., Patterson, M. J. L., Scott, R. B.: Chemotherapy of Hodgkin's disease with cyclophosphamide, vinblastine and procarbazine. Brit. Med. J. **199 II,** 75 (1966).
44. Scott, J. L.: The effect of nitrogen mustard and maintenance chlorambucil in the treatment of advanced Hodgkin's disease. Cancer Chemother. Rep. **27,** 27 (1963).
45. Rapoport, A., Cole, P., Mason, J.: Correlation of survival after initiation of chemotherapy in 142 cases of Hodgkin's disease. Cancer **23,** 377 (1969).
46. Gellhorn, A.: End results of lymphosarcoma and Hodgkin's disease. Proc. III National Cancer Conf., 1957, p. 862.
47. Moxley, J. H. III, DeVita, V. T., Brace, K., Frei, E. III: Intensive combination chemotherapy and X-irradiation in Hodgkin's disease. Cancer Res. **27,** 1258 (1967).
48. Frei, E. III, DeVita, V. T., Moxley, J. H. III, Carbone, P. P.: Approaches to improving the chemotherapy of Hodgkin's disease. Cancer Res. **26,** 1284 (1969).
49. Lacher, M. J., Durant, J. R.: Combined vinblastine and chlorambucil therapy of Hodgkin's disease. Ann. intern. Med. **62,** 468 (1965).
50. DeVita, V. T., Serpick, A.: Combination chemotherapy in the treatment of advanced Hodgkin's disease. Proc. Amer. Ass. Cancer Res. **8,** 13 (1967).
51. Lowenbraun, S., DeVita, V. T., Serpick, A. A.: Combination chemotherapy with nitrogen mustard, vincristine, procarbazine and prednisone in lymphosarcoma and reticulum cell sarcoma. Cancer **25,** 1018 (1970).

Discussion

Treatment of Chronic Lymphocytic Leukemia

RALPH E. JOHNSON

With 1 Figure

The markedly improved survival for patients with acute lymphocytic leukemia has been the consequence of high rates of remission induction combined with maintenance or consolidation programs as discussed by Dr. FREIREICH. In contrast, treatment has failed to materially influence survival for patients with chronic lymphocytic leukemia. This failure almost certainly reflects the inability of conventional therapy to give high quality remissions with any consistency. Dr. GALTON has noted that the usual response to treatment of chronic lymphocytic leukemia is relatively incomplete (Type 2 response in Table 1) and, correspondingly, therapy has not altered the nature of the disease [1].

Five years ago, investigations were begun with total body irradiation in an effort to produce more complete remissions. In preliminary studies, objective responses were observed in patients refractory to standard therapy. Subsequently, attention was directed toward previously untreated patients with progressive, symptomatic disease. Seventeen untreated patients were given small repetitive doses of total body irradiation for approximately four months in a pilot study to induce as complete remissions as possible without causing undue bone marrow toxicity [2]. Eight of these 17 patients had Type 1 responses (Table 1) and another 8 patients had Type 2 responses. Following completion of the initial treatment, the patients were followed without additional therapy to evaluate the duration of unmaintained remission.

As summarized by Fig. 1, those patients with incomplete responses after induction therapy had relatively short (median 4 months) unmaintained remissions. This observation was consistent with the impression that the patients had progressive rather than indolent disease prior to initiation of treatment. As described for acute leukemia [3], the more complete responders had unmaintained remissions of significantly longer duration (median 19 months).

Thus, we now can effect excellent quality remissions with some frequency in patients with chronic lymphocytic leukemia although the influence of this on survival remains to be demonstrated. However, it appears reasonable to assume that the cornerstone for successful therapy in the future will be an effective technique(s)

Table 1. *Criteria for evaluation of therapeutic response in patients with chronic lymphocytic leukemia*

Response	Criteria
Type 1	Requirements include: a) Absolute lymphocyte count below $3000/mm^3$ b) Absolute neutrophile count above $3000/mm^3$ c) Normal hemoglobin (females 12, males 13 Gm/100 ml) d) Platelet count above 50,000 e) Absence of palpable disease (nodes, hepatosplenomegaly) f) Absence of disease-related symptoms g) A minimum decrease of 25% in bone marrow lymphocytosis on the aspirate smear differential count
Type 2	Minimum requirements include: a) 75% reduction in the absolute lymphocyte count b) Partial correction of anemia c) Decrease of measurable disease in all sites d) Definite symptomatic improvement
Type 3	A response which either does not meet the minimal requirements for Type 2 or where there is any sign of progressive disease or symptoms (including iatrogenic)

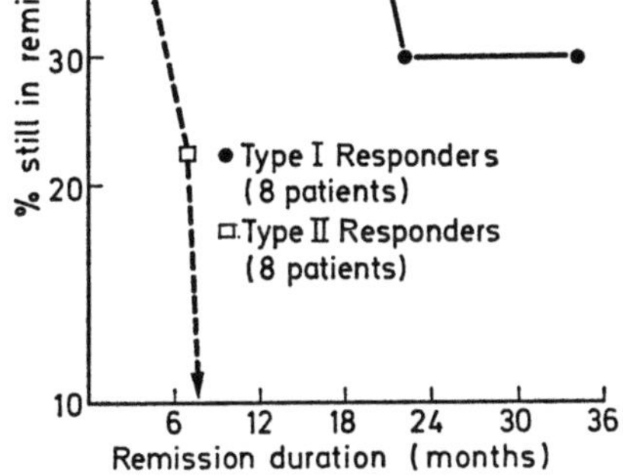

Fig. 1. Duration of unmaintained remissions in chronic lymphocytic leukemia. The duration of remissions were measured from completion of induction therapy with total body irradiation. The observed difference in remission duration between the Type 1 and Type 2 responders is significant ($p < 0.01$) using the Wilcoxon Rank Test

for remission induction. Studies now need to be directed toward (a) refinement of the dose schedules of total body irradiation so that remissions can be achieved with maximum consistency, (b) definition of useful techniques for remission maintenance, and (c) evaluation of remission induction-maintenance programs with respect to improving survival. In light of the tremendous heterogeneity of patients with chronic lymphocytic leukemia, evaluation of the therapeutic efficacy of any treatment will always prove a particularly challenging task.

References

1. SILVER, R. T.: The treatment of chronic lymphocytic leukemia. Seminars Hematology **6**, 344—356 (1969).
2. JOHNSON, R. E.: Total body irradiation of chronic lymphocytic leukemia: incidence and duration of remission. Cancer **25**, 523—530 (1970).
3. JOHNSON, R. E., ZELEN, M., FREIREICH, E. J.: Evaluation of human acute leukemia data using a murine leukemia model system. Cancer **19**, 481—484 (1966).

Immunity to Human Tumor Antigens*

Karl Erik Hellström and Ingegerd Hellström

It has been well established during the last 10—15 years that most (all?) experimentally induced animal tumors possess specific antigens against which an immunity can be demonstrated by *in vivo* and *in vitro* techniques (Old and Boyse, 1964; Sjögren, 1965; Klein, 1966; Hellström and Hellström, 1969 b, 1970 b). Evidence that human neoplasms are antigenic as well has been forthcoming more recently. Some of this evidence will be summarized here, primarily by providing references. No attempts will be made to go into details, since these are covered in two recent review articles (Hellström and Hellström, 1969 b, 1970 b, c; Klein, 1970; Gold, 1970).

Two questions concerning human tumor immunology appear to be obvious: do human neoplasms possess specific antigens absent from normal adult human cells, and is the human body capable of reacting against such antigens, thereby mounting an immunological defense against cancer?

One of the first well-controlled documentations that human cancers have specific antigens was the demonstration by Gold and Freedman (1965) that human colonic carcinomas possess antigens which are absent from adult human tissues, including adult colon. The same antigen was identified in fetal human gut epithelium and has been therefore referred to as a carcinoembryonic antigen (CEA). Approximately fifty percent of patients with colonic carcinomas, particularly those who do not have wide-spread disease, possess detectable serum antibodies to CEA (Gold, 1967). Virtually all of the colon cancer patients have CEA in their serum (Thomson et al., 1969), which indicates that this finding might be used as a basis for immunological diagnosis of colonic carcinomas.

It is so far unknown whether immunological reactions to CEA contribute to the *in vivo* growth of colon carcinomas. The antigen can be detected at the cell surface with immunofluorescence tests (Gold et al., 1968), but since it appears to form part of the glycocalyx rather than being associated with the cell membrane (Gold, 1970), it is possible that CEA is not a regular tumor specific antigen like those detected in experimentally induced animal tumors by transplantation techniques.

Klein et al. (1966) have shown that sera from patients with Burkitt lymphomas contain antibodies that are capable of binding to Burkitt lymphoma cells, as de-

* The studies of the authors referred to in this article have been supported by grants CA-10188 and CA-10189 from National Institutes of Health, by grant T-453 from American Cancer Society, and by contract NIH-69-2061 from National Institutes of Health to the University of Minnesota, subcontracted to us.

tectable by a membrane immunofluorescence assay. Such antibodies also occur in sera from patients who do not have Burkitt lymphomas, but to a much less extent. Normal bone marrow cells from Burkitt lymphoma patients do not react with sera from Burkitt lymphoma patients. Sera from patients who respond well to chemotherapy appear to react better in membrane immunofluorescence tests than sera from patients responding badly which suggests that the antibody response detected might be therapeutically beneficial to the patients (KLEIN et al., 1966). A recent review provides more details on immunity to Burkitt lymphomas, a topic which has been extensively investigated by KLEIN and his colleagues (KLEIN, 1970).

MORTON and co-workers have studied human malignant melanomas and sarcomas by using immunofluorescence and complement fixation assays and have obtained results which are analogous to the Burkitt findings (MORTON et al., 1968, 1969). Sera from patients with malignant melanomas give specific immunofluorescence with melanoma cells, but not with sarcoma cells, while the reverse is true for sera from patients with sarcomas, indicating that the two groups of neoplasms have antigens that are common within each group and different between the groups.

Our own work has been slanted somewhat differently from that so far referred to, since our major interest has been to study to what extent cell-mediated immune reactions can be detected against human tumor antigens and what the mechanisms of the immunological defense against these antigens are. This work has been reviewed recently (HELLSTRÖM and HELLSTRÖM, 1969 b, 1970 b, c), and therefore discussion will be confined to the major findings obtained.

We have used a so-called colony inhibition (CI) assay (HELLSTRÖM, 1967). Target tumor cells are plated onto petri dishes and allowed to attach to their surfaces during incubation overnight. Lymphocyte suspensions are then added to the target cells, the petri dishes incubated, and the number of colonies growing out from the target cells determined 3—5 days later after staining of the petri dishes. Experimental groups which have received lymphocytes from the patients under study are compared with controls exposed to lymphocytes from patients with neoplasms of types other than the target tumors, as well as to lymphocytes from patients who do not have cancer. The percentage reduction in colony numbers in the experimental groups is calculated.

The CI technique was first used to demonstrate cell-mediated immune reactions against a large variety of experimentally induced animal tumors (HELLSTRÖM, 1967; HELLSTRÖM and HELLSTRÖM, 1967, 1969 a, b, 1970 a, b, c; HELLSTRÖM and SJÖGREN, 1967; HELLSTRÖM et al., 1968 a, 1969 a, b, c, 1970 c; HEPPNER, 1969; SJÖGREN, 1970) and to demonstrate cytotoxic (growth inhibitory) antibodies to antigens of solid animal tumors (HELLSTRÖM and SJÖGREN, 1965, 1967, HELLSTRÖM et al., 1968 a, 1969 c). The animal studies were used as models for our later approach to human neoplasms.

The first human tumors studied for cell-mediated immunity with the Cl assay were neuroblastomas, because of evidence suggesting that such tumors might be combated by the patient *in vivo* (EVERSON and COLE, 1966). It was found that lymphocytes from patients with progressively growing neuroblastomas, as well as lymphocytes from patients who were symptom free after therapy, inhibited colony formation of plated neuroblastoma cells, while normal skin fibroblasts from the same patients were not inhibited (HELLSTRÖM et al., 1968 b, 1970 b). The inhibition was independent of whether the lymphocytes were tested on a patient's autochthonous neuroblastoma cells, or on such tumor cells from allogeneic patients, suggesting that neuroblastomas possess cross-reacting tumor antigens.

The finding that lymphocytes from patients free of disease and from patients with progressively growing tumors were equally inhibitory was analogous to observations made on animal tumors (HELLSTRÖM and HELLSTRÖM, 1969 b, 1970 c). It suggested that tumor-bearing human patients—like animals—might contain serum factors, such as blocking antibodies, which can specifically protect a patient's neoplastic cells from immunological destruction.

Experiments have been conducted to test that possibility. They have shown that sera from patients who have metastasizing neuroblastomas can nullify the inhibitory effect of the same patient's immune lymphocytes on neuroblastoma target cells. No such blocking effect has been detected with sera from patients who are symptom-free after therapy for neuroblastoma (HELLSTRÖM et al., 1970 b), which agrees with findings made in animals, showing loss of blocking serum activity following surgical removal or spontaneous regression of tumors (HELLSTRÖM and HELLSTRÖM, 1970 a; HELLSTRÖM et al., 1970 c). These findings suggest that the progressive growth of neuroblastomas *in vivo* may have been made possible by the blocking serum factors, although other, as yet unidentified, factors may also have contributed to the same end.

An unexpected finding was that lymphocytes from certain relatives of neuroblastoma patients, particularly their mothers, were inhibitory to cultivated neuroblastoma cells, derived from the mothers' own or from other children (HELLSTRÖM et al., 1968 b, 1970 b). No blocking effect was detected with serum from these mothers; on the other hand, such sera often contained antibodies cytotoxic to cultivated neuroblastoma cells (HELLSTRÖM et al., 1968 b).

A large number of human tumors other than neuroblastomas have also been studied by the CI technique. The results are very similar to those obtained with neuroblastomas: lymphocytes from tumor-bearing patients inhibit cultivated tumor, but not normal cells, from the same patients, and the degree of inhibition is approximately the same independently of whether the patients are clinically symptom free or have metastatic disease. Sera from the latter group of patients, but not from the former one, are capable of specifically blocking the lymphocyte effect. Cross-reactions have been detected within certain groups of neoplasms, but not between such groups, most notably among tumors of the following types: malignant melanomas, sarcomas, Wilms' tumor, carcinomas of the colon, carcinomas of the breast and carcinomas of the ovary (HELLSTRÖM et al., 1968 c, 1970 a, 1971). Furthermore, BUBENIK et al. (1970 a, b), have shown that human bladder carcinomas have cross-reacting antigens against which lymphocytes from the patients are reactive. Although their assay was similar to the CI technique, individual cells rather than colonies were counted.

The nature of the common tumor antigens detectable by the CI test is still unclear. Recent evidence suggests that the antigens of colon carcinomas may be similar to the carcinoembryonic antigens (CEA) studied by GOLD et al., since lymphocytes from patients with colonic carcinomas inhibit colony formation of fetal human gut cells but not of adult colon mucosa cells or fetal kidney cells (HELLSTRÖM et al., 1970 d). Alternatively, colon carcinomas may have two sets of antigens in common with fetal human gut, one being the CEA of GOLD et al., another being responsible for our CI findings.

Relatively few studies have been conducted to search for cytotoxic humoral antibodies to human tumor antigens. However, there are indications that such antibodies exist against neuroblastomas (HELLSTRÖM et al., 1968 b), colon carcinomas (HELLSTRÖM et al., 1968 c) as well as certain other human neoplasms (unpublished findings); these antibodies are cytotoxic (or growth inhibitory) to target tumor cells plated *in vitro*, if active complement is present in the system.

The findings summarized here indicate that the majority, possibly all, human neoplasms have specific antigens recognized by the tumor-bearing patient's lymphocytes. These lymphocytes can inhibit growth of, and destroy, the neoplastic cells *in vitro*. Our studies have also shown that sera from patients with growing tumors can abrogate that effect. An obvious question is whether this information can be useful for tumor diagnosis, prophylaxis and therapy.

It seems likely that the fact that certain groups of human neoplasms have common antigens can be utilized for development of immunological diagnosis of certain human neoplasms. Attempts to do so might be modeled on the work of THOMSON et al. (1969) on human colon carcinomas. As far as tumor prophylaxis and therapy go, available evidence suggests that two different approaches may be tried, one being to strengthen the cell-mediated immune reactions in a specific or non-specific way so that they are capable of overcoming the blocking effect of serum, and the other being to remove the blocking serum factors and/or to depress the organism's ability to form them. The first approach seems rather obvious, while the latter one might depend upon what the blocking molecules are. At least three possibilities seem to exist: they may be immunoglobulins of either a common (such as IgG) or an unusual type; they may be antigen-antibody complexes; or they may be soluble tumor antigens. The last possibility is unlikely, since the blocking serum activity can be removed by absorption with the target tumor cells. Furthermore, it is detected by incubating the target cells, but not by incubating the lymphocytes, with a blocking serum; in addition, the blocking molecules behave as 7s immunoglobulins on gel filtration (HELLSTRÖM and HELLSTRÖM, 1969 a). If the blocking molecules would prove to be antigen-antibody complexes, the antibody serves as a carrier of a hypothetical "tolerogenic" antigen, capable of depressing the reactivity of otherwise immune lymphocytes, as long as it is present.

Additional mechanisms facilitating the growth of antigenic tumors in the face of an immunity to their antigens have been less studied at least for human neoplasms. One possibility is that tumors established *in vivo* are also protected by coating substances that are more nonspecific than the blocking antibodies and that tumor cells are better protected from immune destruction when belonging to a large mass with an established blood circulation than when isolated *in vitro* or freely suspended in the blood stream. It is also possible that either the expression of the tumor antigens or the sensitivity of neoplastic cells to immune reactions against them may vary with the cell cycle, a possibility that might explain why tumor cells may sometimes remain dormant. Furthermore, tumor cell populations may be subject to immunoselection so that only the least antigenic cells are left growing.

It may be worthwhile mentioning that a specific blocking effect of serum as detected in tumor systems, coexisting with a cell-mediated immunity and compatible with survival of antigenic cells *in vivo*, can be demonstrated also when neoplasia is not involved. BALB/c female mice pregnant with C3H males have been found to possess a cell-mediated immunity to paternally derived C3H alloantigens in their embryos, capable of inhibiting colony formation of plated C3H embryonic cells; sera from the same mice can specifically nullify that effect (HELLSTRÖM et al., 1969 d). Lymphocytes from dogs which have been lethally irradiated and then repopulated with foreign bone marrow have been found to inhibit colony formation of the dogs' own plated skin fibroblasts, which were of recipient origin, as compared to the lymphocytes which came from the repopulating donor grafts, and sera from the same repopulated dogs were found to specifically abrogate the lymphocyte effect (HELLSTRÖM et al., 1970 e). It is tempting to postulate that similar mechanisms may be involved in allograft tolerance, as established either in animals inoculated with foreign bone marrow cells neonatally, or in allophenic mice (HELLSTRÖM and HELLSTRÖM, 1970 c). Further studies in this field may be potentially valuable with respect to tumor therapy and prophylaxis, tissue transplantation and autoimmunity.

Summary

Cell-mediated immunity can be detected against most animal and human tumors by using the so-called colony inhibition test. Lymphocytes from patients having cancer are approximately as inhibitory to the tumor cells as are lymphocytes from individuals whose tumors have been removed. Sera from the first group but not from the latter one contain factors, presumably antibodies or antigen-antibody complexes, that can in a specific way abrogate the tumor cell destruction by lymphocytes immune to their antigens. Since methods now exist by which both cell-mediated immune reaction and their abrogation by blocking serum factors can be assayed, it will be possible to monitor both types of reactions during classical types of tumor therapy as well as during immunotherapy.

References

BUBENIK, J., PERLMANN, P., HELMSTEIN, K., MOBERGER, G.: Immune response to urinary bladder tumours in man. Int. J. Cancer **5**, 39 (1970 a).

— — — — Cellular and humoral immune responses to human urinary bladder carcinomas. Int. J. Cancer **5**, 310 (1970 b).

EVERSON, T. C., COLE, W. H.: Spontaneous Regression of Cancer. Philadelphia: Saunders 1966, 560 pp.

GOLD, P.: The model of colon cancer in the study of human tumor-specific antigens. In: Carcinomas of colon and antecedent epithelium. Ed.: W. J. Burdelle. Springfield: C. C Thomas 1970, p. 131.

— FREEDMAN, S. O.: Specific carcinoembryonic antigens of the human digestive system. J. exp. Med. **122**, 467 (1965).

— Circulating antibodies against carcinoembryonic antigens of the human digestive system. Cancer **20**, 1663 (1967).

— GOLD, M., FREEDMAN, S. O.: Cellular location of carcinoembryonic antigens of the human digestive system. Cancer Res. **28**, 1331 (1968).

HELLSTRÖM, I.: A colony inhibition (CI) technique for demonstration of tumor cell destruction by lymphoid cells in vitro. Int. J. Cancer **2**, 65 (1967).

— EVANS, C. A., HELLSTRÖM, K. E.: Cellular immunity and its serum mediated inhibition in Shope virus-induced rabbit papillomas. Int. J. Cancer **4**, 601 (1969 a).

HELLSTRÖM, I., HELLSTRÖM, K. E.: Cell-bound immunity to autologous and syngeneic mouse tumors induced by methylcholanthrene and plastic discs. Science **156**, 981 (1967).

— Studies on cellular immunity and its serum mediated inhibition in Moloney virus induced mouse sarcomas. Int. J. Cancer **4**, 587 (1969 a).

— Colony inhibition studies on blocking and non-blocking serum effects on cellular immunity to Moloney sarcomas. Int. J. Cancer **5**, 195 (1970 a).

— — BILL, A. H., PIERCE, G. E., YANG, J. P. S.: Studies on cellular immunity to human neuroblastoma cells. Int. J. Cancer **6**, 172 (1970 b).

— — EVANS, C. A., HEPPNER, G. H., PIERCE, G. E., YANG, J. P. S.: Serum mediated protection of neoplastic cells from inhibition by lymphocytes immune to their tumor specific antigens. Proc. nat. Acad. Sci. (Wash.) **62**, 362 (1969 b).

— — PIERCE, G.: In vitro studies of immune reactions against autochthonous and syngeneic mouse tumors induced by methylcholanthrene and plastic discs. Int. J. Cancer **3**, 467 (1968 a).

— — — BILL, A. H.: Demonstration of cell-bound and humoral immunity against neuroblastoma cells. Proc. nat. Acad. Sci. (Wash.) **60**, 1231 (1968 b).

— — — FEFER, A.: Studies on immunity to autochthonous tumors. Proc. Transpl. Soc. **1**, 90 (1969 c).

— — — YANG, J. P. S.: Cellular and humoral immunity to different types of human neoplasms. Nature **220**, 1352 (1968 c).

— — — — Cellular immunity to colon carcinomas in man. In: Carcinomas of Colon and Antecedent Epithelium. Ed.: W. J. BURDETTE. Springfield: C. C. Thomas 176 (1970 a).

— — SHEPHARD, T.: Cell-mediated immunity against antigens common to human colonic carcinomas and fetal gut epithelium. Int. J. Cancer **6**, 346 (1970 d).

— — SJÖGREN, H. O.: Serum mediated inhibition of cellular immunity to methylcholanthrene induced murine sarcomas. Cellular Immunology **1**, 18 (1970 c).

— — — WARNER, G. A.: Demonstration of cell-mediated immunity to human neoplasms of various histological types. Int. J. Cancer (1971).

— — STORB, R., THOMAS, E. D.: Colony inhibition of fibroblasts from chimeric dogs mediated by the dogs' own lymphocytes and specifically abrogated by their own serum. Proc. nat. Acad. Sci. (Wash.) **66**, 65 (1970 e).

— SJÖGREN, H. O.: Demonstration of H-2 isoantigens and polyoma specific tumor antigens by measuring colony formation in vitro. Exp. Cell. Res. **40**, 212 (1965).

— — In vitro demonstration of humoral and cell-bound immunity against common specific transplantation antigen(s) of adenovirus 12-induced mouse and hamster tumors. J. exp. Med. **125**, 1105 (1967).

HELLSTRÖM, K. E., HELLSTRÖM, I.: Cellular immunity against tumor antigens. Advanc. Cancer Res. **12**, 167 (1969 b).

— — Immunological defenses against cancer. Hospital Practice **5**, 45 (1970 b).

— — Immunological enhancement as studied by cell culture techniques. Ann. Rev. Microbiol. **24**, 373 (1970 c).

— — BRAWN, J.: Abrogation of cellular immunity to C3H mouse embryonic cells by serum from BALB/c mothers pregnant by C3H males. Nature **224**, 914 (1969 d).

HEPPNER, G.: Studies on serum-mediated inhibition of cellular immunity to spontaneous mouse mammary tumors. Int. J. Cancer **4**, 608 (1969).

KLEIN, G.: Tumor antigens. Ann. Rev. Microbiol. **20**, 223 (1966).

— Immunological studies on a human tumor — dilemmas of the experimentalist. Israel J. Med Sci. (1970) (in press).

— CLIFFORD, P., KLEIN, E., STJERNSWÄRD, J.: Search for tumor-specific immune reactions in Burkitt lymphoma patients by the membrane immunofluorescence reaction. Proc. nat. Acad. Sci. (Wash.) **55**, 1628 (1966).

MORTON, D. L., MALMGREN, R. A., HOLMES, E. C., KETCHAM, A. S.: Demonstration of antibodies against human malignant melanomas by immunofluorescence. Surgery **64**, 233 (1968).

— — HALL, W. T., SCHIDLOVSKY, G.: Immunologic and virus studies with human sarcomas. Surgery **66**, 152 (1969).

OLD, L. J., BOYSE, E. A.: Immunology of experimental tumors. Ann. Rev. Med. **15**, 167 (1964).
SJÖGREN, H. O.: Transplantation methods as a tool for detection of tumor specific antigens. Progr. exp. Tumor Res. **6**, 289 (1965).
— Immunology in viral carcinogenesis. In: Immunity and Tolerance in Oncogenesis, Fourth Quadrennial Perugia Cancer Conference. Ed.: L. Severi, Perugia University Press, 561 (1961).
THOMSON, D. M. P., KRUPEY, J., FREEDMAN, S. O., GOLD, P.: The radioimmunoassay of circulating carcinoembryonic antigen of the human digestive system. Proc. nat. Acad. Sci. (Wash.) **64**, 161 (1969).

Experimental Approaches to Immunotherapy of Cancer[1]

ALEXANDER FEFER

Recent reports suggesting that human tumors, like animal tumors, may possess tumor-specific transplantation antigens (TSTA) [1—6] have raised the exciting but still theoretical possibility that we might eventually take advantage of these antigens and the immunologic reactions which they evoke for the treatment of human tumors. Unfortunately, we don't know how. Some hints as to direction may be provided by studies in animal tumor immunotherapy models, but their relevance to potential clinical immunotherapy obviously rests on an assumed, but by no means proven, similarity between the immunobiology of animal and human tumors. Nevertheless, in the absence of other leads, and while this similarity is being more convincingly documented, it may be useful to develop immunotherapy models in animals for the study of questions potentially relevant to immunotherapy in man. But the development of such models is still in its early stage and is no simple task, so that Dr. OLD could rightly say in 1964 "Despite the evident antigenicity of a variety of experimental tumors, it is a fact that no immunological maneuver is known that will cause rejection of an established malignant tumor, primary or transplanted, regardless of its size" [7]. One measure of the slow but definite progress in animal tumor immunotherapy is that the statement quoted is no longer totally true. Therefore it is proposed to briefly and somewhat superficially review the principal approaches to experimental immunotherapy as used in animals and to a lesser extent in man, with emphasis on a combination of conventional therapy and adoptive immunity. The references are not intended to be exhaustive and, whenever possible, reviews are given preference.

The first approach is based on the finding that BCG and other nonspecific stimulants of the reticuloendothelial system enhance immunologic reactivity against a variety of antigens including tumor homografts [8]. Likewise, BCG, administered days to weeks before challenge with syngeneic tumor cells often retards and occasionally prevents their subsequent growth, especially if the number of tumor cells inoculated is very low [9—12]. However, BCG has a clinically negligible effect if administered shortly after tumor inoculation and virtually no effect when given to animals with clinically detectable tumors [13]. Similarly, although BCG administered to animals early during the latency period after infection with oncogenic viruses, decreases the incidence of subsequent primary tumors [14], no significant effect has been reported in animals bearing detectable primary tumors.

[1] Some of the author's studies included in this review were supported by Grant CA 10777 from the National Cancer Institute, National Institutes of Health.

By analogy with the animal studies, MATHÉ attempted immunotherapy with BCG in patients with minimal residual disease [15]. Patients with acute leukemia in complete remission after one of three different intensive chemotherapy regimens were treated with BCG by multiple scarifications. The time to relapse was significantly longer in the 8 patients treated with BCG than in the 10 untreated patients. Attempts to confirm these encouraging results with more patients and a uniform induction and consolidation regimen are now in progress.

The second approach to immunotherapy is active immunization with a vaccine prepared from antigenic tumor cells. This is an excellent and classical way to induce resistance to a subsequent tumor transplant in animals [16]. Since each chemically induced tumor possesses largely unique TSTA, the vaccine must be derived from the same tumor as the one used to challenge [7]. On the other hand, since all tumors induced by a given virus possess antigens in common [17], animals immunized with vaccine derived from any tumor induced by a given virus will become resistant to the transplantation of any syngeneic tumor induced by the same virus [18].

Active immunization is also often effective in preventing the development of primary tumors if it is initiated before inoculation of an oncogenic virus [19] or early during the latency period to tumor formation [20]. The immunotherapeutic effect of the vaccine is not, however, always specific [14]. As with BCG, active immunization is usually ineffective if instituted in animals with detectable primary tumors [21, 22]. One exception was reported by EVANS [23] who found that the incidence of regression of Shope papillomas was greatly increased by injecting rabbits bearing papillomas with a vaccine of their own papillomas.

During the past 50 years, patients with various malignancies have been actively immunized with various preparations of their own tumor, e. g. irradiated [24], homogenized [26], conjugated with foreign proteins [27], etc., without convincing clinical benefit. Most recently, MATHÉ [15] treated patients with acute lymphocytic leukemia in remission with multiple injections of formalin or X-ray-inactivated blood from a pool of leukemic donors. Five patients thus treated remained in remission longer than did 10 untreated patients. However, this immunotherapeutic effect probably does not reflect a specific immunization with hypothetical tumor antigens since the 5 patients did no better than did 8 patients treated with BCG or 7 patients treated with both BCG and leukemic cell vaccine. No controlled immunotherapy studies have yet been reported with vaccine prepared from tumor-versus-nontumor tissue.

Results from studies of active immunization in animals raise several additional points about active immunization in man — (a) the use of nonautologous tumor tissue is predicated on a viral rather than chemical etiology for human tumors resulting in antigens shared by all tumors of a given type. Although a viral etiology has not been shown, shared antigens have been detected [1]. (b) The immunogenicity of a tumor vaccine may be destroyed in the course of its preparation. This has been observed in a number of animal tumor systems [7, 23]. The problem may be resolved by testing the ability of the human vaccine in question to absorb specific antibodies or to evoke a delayed hypersensitivity reaction of the type recently studied with Burkitt lymphoma [28]. (c) Active immunization may induce enhancement rather than inhibition of tumor growth [29].

The third approach to immunotherapy is passive transfer of immune serum. Although rejection of antigenic tumor cells is generally thought to be mediated largely by a cellular rather than a humoral immune response and is not usually influenced by serum [16, 30], sporadic but significant evidence of some effect of serotherapy has been reported. Immune serum incubated with graded doses of transplanted tumor cells or administered a couple of days before or after challenge with a small number of tumor cells will retard or inhibit the growth of most lymphoid tumors [31—35] and some non-lymphoid tumors [36, 37]. However, serotherapy is generally not effective against challenge with a large number of tumor cells or against clinically detectable tumors [32, 38]. The only exception has been reported in the primary Moloney sarcoma system in which young mice bearing palpable Moloney sarcoma virus-induced tumors were injected with serum from adult syngeneic or hemisyngeneic mice hyperimmunized with MSV. Thirty-five of 102 tumors treated with immune serum completely regressed, whereas regression was observed in only 3 of 86 untreated tumors and 3 of 85 tumors treated with nonimmune serum [39]. The possibility exists that the limiting factor in serotherapy may be the amount complement circulating in the host. This possibility has not yet been tested.

Serotherapy does present a potential hazard of inducing enhancement rather than inhibition of tumor growth [40]. This has been observed in a large number of tumor systems with sera directed against isoantigens [41] or against TSTA [35, 42, 43]. The probability of this occurring in man is not yet known.

Patients with various tumors have been treated with serum on numerous occasions with generally unimpressive results. Cytotoxic sera directed against the normal isoantigens of the host [44—46] or serum from volunteers immunized with host leukemic cells [47] and therefore directed against both normal tissue and hypothetical tumor antigens has usually induced a significant but rather transient drop in the leukocyte count. However, well-controlled studies showed no significant effect of parental plasma in patients with acute lymphocytic leukemia in remission [48] nor of remission plasma in patients with untreated Burkitt lymphoma [49]. Additional controlled studies are nevertheless indicated with remission sera, or with sera from volunteers immunized with tumor, or with sera from demonstrably reactive relatives, as reported with neuroblastoma [1] and osteogenic sarcoma [3], in patients with a minimal hematologic or nonhematologic tumor load.

The fourth approach to immunotherapy involves the adoptive transfer of lymphocytes. Immune syngeneic lymphocytes incubated with tumor cells (in a ratio of 100—1000 : 1) [16, 34, 50] or administered to animals shortly before [7, 33, 51] or shortly after [34] challenge with a small number of tumor cells will consistently and often impressively inhibit tumor growth, regardless of whether the tumor is a sarcoma or lymphoma of viral or chemical etiology. In order for the lymphocytes to be effective, however, they must have already been immunized to TSTA and they must be viable [16]. Unfortunately, immune syngeneic cells are not usually effective against established transplanted tumors. The principal exception to this generalization emanates from the work of Alexander and his associates [34], who observed temporary regression of 3 out of 4 early transplants of a chemical sarcoma in rats following transfer of immune syngeneic thoracic duct lymphocytes.

Specifically sensitized syngeneic lymphocytes are also quite effective in preventing the development of primary tumors if administered after virus injection during the latency period to tumor formation [30]. Furthermore, immunotherapy with specifically sensitized syngeneic lymphocytes was recently reported to be successful even against established clinically detectable primary tumors induced by MSV [39, 52]. Among the unique features of tumors induced by Moloney sarcoma virus is a high incidence of complete regression presumably mediated by an immunologic reaction of the primary host against TSTA [53]. Accordingly, Moloney sarcoma virus inoculated into immunologically competent adult mice induces tumors which ultimately regress and render the host resistant to subsequent challenge with Moloney sarcoma virus or Moloney sarcoma virus-induced tumor cells, whereas Moloney sarcoma virus inoculated into young mice or into adult mice immunologically suppressed by X-ray or cyclophosphamide (CY) induces tumors almost all of which grow progressively and kill [39, 54].

To determine whether established primary tumors destined to grow progressively could be made to completely regress by treatment with specifically immunized syngeneic lymphocytes, tumors were induced in young mice and in adult mice pretreated with a sublethal but immunosuppressive dose of CY. When tumors became palpable the mice received spleen cells from adult syngeneic mice whose own primary MSV-induced tumors had regressed. Such treatment was modestly effective in young mice [39] and quite effective in adult CY-treated mice [52]. Tumors disappeared in about 40% of young mice given immune cells (as compared with 5% of mice treated with normal cells) and in over 90% of CY-treated adults given immune cells (vs. 7% of such mice given non-immune cells). Since tumor regression in adult mice was also strikingly prevented if CY was administered after the tumor had already become palpable, such tumor-bearing CY-treated mice were also studied with regard to immunotherapy with specifically sensitized cells. The results showed that 70/75 tumors treated with cells from syngeneic mice immunized with MSV completely regressed, whereas only 5/82 tumors regressed after treatment with normal or non-specifically-immunized cells or with nonviable immune cells [52].

Immunotherapy with foreign lymphoid cells specifically sensitized against tumor-specific transplantation antigen has generally been impressively ineffective even against a small number of tumor cells [30, 38, 39, 55]. The failures have usually been attributed to the inability of the foreign lymphoid cells to survive in the immunologically competent host—an explanation predicated on the assumption that immune cells may have to persist in the host for some indeterminant period of time in order to be therapeutically effective against the tumors. This view is supported by studies in which syngeneic lymphoid cells which persist are quite effective whereas identically immunized allogeneic cells are not [30]. The view is also supported by recent immunotherapy experiments utilizing the persistence of donor gamma-globulin in host sera as a marker for the persistence of donor lymphoid cells in the host. Specifically sensitized allogeneic cells were therapeutically effective if they persisted but were ineffective if they were rapidly rejected [39, 52, 55].

Evidence against the necessity of lymphoid cell persistence for therapeutic efficacy is provided chiefly by the earlier work of ALEXANDER [34] who induced temporary regression of established primary sarcomas in rats by infusing thoracic duct lymphocytes from immunized unrelated rats and especially sheep. Since they found that RNA from the sheep lymphoid cells was also effective, all their results are being explained on the basis of a transfer of information to host immunocompetent cells.

These findings, when confirmed, will have major implications for clinical immunotherapy. In the meantime, the question of lymphoid cell persistence and efficacy which is critical for any thinking in clinical immunotherapy must remain open.

Attempts to treat patients with other people's lymphoid cells must be viewed in the light of three apparent prerequisites for successful immunotherapy in animals. (a) The smaller the tumor load the greater the probability of success. (b) The lymphoid cells infused are effective only if they are obtained from donors already immunized against TSTA—unimmunized cells are not effective. (c) Immune allogeneic lymphoid cells must be viable and may have to survive in the host for some time in order to be effective.

If these prerequisites are valid and applicable to man they may explain the lack of significant clinical effect of normal foreign lymphoid cells in patients with a large tumor load [45, 56, 57]. The most extensive studies [58] have involved cross-immunization and cross-transfusion of white cells between patients with the same type of tumor. The cells infused are probably immune but they are likely to be rapidly rejected by the host who has been previously sensitized against donor iso-antigens.

It should be obvious that some of the prerequisites for successful immunotherapy, namely a decreased tumor load and prolonged survival of donor lymphoid cells, may be satisfied by using adoptive immunotherapy as an adjunct to conventional chemotherapy. A simplistic animal immunotherapy model of this kind was recently developed in collaboration with Drs. GLYNN and HALPERN [55]. It involves the treatment of an established systemically-disseminated viral leukemia with a combination of nonlethal, noncurative chemotherapy plus foreign spleen cells from donors specifically sensitized only to TSTA.

Adult BALB/c mice were inoculated subcutaneously with 10^4—10^6 Moloney virus-induced leukemia cells of BALB/c origin. Six days later, mice with palpable tumors and with demonstrable systemic spread, received a sublethal dose of cyclophosphamide (CY) and, 4 hours later, they were injected with 3×10^7 spleen cells from (BALB/c $\times$DBA/2) F_1 mice specifically immunized against Moloney tumor antigens by being exposed to Moloney leukemia cells originating in C57BL/6 mice. Aside from the specificity of the immunization, the essential features of the immunotherapy model are the following: (a) Graft-versus-host disease was avoided. (b) Sublethal CY was used for its antitumor effect—to decrease the tumor load—and for its immunosuppressive activity so as to prevent the host from rejecting the donor lymphoid cells. (c) Persistence of donor lymphoid cells in the host was monitored by documenting the long-term persistence of donor-type gamma-globulin in host sera.

The results of many such experiments show that all mice which were untreated or were treated only with spleen cells from immune or nonimmune donors died with tumor in 10—12 days, and all mice treated with CY alone or with CY plus non-immune spleen cells died in 20—30 days. By contrast, of 142 tumor-bearing mice treated with CY plus immune spleen cells, about 50% survived tumor-free for more than 70 days and 30% survived for the entire observation period of 180—300 days. In short, immunotherapy alone was totally ineffective—either because the tumor load was too great or because the foreign lymphoid cells, in the absence of CY, were too rapidly rejected by the host. Drug alone prolonged survival, but was not curative. The addition of normal unimmunized spleen cells to the drug regimen had no effect, but the combination of drug plus specifically *immune* cells was often curative. A similar approach was also effective against an established slow growing but lethal syngeneic transplanted Moloney sarcoma [39].

Studies in the Moloney leukemia system have been extended [59] to the use of totally allogeneic but H-2-matched spleen cells with similar results. In combination with CY, spleen cells from DBA/2 donors immunized only against tumor antigens or against both tumor antigens and normal host isoantigens are therapeutically effective, whereas cells from unimmunized mice or from mice hyperimmunized only against the host's normal tissue antigens are totally ineffective.

This chemoimmunotherapy approach should theoretically be applicable to other tumors assuming that the tumor is antigenic and somewhat sensitive to the drug used, that the donors are well immunized and that the drug is immunosuppressive. Similar studies are also warranted in tumor-bearing dogs especially since serotyping for histocompatibility antigens is now available.

The analogous approach in patients would involve a patient with minimal tumor receiving a drug with antitumor and immunosuppressive activity plus lymphoid cells from an HL-A-matched sibling. The donor cells should either be already demonstrably reactive against tumor—as has been reported in relatives of patients with neuroblastoma [1] and osteogenic sarcoma [3], or else the donor should be immunized *de novo* with a preparation of the host's tumor or with another patient's tumor of the same type, assuming that the 2 tumors can be demonstrated to share antigens. The principal potential problem clinically is possible graft-versus-host disease— a problem which should receive more investigative attention in experimental animal immunotherapy models.

A more vigorous but potentially feasible approach to tumor immunotherapy involves whole body X-irradiation or drug administration to decrease the tumor load followed by bone marrow transplantation. Since the X-ray or drug will not eradicate the tumor, the infused cells must be able to exert an immunotherapeutic effect against the residual tumor. Attempts to treat animal lymphomas with lethal whole body X-irradiation plus normal syngeneic bone marrow have occasionally been effective in some systems [60], especially if instituted shortly after inoculation of a small number of tumor cells [61] and especially if lymph node cells were also added [62] but ineffective in other systems [63—65], probably reflecting the variable radiosensitivity and relative antigenicity of the tumors studied.

Similarly, patients with acute leukemia in relapse have been treated with high doses of whole body X-ray plus bone marrow from identical twins and have experienced a variable but quite short remission [66]. Thus the clinical results as well as some results in mice showed that although syngeneic bone marrow was effective in preventing death from X-ray, it was immunotherapeutically ineffective against residual tumor.

Recently successful eradication of an established transplanted Moloney leukemia was reported in a significant number of mice by a combination of potentially lethal (but not sublethal) doses of dimethylmyleran plus syngeneic bone marrow and spleen cells [64]. This report broadens the possibilities of syngeneic adoptive immunotherapy to include lethal chemotherapy rather than X-ray—an approach not yet reported in patients.

Lethal levels of whole body X-irradiation plus allogeneic bone marrow and lymphoid cells have also been used to treat animal lymphoid tumors [60, 62, 65], largely in the hope that the resultant graft-versus-host (GVH) reaction would have an anti-tumor effect. All studies have therefore involved marked donor-host histo-incompatibility. Most of the mice died with GVH disease but a few survived tumor-free [60, 62, 65]. Effective treatment of the GVH disease increased the number of tumor-free survivors [65].

Similarly, patients with acute leukemia have been subjected to potentially lethal doses or sublethal levels of whole body X-irradiation plus unmatched allogeneic bone marrow with generally disappointing results. The graft either failed to "take" or induced GVH disease [66, 67]. A few leukemic patients have been treated with allogeneic bone marrow after pretreatment with high doses of cyclophosphamide and with further drug therapy prophylactically for GVH disease [68]. Most patients died rapidly with various complications of the treatment so that the antitumor effect of bone marrow could not be determined.

With the advent of human histocompatibility typing, efforts are now in progress to treat leukemic patients with normal histocompatible bone marrow after high level X-irradiation or with marrow suppressive cyclophosphamide pretreatment. The probability and severity of possible GVH disease and its anti-tumor effect (if any) with histocompatible human bone marrow is not yet known. No analogous animal models are as yet available. Since the early studies of this approach in animals always involved severe donor-host histoincompatibility and tumors of unclear antigenicity, there is much justification for re-examining the bone marrow transplantation approach to immunotherapy in animals with tumors possessing demonstrable TSTA with lesser degrees of donor-host incompatibility, with syngeneic cells sensitized to TSTA, and with allogeneic lymphoid cells specifically immunized against TSTA or against normal host isoantigens or against both. The possible necessity for a small tumor mass, for specifically immunized lymphoid cells, and for persistence of donor cells may thereby be examined.

On the basis of the results reported by the Hellströms [1], two additional approaches to immunotherapy should be attempted in animals and perhaps in man. The first approach is based on the finding that lymphoid cells from virtually every mouse and every patient with virtually any tumor are immunologically reactive against the autologous tumor. Therefore, a patient may be treated with sublethal drug plus re-infusion of his own "immune" lymphocytes in a setting of a decreased tumor load. Such an attempt is now in progress. The second approach is based on the apparent prevalence of antibodies which protect tumor cells against immune lymphocytes *in vitro* [1]. When such antibody is shown to be operative *in vivo* the possibility of removing the antibody and reinfusing the "immune" cells will have to be strongly considered.

My last point is relevant to all the contemplated approaches to clinical immunotherapy. Although much of the evidence implicating immunologic factors in neoplasia in animals is derived from studies of viral leukemias, the overwhelming evidence for the existence of tumor-specific transplantation antigens in *human* tumors is, partly for technical reasons, derived from studies of non-hematologic solid tumors. Therefore, I wonder whether acute leukemia is necessarily the most valid target for clinical immunotherapy. Perhaps we ought to devote more investigative attention to solid, demonstrably antigenic tumors, especially those which are amenable to surgery but which have a high and predictable incidence of subsequent metastatic recurrence.

Summary

The principal approaches to experimental cancer immunotherapy as used in animals and man are reviewed. These are all predicated on the assumed existence of tumor-specific antigens, and include: (1) nonspecific stimulation of immunologic reactivity, (2) active immunotherapy with tumor vaccines, (3) passive serotherapy, and (4) adoptive transfer of lymphocytes or bone marrow. Although every approach has been effective in *some* animal systems if instituted *before* the development of clinically evident tumor, with rare exceptions no approach has been effective against clinically-detectable primary or transplanted tumors. The quantitative relationship between tumor mass and host immunity is therefore critical, and suggests that immunotherapy may ultimately be more effective against established tumors if used not as the *sole* form of therapy but as an *adjunct* to other modes of therapy. Supporting this view are studies in which clinically established murine tumors were eradicated by a combination of noncurative chemotherapy plus lymphoid cells (i. e. chemoimmunotherapy), or by lethal whole body x-irradiation and bone marrow transplantation. Some of the apparent prerequisites for successful immunotherapy in the available animal models are discussed and form the context for a review of the reported attempts at cancer immunotherapy in man.

References

1. Hellström, K. E., Hellström, I.: Cellular immunity against tumor antigens. In: Advances in Cancer Research, Vol. 12. New York: Academic Press 1969, p. 167.
2. Morton, D. L., Malmgren, R. A., Holmes, E. C., Ketchum, A. S.: Demonstration of antibodies against human malignant melanomas by immunofluorescence. Surgery **64**, 233 (1968).
3. — — Human osteosarcomas: Immunologic evidence suggesting an associated infectious agent. Science **162**, 1279 (1968).
4. Klein, G., Klein, E., Clifford, P.: Search for host defences in Burkitt lymphoma: Membrane immunofluorescence tests on biopsies and tissue culture lines. Cancer Res. **27**, 2510 (1967).
5. Bach, M. L., Bach, F. H., Joo, P.: Leukemia-associated antigens in the mixed leukocyte culture test. Science **166**, 1520 (1969).
6. Gold, P., Freedman, F. O.: Demonstration of tumor-specific antigens in human colonic carcinomata by immunological tolerance and absorption techniques. J. Exp. Med. **121**, 439 (1965).
7. Old, L. J., Boyse, E. A.: Immunology of experimental tumors. Ann. Rev. Med. **15**, 167 (1964).
8. — Benaceraf, B., Clarke, D. A., Carswell, E. A., Stockert, E.: The role of the reticuloendothelial system in the host reaction to neoplasia. Cancer Res. **21**, 1281 (1961).
9. Weiss, D. W., Bonhag, R. S., Deome, K. B.: Protective activity of fractions tubercle bacilli against isologous tumors in mice. Nature (Lond.) **190**, 889 (1961).
10. — — Leslie, P.: Studies on the heterologous immunogenicity of a methanol-insoluble fraction of attenuated tubercle bacilli (BCG). II. Protection against tumor isografts. J. exp. Med. **124**, 1039 (1966).
11. Amiel, J. L.: Immunothérapie active non specifique par le BCG de la leucémie virale E♂G_2 chez des réceveurs isogéniques. Rev. franç. Étud. clin. biol. **12**, 912 (1967).
12. Mathé, G.: Immunothérapie active de la leucèmie L1210 appliquée après la greffe tumorale. Rev. franç. Étud. clin. biol. **13**, 881 (1968).
13. Haddow, A., Alexander, P.: An immunological method of increasing the sensitivity of primary sarcomas to local irradiation with x-ray. Lancet **1964 I**, 452.

14. Sjögren, H. O., Ankerst, J.: Effect of BCG and allogeneic tumor cells on adenovirus Type 12 tumor regenesis in mice. Nature (Lond.) **221**, 863 (1969).
15. Mathé, G., Amiel, J. L., Schwarzenberg, L., Schneider, M., Cattan, A., Schlumburger, A. R., Hayat, M., de Vassal, F.: Active immunotherapy for acute lymphoblastic leukemia. Lancet **1969 I**, 697.
16. Klein, G.: Tumor antigens. Ann. Rev. Microbiol. **20**, 223 (1966).
17. Old, L. J., Boyse, E. A.: Antigens of tumors and leukemias induced by viruses. Fed. Proc. **24**, 1009 (1965).
18. Glynn, J. P., McCoy, J. L., Fefer, A.: Cross-resistance to the transplantation of syngeneic Friend, Moloney and Rauscher virus-induced tumors. Cancer Res. **28**, 434 (1968).
19. Fink, M. A., Fauscher, F. J.: Immune reactions to a Murine leukemia virus. I. Induction of immunity to infection with virus in the natural host. J. nat. Cancer Inst. **32**, 1075 (1964).
20. Goldner, H., Girardi, A. J., Larsen, D. M., Hilleman, M. R.: Interruption of SV_{40} virus tumorigenesis using irradiated homologous tumor antigens. Proc. Soc. exp. Biol. (N. Y.) **117**, 851 (1964).
21. Rhodes, E. L.: An attempt to obtain autoimmunity to tumors with Freund's adjuvant and tetanus toxoid. Nature (Lond.) **193**, 1091 (1962).
22. Matsuyama, M., Maekawa, A., Horikawa, H., Suzumori, K., Sogal, K., Iwai, K.: Ineffectiveness of autotransplantation on growth of the methylcholanthrene sarcoma in rats and mice. Nature (Lond.) **197**, 805 (1963).
23. Evans, C. A., Gorman, L. R., Ito, Y., Weiser, R. S.: Antitumor immunity in the Shope papilloma-carcinoma complex of rabbits. I. Papilloma regression induced by homologous and autologous tissue vaccines. J. nat. Cancer Inst. **29**, 277 (1962).
24. Kellock, T. H., Chambers, H., Russ, S.: An attempt to procure immunity to malignant disease in man. Lancet **1922 I**, 217.
25. Wissler, R. W., Craft, K., Kesden, D., Powlisky, B., Dzoga, K.: Inhibition of the growth of the Morris hepatoma (5123) in Buffalo rats using a mixture of Pertussis vaccine and irradiated tumor. In: Advances in Transplantation. Copenhagen: Monksgaard; New York: Williams & Wilkins 1968, p. 538.
26. Graham, J. B., Graham, R. M.: The effect of vaccine on cancer patients. Surg. Gynec. Obstet. **114**, 1 (1962).
27. Czajkowski, N. P., Rosenblatt, M., Wolf, P. L., Vazquez, J.: A new method of active immunization to autologous human tumor tissue. Lancet **1967 II**, 905.
28. Fass, L., Herberman, R. V., Ziegler, J.: Cutaneous hypersensitivity to extracts of Burkitt lymphoma cells. New Engl. J. Med. (in press).
29. McCoy, J. L., Fefer, A., Glynn, J. P.: Influence of infectious virus on the induction of transplantation resistance in the Friend tumor system. Cancer Res. **27**, 2267 (1967).
30. Law, L. W., Ting, R. C., Lecksband, E.: Prevention of virus-induced neoplasms in mice through passive transfer of immunity by sensitized syngeneic lymphoid cells. Proc. nat. Acad. Sci. (Wash.) **57**, 1068 (1967).
31. Varet, B., Levy, J. P., Leclerc, J. C., Senik, A.: Rôle de l'immunité dans le rejet des tumeurs induites par le virus MSV effet des sérums antithymocytes. Int. J. Cancer **3**, 727 (1968).
32. Old, L. J., Stockert, E., Boyse, E. A., Geering, G.: A study of passive immunization against a transplanted G+ leukemia with specific antigens. Proc. Soc. exp. Biol. (N. Y.) **124**, 63 (1967).
33. Mihich, E.: Combined effects of chemotherapy and immunity against leukemia L1210 in DBA/2 mice. Cancer Res. **29**, 848 (1969).
34. Alexander, P.: Immunotherapy of cancer: Experiments with primary tumors and syngeneic tumor grafts. In: Progress in Experimental Tumor Research, Vol. 10. Ed.: F. Homburger. Basel-New York: Karger 1968, p. 22.
35. McCoy, J. L., Fefer, A., Glynn, J. P.: Inhibition and enhancement of syngeneic Friend virus-induced lymphoma cells by passively transferred anti-Friend serum. Exp. Hematol. **16**, 24 (1968).

36. LAW, L. W., TING, R. C., STANTON, M. S.: Some biologic, immunogenic and morphologic effects in mice after infection with a Murine sarcoma virus. I. Biologic and immunogenic studies. J. nat. Cancer Inst. **40**, 1102 (1968).
37. BUBENIK, J., TURANO, A., FADDA, G.: Prevention of carcinogenesis by murine sarcoma virus (Harvey) following injection of immune sera during the latency period. Int. J. Cancer **4**, 648 (1969).
38. EVANS, C. A., WEISER, R. S., ITO, Y.: Antiviral and antitumor immunologic mechanisms operative in the Shope papilloma-carcinoma system. Cold Spr. Harb. Symp. quant. Biol. **27**, 453 (1962).
39. FEFER, A.: Immunotherapy and chemotherapy of Moloney sarcoma virus-induced tumors in mice. Cancer Res. **29**, 2177 (1969).
40. KALISS, N.: Immunological enhancement in tumor homografts in mice. A review. Cancer Res. **18**, 992 (1958).
41. BOYSE, E. A., OLD, L. J., STOCKERT, E.: Immunological enhancement of a leukemia. Nature **194**, 1142 (1962).
42. MÖLLER, G.: The effects on tumor growth in syngeneic recipients of antibodies against tumor-specific antigens in methylcholanthrene-induced mouse sarcomas. Nature **204**, 846 (1964).
43. BUBENIK, J., KOLDOVSKY, P.: Factors influencing the induction of enhancement and resistance to methylcholanthrene-induced tumors in a syngeneic system. Folia biol. (Praha) **11**, 258 (1965).
44. LASZLO, J., BUCKLEY, C. E., III, AMOS, B. D.: Infusion of isologous immune plasma in chronic lymphocytic leukemia. Blood **31**, 104 (1968).
45. DJERASSI, I.: Transfusion of lymphocyte antibody and lymphocytes from multitransfused donors. Clin. pediat. (Bologna) **7**, 272 (1968).
46. HERBERMAN, R., ROGENTINE, G. N., OREN, M. E.: Bioassay of antitumor effects of human alloantisera. Clin. Res. (abstract) **17**, 328 (1969).
47. IZAWA, T., SAKURAI, M., ATSUTA, Y., YOSHIZUMI, P.: Antigenicity of leukemia and antiserum therapy. Ann. paediat. jap. **12**, 346 (1966).
48. ALBO, V., KRIVIT, W., HARTMANN, J.: Fresh plasma as an adjuvant to the chemotherapy of acute lymphatic leukemia in children. Proc. Amer. Ass. Cancer Res. **9**, 2 (1968).
49. FASS, L., HERBERMAN, R. B., ZIEGLER, J., MORROW, R. H.: Evaluation of the effect of remission plasma on untreated patients with Burkitt lymphoma. J. nat. Cancer Inst. **44**, 145 (1970).
50. FEFER, A., MCCOY, J. L., GLYNN, J. P.: Studies on the growth and regression of a transplantable Moloney sarcoma. Cancer Res. **27**, 2207 (1967).
51. BARD, D. S., PILCH, Y. H.: The role of the spleen in the immunity to a chemically induced sarcoma in C3H mice. Cancer Res. **29**, 1125 (1969).
52. FEFER, A.: Immunotherapy of primary Moloney sarcoma virus-induced tumors. Int. J. Cancer **5**, 327 (1970).
53. — MCCOY, J. L., GLYNN, J. P.: Induction and regression of primary Moloney sarcoma virus-induced tumors in mice. Cancer Res. **27**, 1626 (1967).
54. — — PERK, K., GLYNN, J. P.: Immunologic, virologic and pathologic studies of regression of autochthonous Moloney sarcoma virus (MSV)-induced tumors in mice. Cancer Res. **28**, 1577 (1968).
55. GLYNN, J. P., HALPERN, B. L., FEFER, A.: An immunochemotherapeutic system for the treatment of a transplanted Moloney virus-induced lymphoma in mice. Cancer Res. **29**, 515 (1969).
56. WOODRUFF, M. F. A., NOLAN, B.: Treatment of advanced cancer by injection of allogeneic spleen cells. Lancet **1963 II**, 426.
57. SCHWARZENBERG, L., MATHÉ, G., SCHNEIDER, M., AMIEL, J. L., CATTAN, A., SCHLUMBURGER, J. R.: Attempted adoptive immunotherapy of acute leukemia by leukocyte transfusions. Lancet **1966 II**, 365.
58. NADLER, S. H., MOORE, G. E.: Immunotherapy of malignant disease. Arch. Surg. **99**, 376 (1969).
59. FEFER, A.: Unpublished observations.

60. BARNES, D. W. H., LOUTIT, J. F., NEAL, F. E.: Treatment of Murine leukemia with x-rays and homologous bone marrow. Brit. med. J. **1956 II**, 626.
61. TRENTIN, J. J.: Whole body x-ray and bone marrow therapy of leukemia in mice. Proc. Amer. Ass. Cancer Res. (abstract) **2**, 54 (1957).
62. DEVRIES, M. J., VOS, O.: Treatment of mouse lymphosarcoma by total body x-irradiation and by injection of bone marrow and lymph hnode cells. J. nat. Cancer Inst. **21**, 1117 (1958).
63. MATHÉ, G., BEVNASE, J.: Essai de traitement de la leucèmie greffee L1210 par l'irradiation X suivie de transfusions de cellules hématopoietiques normales. Rev. franç. Étud. clin. biol. **442**, 4 (1959).
64. FLOERSHEIM, G. L.: Treatment of Moloney lymphoma with lethal doses of dimethyl myleran combined with injection of hemopoietic cells. Lancet **1969 I**, 228.
65. BORANIC, M.: Transient graft-versus-host reaction in the treatment of leukemia in mice. J. nat. Cancer Inst. **41**, 421 (1968).
66. THOMAS, E. D., HERMAN, E. C., JR., GREENOUGH, W. B., HAGER, E. B., CANNON, J. H., SHALER, O. D., FERREBEE, J. W.: Irradiation and marrow infusion in leukemia. Arch. intern. Med. **107**, 95 (1961).
67. MATHÉ, G., SCHWARZENBERG, L., AMIEL, J. L., SCHNEIDER, M., CATTAN, A., SCHLUMBURGER, J. R., TUBIANA, M., LALANNE, C. L.: Immunogenetics and immunological problems of hemopoietic radio-chimeras in man. Scand. J. Hematol. **4**, 193 (1967).
68. SANTOS, G. W., SENSENBRENNER, LL., BURKE, B. J., COLDIN, O. M., OWENS, A. H., JR., BIAS, W., SLAVIN, R.: Marrow transplant in man utilizing cyclophosphamide. Summary of Baltimore experience. Exp. Hematol. (in press).

Summary of Conference

C. GORDON ZUBROD

It has been a pleasure to take part in this teaching symposium, and as it is now coming to an end, I will try by way of summary, to make a few personal interpretations.

Dr. BAKER pointed out that a substantial fraction of his budget has supported research on the leukemias and lymphomas. Money well spent, if it provides the path to the cure of these diseases, and to the stalking horse (if I may use Dr. BURCHENAL's term) to lead us to the control of other cancers. Our speakers have not only helped us share in their optimism by showing their results but have provided a clear enunciation of the principles involved and detailed blueprints so that all our patients may receive the same benefits.

Diagnosis and Staging

The issues were simply stated by Dr. LUKES and Dr. SHEEHAN. You cannot treat properly unless you know what the disease is, and where it is. In addition, there is a good possibility in Hodgkin's disease that we would do better in planning therapy, if we knew the specific histology—nodular sclerosis, lymphocytic predominance, etc. There is still a need to continue this fine work in order to correlate histology with therapeutic result. There is no question but that staging dictates therapy. Dr. ROSENBERG's paper is a classic in how the physician should use the history, physical and laboratory studies to tie down the exact stage. Even the surgeons have been called upon. I would like to comment on the questions of laparotomy and splenectomy. It is clear that clinical workup in the Rosenberg manner still leaves false positives and false negatives, and that laparotomy can resolve many of these by direct evidence. Laparotomy for staging is fine in the big centers. They have a trained team of surgeons, radiologists and internists who know exactly what is wanted, the dangers and their own limitations. I do not believe this constitutes a general recommendation that all patients be staged in this way or that all patients should have splenectomy. We all hope that from the very careful studies will come a definition of the simplest and safest way to stage and the conditions requiring splenectomy. Drs. JOHNSON and PETERS suggested that all patients except for Stage I and II A should receive total nodal irradiation. Such therapy would make academic the question of the extent of subdiaphragmatic involvement except for the liver. Further work is needed to define the best way of diagnosing and treating involvement of the liver.

The intensive studies on staging and histologic classification have given new insights into the evolution of Hodgkin's disease. From the staging side, we have seen the increasing knowledge on spread within the lymphoid organs, how the mediastinum may be skipped and the route of spread from para-aortic nodes to the spleen and liver. From the histologists we have learned the progression from the lymphocyte rich, Reed-Sternberg poor situation to the lymphocyte depleted—Reed-Sternberg predominant condition. Dr. Lukes sees in this the evidence of prolonged struggle between the malignant cells and the resistant forces of the host. Perhaps in the near future we may have a full understanding of the parts played by the lymphocyte, the histiocyte, nodular sclerosis and fibrosis, and a recognition of how these relate to the loss of skin reactivity and to prognosis and cure.

There emerged from the discussions a need to sharpen the staging criteria for Hodgkin's. New information requires the redoing of the Rye staging criteria, since it is apparent that several large groups have developed separate subclassifications. We cannot afford to return to the Tower of Babel situation that existed prior to the Paris and Rye meetings on Hodgkin's disease.

Radiation Therapy

From Dr. Kaplan's and Dr. Johnson's figures and the work of Dr. Peters and Dr. Easson, it is clear that Hodgkin's disease, Stages I and II A are curable provided tumoricidal doses of 4,000 rad are given in large contiguous fields. For Stage II B there is needed further study of total nodal radiation and probably of combination chemotherapy if total nodal radiation proves to be inadequate. For Stages III A and IV A, there is a 70% five year survival, and for III B and IV B a much lower percentage. The continuing rapid technical advances may indeed allow further improvements. For the other malignant lymphomas, the same principles seem to hold and similar results are being obtained when tumors are limited to lymphoid areas. The full evidence was not presented at this symposium. Unfortunately by the time a physician sees a patient with these lymphomas, there is usually extranodal disease.

Chemotherapy

In Stages III B and IV Hodgkin's disease, Dr. DeVita's combination chemotherapy has given 80% complete remission. Of those reaching complete remission, the median survival is four years. It is too early to reach conclusions about cure, but one can be hopeful that the patients surviving five years after the DeVita regimen will remain largely free of disease as Dr. Kaplan pointed out for those patients who survived five years after radiation. In the other malignant lymphomas, complete remissions are achieved following combination chemotherapy but not so frequently. Of those achieving complete remission, the median survival is also about four years. Clearly there is need for more study of the other malignant lymphomas utilizing both combination chemotherapy and radiation. The question remains open about the best way to combine radiation and chemotherapy for the treatment of lymphomas. It is clearly justified to make careful studies of combination of drugs and radiation to see which modalities give the best cure rate with least hazard to the patient. A conservative view would be that these studies should be confined to Stages III and IV. There seems no need for extension of combination radiation and chemotherapy to Stages I and II unless long term follow-up extended radiation should show a high incidence of acute leukemia. At present there are only a handful of cases occuring six to seven years post irradiation. I am reassured by Dr. PETER's experience, namely, that she has seen only one patient with Hodgkin's who developed acute myelocytic leukemia.

Acute Leukemias

Dr. FREIREICH reviewed the enormous progress that has occurred in the treatment of acute lymphocytic leukemia with the result that almost all children go into complete remission, and the five year survival percentage is rapidly increasing. These results are due to combination chemotherapy, platelet replacement, and the better treatment and prevention of infection. The perfection of laminar flow environments, and of granulocyte, lymphocyte and bone marrow replacement, promise further advances against the main difficulty—infection. In addition, there are available several new highly active agents such as L-asparaginase, daunorubicin and cytosine arabinoside that can now be added to the combination studies. The same principles have been used for acute myelocytic leukemia and although the results have been bleak in the past, the addition of cytosine arabinoside in combination has improved the complete remission rate and length of survival. The exciting but preliminary results with cytosine arabinoside and thioguanine, perhaps offer the opportunity for considerably improved control. The age of the patient makes a good deal of difference with complete remissions below 65 at 70% with no complete remissions in patients over 65. Most of the patients have severe infections and the new supportive therapies offer opportunity for better results in both old and young patients with acute myelocytic leukemia.

Burkitt's Lymphoma

Dr. CARBONE reviewed the history of Burkitt's lymphoma both in Africa and the United States. He emphasized the importance of staging and pointed out that with limited disease a single dose of cyclophosphamide is presumably curative. More intensive therapy is required for advanced stages. The limiting factor is CNS involvement which has not completely yielded to intrathecal methotrexate and cytosine arabinoside.

Chronic Leukemias

Dr. GALTON, in his broad and balanced discussion, concluded that in both types of chronic leukemia, management results in temporary control but not in eradication of the abnormal cells. More intensive therapy of the kind used in the acute leukemias has not really been tried, at least not in the early phases of these diseases. Because of the relatively slow pace of the disease, physicians have understandably been reluctant to use intensive therapy. The physician is caught in this dilemma—the best time to treat tumor is early in the disease, but early intensive treatment for the chronic leukemias risks an early demise from bone marrow failure. It seems to me that soon we will want to consider a fresh approach to the management of the chronic leukemias. Perhaps we won't be convinced of the need for a less conservative therapy until the survival time for the acute leukemias is better than that of the chronic leukemias. When this day comes, I think the approach must be that of the acute leukemias—intensive combination drug treatment early in the disease with maximum use of supportive therapy. Dr. Cronkite showed us his exquisite studies on extracorporeal irradiation of blood from chronic lymphocytic leukemia patients and from calves. With this technique, he has been able to bring new understanding to lymphopoiesis and has demonstrated the existence of a tissue pool of lymphocytes which does not readily exchange with the blood. This apparently prevents the completeness of destruction of abnormal lymphocytes by extracorporeal irradiation. Nevertheless, the technique does allow a significant reduction in the number of leukemic cells in the body and perhaps could be used prior to chemotherapy. Dr. Johnson discussed another possible approach to improved treatment of chronic lymphocytic leukemia; namely, small fractionated doses of total body irradiation. Of 17 patients, eight had complete remission with a median of 19 months. This technique is encouraging, but needs further exploration.

Future Strategy

We have come a long way in the past 15 years in the successful therapy of some of the hematologic neoplasms and it seems clear that at least for acute lymphocytic leukemia, Hodgkin's disease and Burkitt's lymphoma the complete destruction of tumor cells leads to a high frequency of complete remission and ever lengthening survival. The question is what should be the strategy for control of the other leukemias and lymphomas and a number of speakers spelled out the strategic options. Dr. Bruce demonstrated the selective toxicity of drugs for tumor cells. He also defined the critical path to be followed in maximum use of selective toxicity. This involved the quantitative assay of tumor cells able to grow and kill animals. By means of such an assay one can determine the best drugs, schedules and combinations, and can measure relapse. Application of these methods to both transplanted and spontaneous animal tumors revealed the principles of cure. Selectivity depends upon the difference in the sizes of the growth fractions (i. e., the percentage of cells in the proliferative pool) of tumor cells and normal cells. Where the growth fraction of tumor cells is larger than that of normal cells, cure is possible. Where the growth fraction of tumor cells is small, cure is difficult since our mitotically linked drugs have their full effect during the events of the mitotic cycle. For the situation where few of the tumor cells are in the growth fraction, we need drugs with greater selectivity, or drugs that can move resting cells into active cell cycle where drugs can destroy them. Dr. Sartorelli and Dr. Wheeler extended this concept of selective toxicity pointing up the importance of pharmacological variables in reaching and keeping a tumoricidal concentration of drug at the target site. Sartorelli emphasized the need for drugs that would have greater selective binding affinity to active molecular sites in the tumor and he made provocative suggestions on drug combinations that could increase selective toxicity by hitting at different molecular loci within the tumor cell cycle. Dr. WHEELER discussed ways in which alkylating agents could be used more selectively. He emphasized the use of larger doses to have greater effect on the G_2 phase; and the development of agents that will persist longer at target sites. Dr. CLARKSON brought the problem of selective toxicity and growth fractions to clinical application. In theory, the cure of clinical leukemia should be possible by application of Dr. BRUCE's principles. At least in acute myelocytic leukemia this doesn't work except perhaps in a small percentage. The major difference between the leukemias of man and mouse seems to be that in man a larger percentage of cells are in G_1 where they are not susceptible to drugs. This occurs spontaneously, but the administration of drugs can also allow cumulation of cells in G_1. The clinical lesson for the attempted curative chemotherapy of acute myelocytic leukemia would be to get the patients in complete remission by means of combination therapy and then treat intermittently for long periods until all cells in G_1 have cycled through the later events of the cell cycle where drugs are effective. This approach requires that the patient can be protected from infection during the intensive efforts to achieve complete remission.

Immunotherapy

Finally under the strategy for future improvement in selective toxicity we have the suggestions of Drs. HELLSTRÖM and FEFER for immunotherapy. A number of approaches in animals were reviewed, but I'll mention only one. In animal systems, specific antisera can prevent growth of tumors. There is increasing evidence of common tumor specific antigens in human tumors, and so the possibility is open to consider specific immune therapy. Unfortunately these antigens have been found in the solid tumors rather than in the leukemias or lymphomas, although there is some suggestion that Burkitt's lymphoma has a specific antigen. There is a further difficulty as pointed out by Dr. FEFER that established animal tumors cannot be cured by immunotherapy. In the treatment of established clinical tumors, exponential or first order kill is a necessity for cure. Generally immune therapy is arithmetic or zero order in character, and therefore the use of specific immune therapy, while it can confer extraordinary selective toxicity, would necessarily be used as an adjunct to chemotherapy, radiation or surgery.

Conclusion

Some of the diseases we have been discussing, such as Hodgkin's disease and Burkitt's lymphoma, are in large part curable. Some, such as acute lymphoblastic leukemia and the malignant lymphomas, display ever increasing five year survivals. Some, such as acute myelocytic leukemia, are just beginning to yield to chemotherapy. Some, such as the chronic leukemias, have shown little improvement in survival after therapy and a fresh start is needed using the principles successful in the more fulminant leukemias. In all, there are failures of present therapy. The understanding and reversal of these failures will come from the considerations suggested by Dr. Bruce. This means a quantitative assay of the remaining tumor cells in the body, and a measurement of the percent of cells in and out of the proliferative pool. Given these, successful therapeutic strategies can be devised with the tools now at hand although admittedly, more selectively toxic drugs or uses of radiation or the help of immunotherapy would be welcome.

I would like on behalf of the participants and audience, to thank our hosts, the University, Dr. Wissler and Dr. Ultmann, for this splendid teaching symposium. In this setting we are all students and we have had the privilege of seeing how the rapid application of research information to the patient has moved the leukemias and lymphomas from an atmosphere of death and pessimism to one of hope and cure.

Monographs already Published

1 SCHINDLER, R., Lausanne: Die tierische Zelle in Zellkultur. DM 16,—; US $ 4.40
2 Neuroblastomas — Biochemical Studies. Edited by C. BOHUON, Villejuif (Symposium). DM 16,—; US $ 4.40
3 HUEPER, W. C., Bethesda: Occupational and Environmental Cancers of the Respiratory System. DM 34,—; US $ 9.40
4 GOLDMAN, L., Cincinnati: Laser Cancer Research. DM 16,—; US $ 5.00
5 METCALF, D., Melbourne: The Thymus. Its Role in Immune Responses, Leukaemia Development and Carcinogenesis. DM 24,—; US $ 6.60
6 Malignant Transformation by Viruses. Edited by W. H. KIRSTEN, Chicago (Symposium). DM 32,—; US $ 8.80
7 MOERTEL, CH. G., Rochester: Multiple Primary Malignant Neoplasms. Their Incidence and Significance. DM 18,—; US $ 5.00
8 New Trends in the Treatment of Cancer. Edited by L. MANUILA, S. MOLES, and P. RENTCHNICK, Geneva. DM 32,—; US $ 8.80
9 LINDENMANN, J., Zürich, and P. A. KLEIN, Gainesville/Florida: Immunological Aspects of Viral Oncolysis. DM 18,—; US $ 5.00
10 NELSON, R. S., Houston: Radioactive Phosphorus in the Diagnosis of Gastrointestinal Cancer. DM 15,—; US $ 4.20
11 FREEMAN, R. G., and J. M. KNOX, Houston: Treatment of Skin Cancer. DM 15,—; US $ 4.50
12 LYNCH, H. T., Houston: Hereditary Factors in Carcinoma. DM 24,—; US $ 6.60
13 Tumours in Children. Edited by H. B. MARSDEN, and J. K. STEWARD, Manchester. DM 72,—; US $ 18.00
14 ODARTCHENKO, N., Lausanne: Production cellulaire érythropoïétique. DM 28,—; US $ 7.70
15 SOKOLOFF, B., Lakeland/Florida: Carcinoid and Serotonin. DM 24,—; US $ 6.60
16 JACOBS, M. L., Duarte/California: Malignant Lymphomas and their Management. DM 18,—; US $ 5.10
17 Normal and Malignant Cell Growth. Edited by R. J. M. FRY, Argonne, M. L. GRIEM, Argonne, and W. H. KIRSTEN, Chicago (Symposium). DM 56,80; US $ 14.20
18 ANGLESIO, E., Torino: The Treatment of Hodgkin's Disease. DM 24,—; US $ 6.60
19 BANNASCH, P., Würzburg: The Cytoplasm of Hepatocytes during Carcinogenesis. DM 32,—; US $ 8.80
20 Rubidomycin. A new Agent against Leukemia. Edited by J. BERNARD, R. PAUL, M. BOIRON, C. JACQUILLAT, and R. MARAL, Paris. DM 48,—; US $ 13.20
21 Scientific Basis of Cancer Chemotherapy. Edited by G. MATHÉ, Villejuif (Symposium). DM 28,—; US $ 7.00
22 KOLDOVSKÝ, P., Philadelphia: Tumor Specific Transplantation Antigen. DM 24,—; US $ 6.60
23 FUCHS, W. A., Bern, J. W. DAVIDSON, Toronto, and H. W. FISCHER, Ann Arbor: Lymphography in Cancer. DM 76,—; US $ 21.00
24 HAYWARD, J. L., London: Hormonal Research in Human Breast Cancer. DM 34,—; US $ 9.40
25 ROY-BURMAN, P., Los Angeles: Analogues of Nucleic Acid Components. Mechanisms of Action. DM 28,—; US $ 7.70
26 Tumors of the Liver. Edited by G. T. PACK and A. H. ISLAMI, New York. DM 56,—; US $ 15.40

27 SZYMENDERA, J., Warsaw: Bone Mineral Metabolism in Cancer. DM 32,—; US $ 8.80

28 MEEK, E. S., Bristol: Antitumour and Antiviral Substances of Natural Origin. DM 16,—; US $ 4.40

29 Aseptic Environments and Cancer Treatment. Edited by G. MATHÉ, Villejuif (Symposium). DM 22,—; US $ 6.10

30 Advances in the Treatment of Acute (Blastic) Leukemias. Edited by G. MATHÉ, Villejuif (Symposium). DM 38,—; US $ 10.50

31 DENOIX, P., Villejuif: Treatment of Malignant Breast Tumors: Indications and Results. DM 48,—; US $ 13.20

32 NELSON, R. S., Houston: Endoscopy in Gastric Cancer. DM 48,—; US $ 13.20

33 Experimental and Clinical Effects of L-Asparaginase. Edited by E. GRUNDMANN, Wuppertal-Elberfeld, and H. F. OETTGEN, New York (Symposium). DM 58,—; US $ 16.—

34 ENDO, H., Fukuoka, T. ONO, Tokyo, T. SUGIMURA, Tokyo: Chemistry and Biological Actions of 4-Nitroquinoline 1-oxide. DM 36,—; US $ 9.90

35 PENN, I., Denver: Malignant Tumors in Organ Transplant Recipients. DM 24,—; US $ 6.60

36 Current Concepts in the Management of Leukemia and Lymphoma. Edited by J. E. ULTMANN, M. L. GRIEM, W. H. KIRSTEN, and R. W. WISSLER, Chicago (Symposium) DM 48,—; US $ 13.20

Special Supplement: Biology of Amphibian Tumors. Edited by M. MIZELL, New Orleans. DM 86,—; US $ 24.00

In Production

37 CHIAPPA, S., R. MUSUMECI, and C. USLENGHI, Milano: Endolymphatic Radiotherapy in Malignant Lymphomas. DM 48,—; US $ 13.20

In Preparation

ACKERMANN, N. B., Boston: Use of Radioisotopic Agents in the Diagnosis of Cancer

BOIRON, M., Paris: The Viruses of the Leukemia-Sarcoma Complex

CAVALIERE, R., A. ROSSI-FANELLI, B. MONDOVI, and G. MORICCA, Roma: Selective Heat Sensitivity of Cancer Cells

GRUNDMANN, E., Wuppertal-Elberfeld: Morphologie und Cytochemie der Carcinogenese

IRLIN, I. S., Moskva: Mechanisms of Viral Carcinogenesis

LANGLEY, F. A., and A. C. CROMPTON, Manchester: Epithelial Abnormalities of the Cervix Uteri

MATHÉ, G., Villejuif: L'Immunothérapie des Cancers

MERKOW, L., and M. SLIFKIN, Pittsburgh: Oncogenic Simian Adenoviruses

PARKER, J., and R. J. LUKES, Los Angeles: Lymphocyte Transformation in Neoplastic Disease

WEIL, R., Lausanne: Biological and Structural Properties of Polyoma Virus and its DNA

WILLIAMS, D. C., Oxted, Surrey: The Basis for Therapy of Hormon Sensitive Tumours

WILLIAMS, D. C., Oxted, Surrey: The Biochemistry of Metastasis

1

MIX
Papier aus verantwortungsvollen Quellen
Paper from responsible sources
FSC® C105338

If you have any concerns about our products,
you can contact us on
ProductSafety@springernature.com

In case Publisher is established outside the EU,
the EU authorized representative is:
Springer Nature Customer Service Center GmbH
Europaplatz 3, 69115 Heidelberg, Germany

Printed by Libri Plureos GmbH
in Hamburg, Germany